theclinics.com

ENDOCRINOLOGY AND METABOLISM CLINICS OF NORTH AMERICA

Endocrine Disorders During Pregnancy

GUEST EDITOR
Susan J. Mandel, MD, MPH

CONSULTING EDITOR
Derek LeRoith, MD, PhD

March 2006 • Volume 35 • Number 1

SAUNDERS

An Imprint of Elsevier, Inc.
PHILADELPHIA   LONDON   TORONTO   MONTREAL   SYDNEY   TOKYO

W.B. SAUNDERS COMPANY
A Division of Elsevier Inc.

1600 John F. Kennedy Boulevard • Suite 1800 • Philadelphia, Pennsylvania 19103-2899

http://www.theclinics.com

ENDOCRINOLOGY AND METABOLISM	Volume 35, Number 1
CLINICS OF NORTH AMERICA	ISSN 0889-8529
March 2006	ISBN 1-4160-3517-6

Editor: Joe Rusko

The ideas and opinions expressed in *Endocrinology and Metabolism Clinics of North America* do not necessarily reflect those of the Publisher. The Publisher does not assume any responsibility for any injury and/or damage to persons or property arising out of or related to any use of the material contained in this periodical. The reader is advised to check the appropriate medical literature and the product information currently provided by the manufacturer of each drug to be administered to verify the dosage, the method and duration of administration, or contraindications. It is the responsibility of the treating physician or other health care professional, relying on independent experience and knowledge of the patient, to determine drug dosages and the best treatment for the patient. Mention of any product in this issue should not be construed as endorsement by the contributors, editors, or the Publisher of the product or manufacturers' claims.

Endocrinology and Metabolism Clinics of North America (ISSN 0889-8529) is published quarterly by Elsevier Inc. Corporate and editorial offices: 1600 John F. Kennedy Boulevard, Suite 1800, Philadelphia, PA 19103-2899. Accounting and circulation offices: 6277 Sea Harbor Drive, Orlando, FL 32887-4800. Periodicals postage paid at Orlando, FL 32862, and additional mailing offices. Subscription prices are USD 175 per year for US individuals, USD 295 per year for US institutions, USD 90 per year for US students and residents, USD 220 per year for Canadian individuals, USD 355 per year for Canadian institutions, USD 240 per year for international individuals, USD 355 per year for international institutions and USD 125 per year for Canadian and foreign students/residents. To receive student/resident rate, orders must be accompanied by name of affiliated institution, date of term, and the *signature* of program/residency coordinator on institution letterhead. Orders will be billed at individual rate until proof of status is received. Foreign air speed delivery is included in all *Clinics* subscription prices. All prices are subject to change without notice. POSTMASTER: Send address changes to *Endocrinology and Metabolism Clinics of North America*, W.B. Saunders Company, Periodicals Fulfillment, Orlando, FL 32887-4800. **Customer Service: (+1) 800-654-2452 (US). From outside of the US, call (+1) 407-345-4000; e-mail: hhspcs@harcourt.com.**

Reprints. For copies of 100 or more, of articles in this publication, please contact the Commercial Rights Department, Elsevier Inc., 360 Park Avenue South, New York, NY 10010-1710; phone: (+1) 212-633-3813; fax: (+1) 212-462-1935; e-mail: reprints@elsevier.com.

Endocrinology and Metabolism Clinics of North America is covered in *Index Medicus, EMBASE/Excerpta Medica, Current Contents/Clinical Medicine, Current Contents/Life Sciences, Science Citation Index, ISI/BIOMED, BIOSIS,* and *Chemical Abstracts.*

Printed in the United States of America.

CONSULTING EDITOR

DEREK LeROITH, MD, PhD, Chief, Division of Endocrinology, Metabolism, and Bone Diseases, Mount Sinai School of Medicine, New York, New York

GUEST EDITOR

SUSAN J. MANDEL, MD, MPH, Associate Professor (Medicine and Radiology); and Associate Chief, Clinical Affairs, Division of Endocrinology, Diabetes, and Metabolism, University of Pennsylvania School of Medicine, Philadelphia, Pennsylvania

CONTRIBUTORS

GHADA EL-HAJJ FULEIHAN, MD, MPH, Professor (Medicine); and Director, Calcium Metabolism and Osteoporosis Program, American University of Beirut Medical Center, Beirut, Lebanon

LOIS JOVANOVIC, MD, Clinical Professor (Medicine), Keck School of Medicine, University of Southern California at Los Angeles, Los Angeles; Adjunct Professor (Biomolecular Science and Engineering), University of California at Santa Barbara; Chief Executive Officer; and Chief Scientific Officer, Sansum Diabetes Research Institute, Santa Barbara, California

CHRISTOPHER S. KOVACS, MD, FRCPC, FACP, Professor (Medicine, Obstetrics and Gynecology, and Basic Medical Sciences), Faculty of Medicine–Endocrinology, Memorial University of Newfoundland, Health Sciences Center, St. John's, Newfoundland, Canada

ODED LANGER, MD, PhD, Professor and Chairman, Department of Obstetrics and Gynecology, St. Luke's–Roosevelt Hospital Center, University Hospital of Columbia University, New York, New York

SHANE O. LeBEAU, MD, Clinical Assistant Professor, Division of Endocrinology and Metabolism, Department of Medicine, University of Pittsburgh Medical Center, Pittsburgh, Pennsylvania

JOHN R. LINDSAY, MD, Endocrinology Fellow, Reproductive Biology and Medicine Branch, National Institute of Child Health and Human Development, National Institutes of Health, Bethesda, Maryland

SUSAN J. MANDEL, MD, MPH, Associate Professor (Medicine and Radiology); and Associate Chief, Clinical Affairs, Division of Endocrinology, Diabetes, and Metabolism, University of Pennsylvania School of Medicine, Philadelphia, Pennsylvania

MARK E. MOLITCH, MD, Professor, Division of Endocrinology, Metabolism, and Molecular Medicine, Department of Medicine, Northwestern University Feinberg School of Medicine, Chicago, Illinois

YUICHIRO NAKAI, MD, Endocrinology and Metabolism Fellow, Department of Medicine, University of California Davis Health Systems, Sacramento, California

JOHN E. NESTLER, MD, William G. Blackard Professor of Medicine; Chair, Division of Endocrinology and Metabolism; and Vice Chair, Department of Internal Medicine, Medical College of Virginia, Virginia Commonwealth University, Richmond, Virginia

LYNNETTE K. NIEMAN, MD, Senior Investigator, Reproductive Biology and Medicine Branch, National Institute of Child Health and Human Development, National Institutes of Health, Bethesda, Maryland

ERROL R. NORWITZ, MD, PhD, Associate Professor, Department of Obstetrics, Gynecology, and Reproductive Sciences, Yale University School of Medicine, New Haven, Connecticut

JOONG SHIN PARK, MD, PhD, Associate Professor, Department of Obstetrics and Gynecology, Seoul National University College of Medicine, Seoul, Korea

SHRITA M. PATEL, MD, Postdoctoral Fellow, Division of Endocrinology, Diabetes, and Metabolism; and Postdoctoral Fellow, Center for Clinical Epidemiology and Biostatistics, University of Pennsylvania School of Medicine, Philadelphia, Pennsylvania

ELLEN W. SEELY, MD, Associate Professor (Medicine), Endocrinology, Diabetes, and Hypertension Division, Harvard Medical School, Brigham and Women's Hospital, Boston, Massachusetts

REBECCA SIMMONS, MD, Associate Professor (Pediatrics), Department of Pediatrics, Children's Hospital of Philadelphia; and University of Pennsylvania, Philadelphia, Pennsylvania

VICTORIA SNEGOVSKIKH, MD, Postdoctoral Fellow, Department of Obstetrics, Gynecology, and Reproductive Sciences, Yale University School of Medicine, New Haven, Connecticut

CAREN G. SOLOMON, MD, MPH, Assistant Professor (Medicine), Divisions of General Medicine and Women's Health, Harvard Medical School, Brigham and Women's Hospital, Boston, Massachusetts

CONTENTS

Endocrinology of Parturition 173
Victoria Snegovskikh, Joong Shin Park, and Errol R. Norwitz

Reproductive success is critical for survival of the species. The timely onset of labor and delivery is an important determinant of perinatal outcome. Both preterm birth (defined as delivery before 37 weeks' gestation) and post-term pregnancy (defined as pregnancy continuing beyond 42 weeks) are associated with a significant increase in perinatal morbidity and mortality. The factors responsible for the timing of labor in the human are complex and, as yet, are not completely understood. This article reviews the current understanding of the parturition cascade responsible for the spontaneous onset of labor at term and discusses preterm labor and post-term pregnancy.

Developmental Origins of Adult Metabolic Disease 193
Rebecca Simmons

The combined epidemiologic, clinical, and animal studies clearly demonstrate that the intrauterine environment influences growth and development of the fetus and the subsequent development of adult diseases. There are critical specific windows during development, often coincident with periods of rapid cell division, during which a stimulus or insult may have long-lasting consequences on tissue or organ function after birth. Birth weight is only one marker of an adverse fetal environment, and confining studies to this population only may lead to erroneous conclusions regarding etiology. Studies using animal models of uteroplacental insufficiency suggest that mitochondrial dysfunction and oxidative stress play an important role in the pathogenesis of the fetal origins of adult disease.

FORTHCOMING ISSUES

RECENT ISSUES

ELSEVIER
SAUNDERS

Endocrinol Metab Clin N Am
35 (2006) xi–xii

ENDOCRINOLOGY
AND METABOLISM
CLINICS
OF NORTH AMERICA

Foreword

Endocrine Disorders During Pregnancy

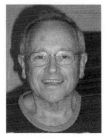

Derek LeRoith, MD, PhD
Consulting Editor

In the present issue of *Endocrinology and Metabolism Clinics of North America*, Dr. Mandel has compiled articles by experts on a topic involving endocrine disorders during pregnancy.

In the article on the gestational diabetes, Dr. Langer points out that diabetes is the commonest medical complication of pregnancy. On the important topic of therapy he further describes the issues of using insulin analogs and oral agents in pregnancy. The article by Jovanovic and Nakai cover similar aspects but focus more on the pregnant Type 1 diabetic patient.

Dr. Nestler approaches the patient with polycystic ovarian syndrome (PCOS); one of the commonest causes of infertility. As is now commonly appreciated, PCOS is associated with insulin resistance and often has features related to this metabolic disorder. Therapy with metformin (a biguanide) or thiazolidinediones reduces insulin resistance, restores menstruation, and often is associated with restoration of fertility.

Hypertensive disorders and pregnancy ranging from essential hypertension to the more serious condition of preeclampsia and eclampsia are well-covered in practical terms in the article by Dr. Seely.

Adult endocrinologic disorders during pregnancy are discussed in this issue and include pituitary, adrenal, thyroid and calcium disorders.

Dr. Molitch discusses pituitary disorders and describes the diagnosis and management of prolactinomas, acromegaly, pituitary Cushing's disease, hypopituitary and hypophysitis, reminding the reader of the pitfalls of hormonal measurements that are altered by the pregnant state.

In the article by Drs. Lindsay and Nieman on adrenal disorders, there is an excellent account of some endocrine conditions that are rare in pregnancy including Cushing's disease, pheochromocytoma, primary aldosteronism, and Addison's disease. The authors describe the pitfalls in clinical diagnosis and testing as well as management that will be extremely informative for many clinicians.

There are quite significant changes in calcium and bone metabolism during pregnancy and lactation including changes in intestinal calcium absorption and calcium release from the skeleton. All of these are necessary for fetal and neonatal development. As discussed by Drs. Kovacs and Fuleihan the long-term consequences to the mother are minimal. However, once again these marked changes in many of the parameters make the diagnosis and management of the various disease syndromes in pregnancy more complicated. While hyper and hypoparathyroidsm and other metabolic bone conditions are relatively rare, they need particular attention as described in this article.

Drs. Mandel and LeBeau discuss thyroid disorders in pregnancy, covering the effect of pregnancy on thyroid function and thyroid hormone measurements. Conversely, thyroid metabolism affects pregnancy, and thyroid disorders in pregnancy need particular care due to the effects on the pregnancy, the fetus, and the newborn.

Finally, there are two excellent articles that round off the topic; one covered by Dr. Norwitz on the endocrinology of parturition and the other by Dr. Simmons on fetal imprinting and its effects on the endocrine system. These articles bring the reader information that will have practical importance in the not too distant future.

Like Dr. Mandel, who has succeeded a timely and important issue, I believe that the reader will find this issue both extremely informative and practical.

Derek LeRoith, MD, PhD
Division of Endocrinology, Metabolism, and Bone Diseases
Mount Sinai School of Medicine
New York, NY, USA

ENDOCRINOLOGY
AND METABOLISM
CLINICS
OF NORTH AMERICA

ELSEVIER
SAUNDERS

Endocrinol Metab Clin N Am
35 (2006) xiii–xiv

Preface

Endocrine Disorders During Pregnancy

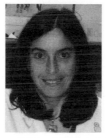

Susan J. Mandel, MD, MPH
Guest Editor

It has been 11 years since the last publication of an issue of the *Endocrinology and Metabolism Clinics of North America* that focused on endocrine disorders during pregnancy. In the preface, Lois Jovanovic, guest editor of and contributing author in that issue, wrote that there were three endocrine components to mammalian pregnancy: fetal, placental, and maternal endocrinology. And, of these, she observed, the maternal was the most understood and the focus of many of the articles contained in that issue. Fortunately, in the ensuing 11 years, we have learned much about the other two components, specifically the influences of maternal endocrine disorders on the feto–placental unit.

In this issue, I have selected topics that cover each of the main subspecialties (adrenal, pituitary, diabetes, thyroid, and calcium/bone) within adult endocrinology. For each area, the authors have delineated the current understanding of its physiology and pathophysiology during gestation as well as outlined the maternal therapy to optimize pregnancy outcome. In addition, I have included an article on the impact of polycystic ovarian syndrome on fertility, relevant because of its prevalence and the availability of therapy. Cardiovascular endocrinology, a newer subspecialty within our discipline, is well-represented by the article on pregnancy and hypertensive disorders. There are two other "nontraditional" articles. Recently, we have gained understanding of the effects of the intrauterine milieu on the future endocrine development of the child and this is presented in the section on imprinting. Lastly, the conclusion of pregnancy, parturition, represents a complex hormonal interplay that is described in the article on endocrinology of parturition.

I have had the pleasure and honor of working with renowned experts in their respective fields and in large part because of them, it has been a privilege to serve as the Guest Editor of this issue of the *Endocrinology and Metabolism Clinics of North America*. I thank my colleagues for their outstanding contributions to this volume, which is a valuable and timely addition to its field.

Susan J. Mandel, MD, MPH
Division of Endocrinology, Diabetes, and Metabolism
University of Pennsylvania School of Medicine
415 Curie Boulevard
611 CRB
Philadelphia, PA 19104, USA

E-mail address: smandel@mail.med.upenn.edu

ELSEVIER
SAUNDERS

Endocrinol Metab Clin N Am
35 (2006) 1–20

ENDOCRINOLOGY
AND METABOLISM
CLINICS
OF NORTH AMERICA

Adrenal Disorders in Pregnancy

John R. Lindsay, MD, Lynnette K. Nieman, MD*

Reproductive Biology and Medicine Branch, National Institute of Child Health and Human Development, National Institutes of Health, Bethesda MD, USA

The hypothalamic-pituitary-adrenal (HPA) axis and the renin-angiotensin system (RAS) are up-regulated during normal pregnancy. Pregnancy represents a state of relative hypercortisolism, resulting from the interaction of the maternal HPA axis and the fetal-placental unit. Consistent with a physiologic role, the RAS maintains normal sodium balance and volume homeostasis. In normal gestation, hypercortisolism and relative hyperaldosteronism are not usually clinically apparent. In contrast, adrenal disorders that do occur during pregnancy contribute to significant maternal and fetal morbidity. This article reviews the natural history, causes, diagnosis, and treatment of adrenal causes of Cushing's syndrome, adrenocortical hypofunction, primary hyperaldosteronism, and the management of adrenal pheochromocytoma in pregnancy.

Cushing's syndrome in pregnancy

The clinical presentation of Cushing's syndrome in pregnancy is similar to that in the general population, except for the preservation of menses before conception. The cause, however, differs between the pregnant and nonpregnant state because adrenal causes of Cushing's syndrome account for over 60% of 122 previous reports in pregnancy, in contrast with 15% in nonpregnant women [1,2]. Solitary adrenal adenomas are the most common cause, whereas adrenal carcinoma accounts for approximately 10% of cases [3,4]. Pheochromocytoma causing ectopic Cushing's syndrome was reported on two occasions. Its rarity may be explained by the anovulation that usually accompanies severe hypercortisolism [3,5]. Primary pigmented

---

* Corresponding author. Reproductive Biology and Medicine Branch, National Institute of Child Health and Human Development, National Institutes of Health, Building 10, CRC Room 1-3140, Bethesda MD 20892-1109.

E-mail address: niemanl@mail.nih.gov (L.K. Nieman).

0889-8529/06/$ - see front matter Published by Elsevier Inc.
doi:10.1016/j.ecl.2005.09.010

nodular adrenal disease and adrenocorticotropic hormone (ACTH)-inde-
pendent hyperplasia, caused possibly by aberrant receptor stimulation, accounted for eight cases of the pregnancies [1]. The overall increased
incidence of adrenal Cushing's syndrome suggests that anovulation may
be less prevalent in this cause or that unrecognized, illicit luteinizing hor-
mone/human chorionic gonadotropin receptor expression was considered
to be adrenal adenoma [6,7]. In the latter setting, Cushing's syndrome would
not be triggered until pregnancy is established.

Cushing's syndrome in gestation is associated with maternal morbidity,
including preeclampsia, hypertension, diabetes, wound breakdown, oppor-
tunistic infections, and fracture [4,8]. Maternal death was reported in two
cases [5,9]. Hypercortisolism effects on the fetus include increased rates of
spontaneous abortion, perinatal death, premature birth, and intrauterine
growth retardation [2,4]. As a result of this fetal and maternal morbidity,
early diagnosis and treatment of Cushing's syndrome in pregnancy are critical. However, the physiologic changes of pregnancy complicate this goal.
Plasma cortisol, cortisol-binding protein (CBG), and urinary free cortisol
(UFC) increase during the second and third trimesters (Fig. 1) [10,11]. There
are no formal studies of how the usual diagnostic criteria should be modified
to allow for pregnancy-induced hypercortisolism.

Screening and differential diagnosis of Cushing's syndrome

The interpretation of screening tests for hypercortisolism is more difficult
in pregnancy, particularly in the second and third trimesters. In the first trimester, cortisol excretion is similar to that of nonpregnant women. It then
increases up to threefold by term, to overlap values seen in pregnant women
with Cushing's syndrome [10]. As a result, it is likely that only the UFC values in the second and third trimester greater than three times the upper limit
of normal can be interpreted as indicating Cushing's syndrome. Unfortunately, there are limited data on the upper range of UFC in normal pregnancy, using modern antibody-based assays, and no reports of UFC
measured by structural assays such as mass spectrometry. Plasma cortisol
diurnal variation is preserved in normal pregnancy, albeit with a higher
nighttime nadir. Although the loss of diurnal variation is characteristic of
Cushing's syndrome, diagnostic thresholds for evening plasma or salivary
cortisol levels in pregnant patients have not been developed [1,10]. Furthermore, the suppression of serum and urinary cortisol by dexamethasone is
blunted in pregnancy (Fig. 2). Thus, this screening test has an increased potential for false-positive results in pregnancy. Although the evidence is limited, the present authors suggest a combination of greater than threefold
elevation of UFC and elevated midnight salivary cortisol as a diagnostic
strategy for the identification of Cushing's syndrome in pregnancy [12,13].

The first step in the differential diagnosis is to discriminate between
ACTH-independent and ACTH-dependent hypercortisolism, which may

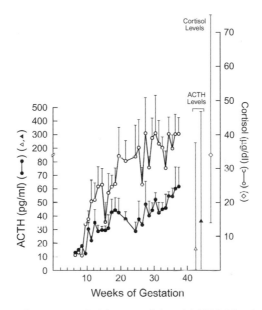

Fig. 1. Serial increases in serum cortisol (*open circles*) and ACTH (*closed circles*) during pregnancy in normal controls throughout pregnancy. This graph was modified from the series of five normal pregnant women studied by Carr and colleagues (1981). The bars adjacent to the right axis are summary data derived from a recent series [1] to denote the range of serum cortisol observed in Cushing's syndrome in pregnancy (*open diamonds*, median and range; n = 52); ACTH values for Cushing's disease (*closed triangles*, median and range, n = 18); and adrenal Cushing's syndrome (*open triangles*, median and range, n = 17). (*Modified from* Carr BR, Parker CR Jr, Madden JD, et al. Maternal plasma adrenocorticotropin and cortisol relationships throughout human pregnancy. Am J Obstet Gynecol 1981;139(4):416–22.)

be achieved by measuring plasma ACTH levels [14]. A two-site immunometric assay is preferred to radioimmunoassay, unless the latter can reliably discriminate low or suppressed ACTH levels (≤ 10 pg/mL [2.2 pmol/L]) [14,15]. To avoid falsely low results, it is important to collect the sample in prechilled ethylenediaminetetraacetic acid tubes, transport it to an ice bath, and prepare it promptly by refrigerated centrifugation and plasma separation.

In the nonpregnant population, plasma ACTH suppression (≤ 5 pg/mL [1.1 pmol/L]) identifies ACTH-independent primary adrenal causes of Cushing's syndrome. However, in a recent review of Cushing's syndrome in pregnancy, mean plasma ACTH levels were nonsuppressed in approximately half of those patients who had primary adrenal disorders, perhaps because of continued stimulation of the maternal HPA axis by placental CRH or because of placental secretion of ACTH [1,16]. As a result, the recommended diagnostic ACTH thresholds in the general population may lead to inaccurate diagnoses in pregnancy [15].

If plasma ACTH is suppressed, no further biochemical testing is needed, and imaging of the adrenal glands, discussed below, then will localize the

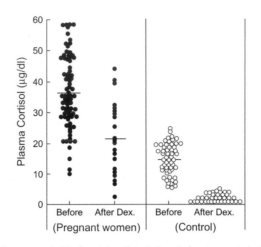

Fig. 2. Change in plasma cortisol before (*closed circles*) and after (*open circles*) the administration of 1 mg of dexamethasone (Dex) in pregnant women. Blood was drawn at 8 AM. A single dose of dexamethasone was administered orally at 11 PM, and blood was drawn at 8 AM on the following day. (*From* Odagiri E, Ishiwatari N, Abe Y, et al. Hypercortisolism and the resistance to dexamethasone suppression during gestation. Endocrinol Jpn 1988;35:685–90; with permission.)

abnormality to a unilateral adrenal adenoma or carcinoma or rare bilateral adrenal disorders. A normal or elevated plasma ACTH level ($\geq$15 pg/mL [3.3 pmol/L]) is consistent with an ACTH-producing tumor (keeping in mind the caveats discussed above) [15]. Although the high-dose dexamethasone suppression test (HDST) has not been formally validated in pregnancy, it may have added value for the differential diagnosis of adrenal Cushing's syndrome, given the difficulties in the interpretation of plasma ACTH and the increased prevalence of adrenal disorders. Using a criterion of 80% suppression of serum cortisol, none of seven cases who had ACTH-independent Cushing's syndrome showed suppression in a recent small series. However three of seven cases of Cushing's disease would have been misclassified because they also failed to suppress [1].

The CRH stimulation test is useful primarily for the differential diagnosis of ACTH-dependent Cushing's syndrome. Ovine CRH (the analog available in the United States) is a category C drug approved by the US Food and Drug Administration (FDA). Therefore, the present authors advocate that its use be reserved for patients in whom adrenal disorders are unlikely after initial testing.

Patients with borderline or low plasma ACTH or without suppression on HDST are likely to have an adrenal cause, and such cases warrant adrenal imaging. Ultrasonographic (US) imaging has a reported sensitivity for detection of adrenal lesions of 89% to 97%, and its use is not limited by pregnancy [17]. The advantages of US are that it is noninvasive, rapid, inexpensive, and readily available. However, MRI may be preferred, particularly if an ACTH-producing pheochromocytoma is being considered, because its appearance on T2-weighted imaging is bright. MRI also may provide better imaging resolution preoperatively. (Because gadolinium contrast is an FDA category C agent, it is not given to pregnant women at the authors' institution.) MRI alone is contraindicated in the first trimester because of unknown potential teratogenic effects, but it is considered safe after 32 weeks. In the middle trimester, the potential benefits of MRI must be weighed against its possible risks. A suggested algorithm for the differential diagnosis of Cushing's syndrome is shown in Fig. 3.

Treatment

There does not appear to be a rationale for supportive care as the only treatment of Cushing's syndrome in pregnancy. The live birth rate after unilateral or bilateral adrenalectomy is approximately 87% [1]. In contrast, the prognosis for the fetus remains guarded when hypercortisolism persists. Although placental degradation of cortisol appears to protect the fetus from glucocorticoid excess, the high incidence of adverse fetal outcomes probably reflects placental and maternal abnormalities. Thus, the present authors recommend surgical treatment of Cushing's syndrome in the second trimester of pregnancy, with medical treatment as a second choice.

The surgical approach is not altered by pregnancy, and the goal is to remove the tumor causing the condition. Thus, transsphenoidal surgery is recommended for pituitary ACTH-producing tumors (see elsewhere in this issue), specific resection for ectopic ACTH-producing tumors, and unilateral

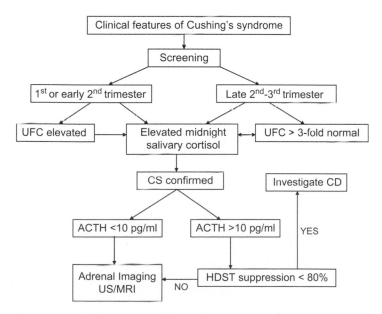

Fig. 3. Diagnostic algorithm for the differential diagnosis of Cushing's syndrome (CS) in pregnancy.

or bilateral adrenalectomy for primary adrenal disorders. Unless otherwise contraindicated, a laparoscopic approach for adrenalectomy is standard. Bilateral adrenalectomy remains an option for patients needing an immediate cure of Cushing's syndrome in whom the primary tumor is occult, inoperable, or metastatic, just as for nonpregnant patients.

Primary medical therapy has been reported in approximately 20 women with Cushing's syndrome resulting from a range of causes [18,19]. Metyrapone was used in about half the women, and, whereas it was well tolerated generally, the side effects included hypertension and progression to preeclampsia [20–22]. Therefore metyrapone is best reserved as an interim treatment, pending definitive surgical treatment [20]. Ketoconazole is an FDA category C agent and has been used successfully in three pregnancies despite known teratogenic effects at high dosages in rats but not in rabbits [1,18]. Given the potential risks, in the present authors' opinion, ketoconazole should be reserved for individuals who need emergent medical therapy but cannot tolerate metyrapone [18]. Cyproheptadine is not effective in nonpregnant individuals and thus is not recommended [23]. Fetal masculinization precludes the use of aminoglutethimide [24]. Similarly, mitotane is contraindicated because it crosses the placenta and is teratogenic [25].

Primary adrenal insufficiency in pregnancy

Primary adrenal insufficiency (AI) can present acutely or with a more insidious set of chronic symptoms. Primary AI (so-called Addison's disease) is characterized by the impairment of aldosterone or cortisol secretion and adrenocortical atrophy arising from insensitivity to ACTH and angiotensin II stimulation. The exact prevalence of AI occurring in pregnancy is unknown. In a series reported by Albert and colleagues [26] from Tromso, Norway, the estimated incidence of AI in pregnancy was 1 per 3000 births between 1976 and 1987.

Isolated autoimmune adrenalitis is the most common cause of primary AI in developed countries. Although the glands are small in autoimmune primary adrenal disease, they are large in tuberculous or fungal infection, bilateral metastases, hemorrhage, or infarction. Less common causes of AI, autoimmune polyglandular syndrome type 2 (APS-2) and Schmidt's syndrome (primary autoimmune hypoadrenalism, type 1 diabetes mellitus, thyroid autoimmune disease), were reported in at least seven pregnancies [27]. In APS-2, the appropriate management of hypothyroidism and diabetes during gestation poses a particular challenge beyond that of isolated hypoadrenalism [27].

Maternal and fetal morbidity and mortality

AI in pregnancy was associated with maternal mortality rates of 35% in the 70-year period before 1930, which improved to 18% between 1940 and

1947 [28]. The present authors believe there have been no reports of maternal deaths from AI in pregnancy since the 1950s, with the introduction of cortisone, earlier diagnosis, and improved antenatal care. However, a reported case of maternal death at 8 months after delivery illustrates the importance of careful postpartum follow-up [26]. Some cases that were not diagnosed during pregnancy had normal maternal and fetal outcomes, suggesting that women with unrecognized AI benefit from transplacental passage of cortisol from the fetus. Therefore, AI may only become apparent in the immediate postpartum period [29]. In women known to have the disease, careful titration of glucocorticoid and mineralocorticoid replacement are required to avoid an adrenal crisis and potential side effects, including hypertension and exacerbation of preeclampsia [26,30].

Gestational AI has been associated with high rates of intrauterine growth retardation, low birth weight [31,32], and fetal mortality [33]. A recent Italian series reported improved miscarriage rates (16 of 104 pregnancies) compared with intrauterine death rates in the 1950s of 40% to 50% [34]. Most of the earlier reports consisted of previously unrecognized cases or preceded the availability of modern glucocorticoid regimens [35]. These differences have led to the speculation that, treated properly, women do not have increased complications of gestation. There does not appear to be an increased risk of preterm abortion or congenital anomalies resulting from AI alone, when patients are treated adequately [36]. However, when AI is associated with other autoimmune conditions, including positive circulating anticardiolipin antibodies, lupus anticoagulant, and diabetes, there may be additional risks of preterm abortion [37–39].

Diagnosis

Clinical and laboratory features

Most cases of primary AI are diagnosed before pregnancy. During gestation, a new diagnosis should be considered in a case with classic symptoms of excessive fatigue, malaise, weight loss, vomiting, orthostasis, abdominal pain, hyperpigmentation, or biochemical disturbance [30,39,40]. Hypoglycemia, salt craving, malaise, seizures, or even coma should prompt testing of the HPA axis in pregnancy. Persistent vomiting can be mistaken for hyperemesis gravidarum, potentially leading to a fatal outcome if left undiagnosed [40]. Biochemical disturbance with hyponatremia is characteristic; however, this is usually more severe than the mild hyponatremia (5-mmol/L decrease) that occurs in normal pregnancy. Severe hyponatremia or metabolic acidosis is associated with poor outcomes, including fetal death [33]. Hyperkalemia was reported to be absent in several cases of newly diagnosed primary AI during pregnancy. This may reflect the increase in the RAS, rather than the severity of adrenocortical dysfunction [33,40].

Screening tests and differential diagnosis of adrenal insufficiency

Testing consists of assessing the functional integrity of the HPA axis followed by a search for the underlying cause of AI. In an unstable patient, empirical glucocorticoid therapy is recommended when the clinical suspicion for adrenal crisis is high, just as in nonpregnant patients [30]. Samples for plasma cortisol and ACTH should be obtained before treatment, whenever possible. The existing tests of HPA reserve have not been validated formally in pregnancy. The present authors do not recommend using metyrapone stimulation or insulin tolerance tests in pregnancy because of the potential risks to the fetus of precipitating maternal adrenal crisis. The CRH stimulation test is useful for differentiating between tertiary and secondary AI in nonpregnant patients, but it cannot be relied on for a diagnosis in pregnancy because cortisol and ACTH responses to CRH are blunted [41].

A low early morning plasma cortisol level (≤ 3.0 μg/dL [83 nmol/L]) confirms AI in the setting of a typical clinical presentation [42]. In the first and early second trimesters, the diagnosis can be excluded in a clinically stable patient if basal plasma cortisol levels are greater than 19 μg/dL (525 nmol/L) [42,43]. Because of the normal increase in cortisol and CBG in the late second and third trimesters, the present authors recommend formal dynamic testing of the HPA axis at those times.

The standard cosyntropin (1–24 corticotropin) test (SCT) is performed by administering a supraphysiologic dose of 250 μg, intramuscularly (IM) or intravenously (IV), and measuring plasma cortisol levels after 30 and 60 minutes. Cosyntropin is licensed by the FDA as category C. The test may be performed at any time of the day, and the 30-minute cutoff point is considered the most consistent measure for diagnosis [44]. In the nonpregnant population, cortisol cutoff points for the diagnosis of AI range from 18 μg/dL to 25.4 μg/dL (497–700 nmol/L) [45–47]. The standard test performs well in nonpregnant patients who have primary AI, with high sensitivity and specificity (97% and 95%, respectively) [48], but it is less sensitive for the detection of early hypopituitarism [49]. Although conventional nonpregnant criteria generally have been applied in pregnancy, in one series [50], plasma cortisol responses to standard cosyntropin testing in normal pregnant women ranged from 60% to 80% above nonpregnant responses in the second and third trimesters. As a result, there is insufficient information to determine appropriate pregnancy-specific cutoff points.

McKenna and colleagues [42] recently examined responses to the 1-μg low-dose cosyntropin test (LCT) for diagnosis of secondary AI in women at 24–34 weeks of gestation. Using a threshold above 30 μg/dL (828 nmol/L) following LCT, the test had high sensitivity for the diagnosis of AI. Significantly, in most cases, the diagnosis of AI could be predicted by an 8 AM plasma cortisol level of less than 3 μg/dL (83 nmol/L). Furthermore, the low-dose test is more difficult to perform than the SCT with regard to preparation, dilution, and ensuring an accurate dose administration [42].

Although criteria for diagnosing AI in pregnancy have not been developed, the previously reported 8 AM third-trimester plasma cortisol levels and responses to the SCT in normal pregnant women and the results from the low-dose cosyntropin stimulation testing cited above provide useful information. Taken together, the present authors consider basal or ACTH-stimulated plasma cortisol levels in the third trimester greater than 30 µg/dL (828 nmol/L) sufficient to exclude AI [42].

Tests used for the differential diagnosis

Plasma ACTH levels differentiate primary (elevated) from secondary adrenal failure (low or normal) and can help to confirm primary AI in non-pregnant patients who have borderline plasma cortisol levels. An ACTH level above 100 pg/mL (22 pmol/L) is generally consistent with primary AI, even in late pregnancy [43]. However, ACTH levels fluctuate widely day-to-day, and a single value cannot be relied on for the diagnosis of either primary or secondary AI.

Approximately 90% of nonpregnant patients who have idiopathic AI are positive for 21-hydroxylase antibodies, and antibodies to 17-α-hydroxylase and side-chain cleavage enzymes are positive in approximately 30% of patients [51]. The presence of adrenal antibodies provides confirmatory evidence for an autoimmune cause, but it cannot be relied on for diagnosing AI, given the 10% prevalence of negative test results in patients proven to have AI. The presence of mineralocorticoid deficiency is highly suggestive of primary AI arising from adrenocortical atrophy, and in this setting, plasma aldosterone-to-renin ratios are low in association with elevated plasma renin activity [52].

Patients who have an autoimmune cause do not require imaging. Imaging of the adrenal glands can detect the large glands associated with other causes, such as tuberculous or fungal infection, bilateral metastases, hemorrhage, or infarction [39,53,54]. US imaging is safe but may have limited resolution. Non-gadolinium-enhanced MRI is preferred to CT in pregnancy. Although MRI provides excellent soft tissue enhancement and has improved resolution compared with ultrasound [55], deferring adrenal imaging until the postpartum period should be considered if the patient is clinically stable.

Treatment

The optimal antenatal management of AI occurs in a multidisciplinary clinic that includes an endocrinologist. The primary roles for the endocrinologist are to provide a diagnosis, monitor the adequacy of corticosteroid or mineralocorticoid replacement regimens during gestation, crisis, and labor, and to ensure continuity during the postpartum period. Prepregnancy counseling should be conducted routinely in women of childbearing age. Women should be educated regarding the principles of self-administration of intramuscular hydrocortisone (50–100 mg) for pregnancy-associated emesis before urgent medical assessment. All patients should wear a medic alert bracelet or necklace for identification during an emergency.

Physiologic glucocorticoid and mineralocorticoid treatment appears to be safe during pregnancy [56]. The most critical periods in pregnancy when the adequacy of glucocorticoid replacement regimens may affect outcomes are in undiagnosed cases during the first trimester when symptoms of adrenal crisis can be mistaken for pregnancy-associated emesis and during the stress of labor and delivery [33].

Several glucocorticoid regimens are available for chronic replacement during pregnancy. Hydrocortisone is the present authors' preferred choice, at a replacement dose of 12 mg/m^2 to 15 mg/m^2 of body surface area [57]. Two thirds of the daily dose is given when the patient awakens, with the remainder given in the afternoon to mimic normal diurnal variation. Although this dose may lead to over-replacement in a proportion of nonpregnant cases, in the absence of more detailed studies during pregnancy, this approach seems reasonable [58]. Glucocorticoid replacement regimens usually remain stable during gestation, even until late in the third trimester. Prednisone or prednisolone may be used as alternative glucocorticoid regimens. Prednisone and cortisone acetate are not useful for the emergency management of adrenal crisis because they require the reduction of a ketone group to a hydroxyl group on carbon-11 to active metabolites. Furthermore, they are longer acting compared with hydrocortisone and less suitable for physiologic replacement [59].

Oral fludrocortisone, 0.1 mg daily (ranging between 0.05 mg and 0.2 mg), is standard mineralocorticoid replacement and has largely replaced salt tablet regimens [59]. Fludrocortisone dosages are usually stable through pregnancy but occasionally may need to be reduced during the third trimester to avoid the side effects of edema or exacerbation of hypertension [60].

The acute treatment of adrenal crisis includes prompt, rapid glucocorticoid replacement with hydrocortisone, 100 mg to 200 mg IV, as a single bolus. Thereafter a bolus of 50 mg to 100 mg is given every 6 to 8 hours during the acute period, based on maximal cortisol production rates of 200 mg/d to 400 mg/d [30]. Women with hypoglycemia should receive 5% dextrose infusions, and those with hypotension should receive 0.9% saline. Because hydrocortisone at these dose levels contains adequate mineralocorticoid activity, fludrocortisone is not indicated in the acute period and has been associated with the side effects of pulmonary edema caused by salt and water retention [30]. A transfer to routine oral therapy is warranted when acute symptoms have settled or when the patient is tolerating oral fluids.

During labor and the postpartum period

Routine glucocorticoid and mineralocorticoid replacement therapy can be continued until the onset of labor, provided that the patient has no symptoms of under-replacement. Normal vaginal delivery is a reasonable expectation for women with AI. Caesarian (C)-section is considered for indications similar to those in a nonpregnant individual [26]. During labor, the patient's normal dose of hydrocortisone is doubled, provided that oral intake is tolerated. Alternatively, a single dose of hydrocortisone, 50 mg IV, may be considered during the second stage of labor [34]. Before caesarian section is performed, however, stress doses of hydrocortisone, 100 mg IV or IM, are given at the onset and continued at 6- to 8-hour intervals after delivery [57]. The doses of hydrocortisone can then be tapered over 48 hours to a regular replacement dose [57,59].

After delivery, all women should recommence mineralocorticoid or corticosteroid replacement within the first 24 to 48 hours, usually at the dose used before gestation. Stress coverage may be required during recovery from surgery or intercurrent illness. The assessment of the HPA axis is usually not necessary for infants whose mothers with AI received appropriate physiologic glucocorticoid replacement. However, infants born to mothers receiving pharmacologic doses of agents that cross the placenta (such as dexamethasone) require more formal assessment to exclude AI. Physiologic glucocorticoid replacement can continue during breast-feeding because less than 0.5% of the absorbed dose is excreted per liter of breast milk [32,56].

Hypertension in pregnancy

Normal gestation is associated with a fall in blood pressure toward the end of the first trimester, reaching a nadir between 22 and 24 weeks. Hypertension during pregnancy, defined by an absolute systolic or diastolic blood pressure exceeding 140 or 90 mmHg, respectively, complicates approximately 15% of pregnancies [61]. Increased vascular distensibility and reduced peripheral vascular resistance occurring in pregnancy are accompanied by physiologic changes, including sodium retention, increased extracellular fluid, and up-regulation of the RAS [62].

Hyperaldosteronism

The prevalence of primary hyperaldosteronism (PA) in nonpregnant hypertensive subjects varies between 1% and 12%, depending on the patient population, diagnostic methods used, and confirmation by surgery [63]. In contrast, PA is rare in pregnancy, with approximately 31 cases reported worldwide since the original description by Crane in 1964 [64,65]. The majority of reported cases arise as a result of adrenal adenoma or hyperplasia. However, there are rare reports of glucocorticoid-remediable hyperaldosteronism in pregnancy [66].

Plasma renin activity increases early in the first trimester of normal pregnancy, reaching values almost three- to seven-fold greater than the normal range by the third trimester [67,68]. The fetal-placenta unit is an additional important site of RAS activity [67,69]. Plasma aldosterone concentrations increase 5- to 20-fold between the first and third trimesters, in association with the enlargement of the zona fasiculata [70]. Corticosterone, deoxycortisol, and cortisone parallel the two- to threefold rise seen in cortisol during gestation [70]. Although the RAS is markedly stimulated during pregnancy, both renin and aldosterone respond physiologically, albeit at an altered set point [71]. Aldosterone responses to salt loading, posture, diuretics, volume depletion, and the administration of mineralocorticoid suggest that the RAS is under tight physiologic control [62,72].

PA in pregnancy is associated typically with hypertension and associated with hypokalemia in a high proportion of cases (16/29) in a recent review by Okawa and colleagues [64,73]. Patients may present with symptoms that include headache, fatigue, weakness, dizziness, and muscle cramps [74]. In a series of 27 cases progressing to delivery, pregnancy was characterized by moderate to severe hypertension in 85% and proteinuria in 52% of patients [64]. Placental abruption complicated the clinical course of several cases, and two intrauterine fetal deaths occurred [65,75]. High rates of preterm delivery (52%) were partially attributable to emergent delivery for cases with uncontrolled hypertension [75]. Hypertension may improve during gestation in PA because elevated progesterone levels have antimineralocorticoid effects at the renal tubule [73].

The diagnosis and treatment of PA present particular challenges in the setting of pregnancy. PA during pregnancy is characterized by elevated aldosterone and suppressed plasma renin. Although pregnancy-specific cutoffs for PA have not been validated, the range of plasma aldosterone in one series was 129 pg/mL to 1093 pg/mL [64]. The peak mean third trimester pregnancy levels for plasma renin activity and aldosterone were 5.8 ng/mL/h and 594 pg/mL, respectively, in the series by Wilson and colleagues [68]. Thus, the physiologic rise in aldosterone in normal pregnancy overlaps the values seen with PA, making the diagnosis of PA more difficult. However, suppressed renin in the setting of hyperaldosteronism is diagnostic of PA.

The confirmation of PA during gestation with dynamic testing using intravenous saline may not be helpful, given the potential risks to the fetus and the lack of normative data [76]. Although posture testing can sometimes differentiate unilateral adenoma from bilateral hyperplasia, the diagnostic accuracy of this technique remains controversial, even in nonpregnant patients. The differential diagnostic strategy for PA in the nonpregnant population consists of adrenal CT and adrenal vein sampling to localize an adenoma and discriminate it from bilateral adrenal hyperplasia. In pregnancy, imaging with MRI or ultrasonography is preferable to CT, with the appropriate precautions and limitations outlined above. In the present authors' experience, adrenal vein sampling has not been attempted during pregnancy. It is not clear that the potential risk from fluoroscopy during the procedure would outweigh the potential benefit. In nonpregnant cases under the age of 40 years, it is generally considered appropriate to proceed to unilateral adrenalectomy for patients who have unilateral adrenal macronodules ($\geq$ 1 cm) and a normal contralateral gland. However, there are no published guidelines for localization based on adenoma size alone in pregnancy. In the absence of definitive imaging findings, deferring additional diagnostic tests and surgery to the postpartum period may be more appropriate.

Adrenalectomy in the second trimester may be considered for cases with PA caused by adrenal adenoma. Adrenalectomy has been reported in four cases of PA caused by adenoma during pregnancy [77–79]. In each instance, the blood pressure normalized after surgery. The benefits of successful surgery include normalization of blood pressure, which can be expected in approximately two thirds of nonpregnant cases, together with the normalization of serum potassium in a majority of cases. These benefits have to be balanced against the potential risks of surgery or medical therapy in pregnancy. At least two cases illustrate successful medical management pending definitive localization or adrenalectomy in the postpartum period [73,80].

Medical therapy is indicated for cases that have adrenal adenoma that are identified late in gestation or those who have adrenal hyperplasia. Therapeutic options in nonpregnant patients include spironolactone or amiloride for specific aldosterone blockade. However, spironolactone is contraindicated in pregnancy because it has been associated with incomplete virilization of the male rat and has the potential for feminization of a male infant [81]. Amiloride, which is FDA class C, has been used safely in Bartter syndrome in pregnancy, with no reported teratogenicity [82]. The antihypertensive agents considered safe in pregnancy such as methyldopa may have limited efficacy in treating PA. The additional disadvantages of these and other agents are the ongoing requirements for high potassium supplementation. Angiotensin converting enzyme inhibitors are contraindicated in pregnancy. Although calcium channel blockers are relatively safe in pregnancy, they may have limited efficacy in the setting of hyperaldosteronism [76].

Pheochromocytoma in pregnancy

Pheochromocytoma accounts for approximately 0.1% cases of hypertension in the general population. There have been at least 200 cases diagnosed in pregnancy, and the estimated prevalence at term is approximately 1 in 54,000 [83,84]. Pheochromocytoma is associated with sustained or paroxysmal episodes of hypertension, pallor, headaches, and palpitations [84]. Other presentations include chest pain, dyspnea, abdominal pain, seizure, or even sudden death [85]. Although antenatal diagnosis is associated with improved outcomes, pheochromocytoma can be missed because of unexpectedly normal blood pressure during gestation [83,85]. A recent case illustrated the course of a women who was managed emergently after being diagnosed during labor [86]. However, a delayed diagnosis has been associated with maternal death caused by cerebral edema associated with cardiogenic shock [85].

Untreated pheochromocytoma is associated with increased fetal and maternal morbidity and mortality. The maternal mortality rate was 48% before 1969 and 26% in the 1970s, and subsequently it fell to 17% [87–89]. Since 1990, approximately 85% of cases have been diagnosed antenatally, perhaps because of increased awareness [84]. In one series, antenatal diagnosis reduced the maternal mortality and the fetal loss rate to less than 1% and 15%, respectively [88]. A hypertensive crisis may be precipitated by abdominal palpitation [84], drugs, including metoclopramide [87], or labor. Pheochromocytoma should be actively sought for in patients who have affected family members with von Hippel-Lindau or multiple endocrine neoplasia 2 syndromes [90]. The lack of proteinuria in pheochromocytoma may differentiate pheochromocytoma from hypertension associated with preeclampsia. Other potential differential diagnoses include anxiety, cocaine use, pulmonary embolism, and alcohol withdrawal [84].

Catecholamine production generally remains stable during gestation [91]. Screening for pheochromocytoma was traditionally undertaken by assessing elevated 24-hour urinary epinephrine and norepinephrine excretions. Because tumor secretion may be episodic, these methods have been largely superseded by more sensitive and specific techniques. Fractionated urinary metanephrines and plasma metanephrines are more sensitive for the diagnosis of pheochromocytoma in nonpregnant patients, but their value in pregnancy has yet to be evaluated fully [92]. Dynamic testing with clonidine has not been validated in pregnancy [93]. Adrenal imaging is performed when the diagnosis is confirmed biochemically using existing nonpregnant reference ranges. MRI (without gadolinium) has better specificity than ultrasonography and is preferred to CT to minimize exposure to ionizing radiation. Pheochromocytoma is typically bright on T2-weighted MRI, with a sensitivity of 93% to 100% [94]. Metaiodobenzylguanidine-, fluorine-18 ([^{18}F])-dopa–, and [^{18}F]-dopamine–labeled positron emission tomography scanning methods are highly specific, functional imaging modalities that may be considered for localization in the postpartum period and have additional utility for assessing extra-adrenal disease, which occurs in approximately 10% of cases [94].

Adrenalectomy is the preferred definitive treatment of pheochromocytoma following adequate α- and β-blockade for at least 2 weeks before surgery. Primary medical therapy is indicated for cases diagnosed after 24 weeks gestation because of the attendant difficulties and risks of surgery performed at that time. α-Blockade with phenoxybenzamine, 10 mg to 20 mg twice daily, is begun initially, with titration to a dose of approximately 1 mg/kg/d until hypertension is controlled. After several days of α-blockade, β-blockers are added to minimize reflex tachycardia, despite their possible association with intrauterine growth retardation [88]. When used as monotherapy, unopposed β-blockade leads to vasoconstriction and potential hypertensive crisis and should be avoided. Metyrosine is a specific inhibitor of cathecholamine synthesis through its effect on tyrosine hydroxylase. Although it is an FDA category C agent, metyrosine was previously used in one patient with malignant pheochromocytoma without complication [95]. There are insufficient data to recommend its routine use in pregnancy, but it may be considered for short-term emergency use in cases late in the third trimester with refractory hypertension or arrhythmia [95]. Phentolamine, 1 mg to 5 mg, is the agent of choice for the treatment of a hypertensive crisis [86].

The optimal timing of adrenalectomy is late in the first or early in the second trimester. In the third trimester, a combined caesarian section followed by adrenalectomy for cases managed conservatively with medical therapy may be considered. Vaginal delivery is not recommended because of the potential for exacerbating a hypertensive crisis. A close liaison with the anesthesiologist is imperative before adrenalectomy, C-section, or labor.

Pregnancy and congenital adrenal hyperplasia

The prenatal diagnosis and treatment of 21-hydroxylase (CYP21 gene)–deficiency are options for couples who have a previously affected infant and may be requested by an index case before attempting pregnancy. Genetic counseling is guided by molecular investigation of the family, ideally by CYP21 genotyping of the affected individuals and an evaluation of the parents to exclude a new mutation in the child. Biochemical testing of the partner of an affected individual can identify a potential heterozygote, in which case genotyping should be performed [96].

Couples at risk for an affected infant may choose to undergo prenatal treatment with dexamethasone coupled with prenatal diagnosis. The goal of the treatment is to inhibit fetal ACTH and so prevent hyperandrogenism and virilization of an affected female fetus. Thus, dexamethasone, at a divided daily dose of 20 μg/kg of prepregnancy weight, is started when pregnancy is diagnosed. Dexamethasone is the agent of choice because it is not a ready substrate for 11-β-hydroxysteroid dehydrogenase type 2. Chorionic villous sampling is performed at 9 to 11 weeks for the evaluation of the fetus' sex and CYP21 gene. Dexamethasone is discontinued if the fetus is male or an unaffected female. As a result of this strategy, treatment would continue in only one of eight pregnancies. The initiation of therapy before 9 weeks has resulted in normal genitalia in 11 of 25 affected females and only mild virilization in another 11, but later treatment or the use of a lower dose of dexamethasone has resulted in virilization in 23 of 24 affected infants [97].

There are relatively few data on the long-term risks of prenatal dexamethasone treatment for affected or unaffected fetuses. One recent study showed that 174 children (including 48 who had CAH) who received dexamethasone did not differ in cognitive or motor development from 313 unexposed children, based on a maternal survey [98]. However, these children were 1 to 12 years old, and there are no data on long-term follow-up. Significant maternal side effects, including weight gain, edema, abnormal glucose tolerance, and hypertension, occur in up to 50% of women treated until delivery.

A recent consensus statement has emphasized the ethical issues related to the unnecessary treatment of unaffected female or male fetuses, the unknown risks to the infants, and the maternal risks. The statement counsels that only an experienced team should direct this therapy and that optimally patients should provide written informed consent and be enrolled in a research protocol approved by an ethics committee. Additionally, the report recommends prospective and long-term follow-up of all children receiving prenatal treatment [99].

Summary

Adrenal disorders occurring in pregnancy are rare but are associated with significant maternal and fetal morbidity. The diagnosis of adrenocortical and medullary dysfunction is more challenging than in the general population because of overlapping clinical and biochemical features of normal pregnancy. This article illustrates the pitfalls and challenges involved in the differential diagnosis and treatment during gestation. Increased suspicion for the diagnosis of adrenal disorders during pregnancy would likely facilitate early treatment and result in improved outcome for both the mother and fetus.

References

[1] Lindsay JR, Jonklaas J, Oldfield EH, et al. Cushing's syndrome during pregnancy: personal experience and review of the literature. J Clin Endocrinol Metab 2005;90(5):3077–83.
[2] Buescher MA, McClamrock HD, Adashi EY. Cushing syndrome in pregnancy. Obstet Gynecol 1992;79(1):130–7.
[3] Guilhaume B, Sanson ML, Billaud L, et al. Cushing's syndrome and pregnancy: aetiologies and prognosis in twenty-two patients. Eur J Med 1992;1(2):83–9.
[4] Aron DC, Schnall AM, Sheeler LR. Cushing's syndrome and pregnancy. Am J Obstet Gynecol 1990;162(1):244–52.
[5] Oh HC, Koh JM, Kim MS, et al. A case of ACTH-producing pheochromocytoma associated with pregnancy. Endocr J 2003;50(6):739–44.
[6] Wy LA, Carlson HE, Kane P, et al. Pregnancy-associated Cushing's syndrome secondary to a luteinizing hormone/human chorionic gonadotropin receptor-positive adrenal carcinoma. Gynecol Endocrinol 2002;16(5):413–7.
[7] Lacroix A, Hamet P, Boutin JM. Leuprolide acetate therapy in luteinizing hormone-dependent Cushing's syndrome. N Engl J Med 1999;341(21):1577–81.
[8] Sheeler LR. Cushing's syndrome and pregnancy. Endocrinol Metab Clin North Am 1994; 23(3):619–27.
[9] Koerten JM, Morales WJ, Washington SR III, et al. Cushing's syndrome in pregnancy: a case report and literature review. Am J Obstet Gynecol 1986;154(3):626–8.
[10] Carr BR, Parker CR Jr, Madden JD, et al. Maternal plasma adrenocorticotropin and cortisol relationships throughout human pregnancy. Am J Obstet Gynecol 1981;139(4):416–22.

[11] Evans JJ, Sin IL, Duff GB, et al. Estrogen-induced transcortin increase and progesterone and cortisol interactions: implications from pregnancy studies. Ann Clin Lab Sci 1987;17(2): 101–5.

[12] Putignano P, Toja P, Dubini A, Giraldi FP, et al. Midnight salivary cortisol versus urinary free and midnight serum cortisol as screening tests for Cushing's syndrome. J Clin Endocrinol Metab 2003;88(9):4153–7.

[13] Gafni RI, Papanicolaou DA, Nieman LK. Nighttime salivary cortisol measurement as a simple, noninvasive, outpatient screening test for Cushing's syndrome in children and adolescents. J Pediatr 2000;137(1):30–5.

[14] Raff H, Findling JW. A new immunoradiometric assay for corticotropin evaluated in normal subjects and patients with Cushing's syndrome. Clin Chem 1989;35(4):596–600.

[15] Arnaldi G, Angeli A, Atkinson AB, et al. Diagnosis and complications of Cushing's syndrome: a consensus statement. J Clin Endocrinol Metab 2003;88(12):5593–602.

[16] Magiakou MA, Mastorakos G, Rabin D, et al. The maternal hypothalamic-pituitary-adrenal axis in the third trimester of human pregnancy. Clin Endocrinol (Oxf) 1996;44(4): 419–28.

[17] Bowerman RA, Silver TM, Jaffe MH, et al. Sonography of adrenal pheochromocytomas. AJR Am J Roentgenol 1981;137(6):1227–31.

[18] Berwaerts J, Verhelst J, Mahler C, Abs R. Cushing's syndrome in pregnancy treated by ketoconazole: case report and review of the literature. Gynecol Endocrinol 1999;13(3): 175–82.

[19] Hana V, Dokoupilova M, Marek J, et al. Recurrent ACTH-independent Cushing's syndrome in multiple pregnancies and its treatment with metyrapone. Clin Endocrinol (Oxf) 2001;54(2):277–81.

[20] Connell JM, Cordiner J, Davies DL, et al. Pregnancy complicated by Cushing's syndrome: potential hazard of metyrapone therapy: case report. Br J Obstet Gynaecol 1985;92(11): 1192–5.

[21] Close CF, Mann MC, Watts JF, et al. ACTH-independent Cushing's syndrome in pregnancy with spontaneous resolution after delivery: control of the hypercortisolism with metyrapone. Clin Endocrinol (Oxf) 1993;39(3):375–9.

[22] Gormley MJ, Hadden DR, Kennedy TL, et al. Cushing's syndrome in pregnancy–treatment with metyrapone. Clin Endocrinol (Oxf) 1982;16(3):283–93.

[23] Khir AS, How J, Bewsher PD. Successful pregnancy after cyproheptadine treatment for Cushing's disease. Eur J Obstet Gynecol Reprod Biol 1982;13(6):343–7.

[24] Hanson TJ, Ballonoff LB, Northcutt RC. Amino-glutethimide and pregnancy [letter]. JAMA 1974;230(7):963–4.

[25] Leiba S, Weinstein R, Shindel B, et al. The protracted effect of o, p'-DDD in Cushing's disease and its impact on adrenal morphogenesis of young human embryo. Ann Endocrinol (Paris) 1989;50(1):49–53.

[26] Albert E, Dalaker K, Jorde R, Berge LN. Addison's disease and pregnancy. Acta Obstet Gynecol Scand 1989;68(2):185–7.

[27] Stechova K, Bartaskova D, Mrstinova M, et al. Pregnancy in a woman suffering from type 1 diabetes associated with Addison's disease and Hashimoto's thyroiditis (fully developed autoimmune polyglandular syndrome type 2). Exp Clin Endocrinol Diabetes 2004;112(6): 333–7.

[28] Cohen M. Addison's disease complicated by toxemia of pregnancy. Arch Intern Med 1948; 81:879–87.

[29] Drucker D, Shumak S, Angel A. Schmidt's syndrome presenting with intrauterine growth retardation and postpartum addisonian crisis. Am J Obstet Gynecol 1984;149(2):229–30.

[30] Seaward PG, Guidozzi F, Sonnendecker EW. Addisonian crisis in pregnancy: case report. Br J Obstet Gynaecol 1989;96(11):1348–50.

[31] Osler M, Pedersen J. Pregnancy in a patient with Addison's disease and diabetes mellitus. Acta Endocrinol (Copenh) 1962;41:79–87.

[32] O'Shaughnessy RW, Hackett KJ. Maternal Addison's disease and fetal growth retardation: a case report. J Reprod Med 1984;29(10):752–6.

[33] Gradden C, Lawrence D, Doyle PM, et al. Uses of error: Addison's disease in pregnancy. Lancet 2001;357(9263):1197.

[34] Ambrosi B, Barbetta L, Morricone L. Diagnosis and management of Addison's disease during pregnancy. J Endocrinol Invest 2003;26(7):698–702.

[35] Allemang WH. Pregnancy in the absence of adrenal cortical function. Can Med Assoc J 1961;85:118–22.

[36] Donnelly JC, O'Connell MP, Keane DP. Addison's disease, with successful pregnancy outcome. J Obstet Gynaecol 2003;23(2):199.

[37] Grottolo A, Ferrari V, Mariano M, Zambruni A, et al. Primary adrenal insufficiency, circulating lupus anticoagulant and anticardiolipin antibodies in a patient with multiple abortions and recurrent thrombotic episodes. Haematologica 1988;73(6):517–9.

[38] Vengrove MA, Amoroso A. Reversible adrenal insufficiency after adrenal hemorrhage. Ann Intern Med 1993;119(5):439.

[39] Guibal F, Rybojad M, Cordoliani F, et al. Melanoderma revealing primary antiphospholipid syndrome. Dermatology 1996;192(1):75–7.

[40] George LD, Selvaraju R, Reddy K, Stout TV, et al. Vomiting and hyponatraemia in pregnancy. BJOG 2000;107(6):808–9.

[41] Schulte HM, Weisner D, Allolio B. The corticotrophin releasing hormone test in late pregnancy: lack of adrenocorticotrophin and cortisol response. Clin Endocrinol (Oxf) 1990; 33(1):99–106.

[42] McKenna DS, Wittber GM, Nagaraja HN, et al. The effects of repeat doses of antenatal corticosteroids on maternal adrenal function. Am J Obstet Gynecol 2000;183(3):669–73.

[43] Grinspoon SK, Biller BM. Clinical review 62: laboratory assessment of adrenal insufficiency. J Clin Endocrinol Metab 1994;79(4):923–31.

[44] Nieman LK. Dynamic evaluation of adrenal hypofunction. J Endocrinol Invest 2003; 26(Suppl 7):S74–82.

[45] May ME, Carey RM. Rapid adrenocorticotropic hormone test in practice: retrospective review. Am J Med 1985;79(6):679–84.

[46] Speckart PF, Nicoloff JT, Bethune JE. Screening for adrenocortical insufficiency with cosyntropin (synthetic ACTH). Arch Intern Med 1971;128(5):761–3.

[47] Dickstein G. Hypothalamo-pituitary-adrenal axis testing: nothing is sacred and caution in interpretation is needed. Clin Endocrinol (Oxf) 2001;54(1):15–6.

[48] Dorin RI, Qualls CR, Crapo LM. Diagnosis of adrenal insufficiency. Ann Intern Med 2003; 139(3):194–204.

[49] Courtney CH, McAllister AS, McCance DR, et al. Comparison of one week 0900 h serum cortisol, low and standard dose synacthen tests with a 4 to 6 week insulin hypoglycaemia test after pituitary surgery in assessing HPA axis. Clin Endocrinol (Oxf) 2000;53(4):431–6.

[50] Nolten WE, Lindheimer MD, Oparil S, et al. Desoxycorticosterone in normal pregnancy: I. sequential studies of the secretory patterns of desoxycorticosterone, aldosterone, and cortisol. Am J Obstet Gynecol 1978;132(4):414–20.

[51] Nigam R, Bhatia E, Miao D, et al. Prevalence of adrenal antibodies in Addison's disease among north Indian Caucasians. Clin Endocrinol (Oxf) 2003;59(5):593–8.

[52] Symonds EM, Craven DJ. Plasma renin and aldosterone in pregnancy complicated by adrenal insufficiency. Br J Obstet Gynaecol 1977;84(3):191–6.

[53] Ilbery M, Jones AR, Sampson J. Lupus anticoagulant and HELLP syndrome complicated by placental abruption, hepatic, dermal and adrenal infarction. Aust N Z J Obstet Gynaecol 1995;35(2):215–7.

[54] Kelestimur F. The endocrinology of adrenal tuberculosis: the effects of tuberculosis on the hypothalamo-pituitary-adrenal axis and adrenocortical function. J Endocrinol Invest 2004;27(4):380–6.

[55] Levine D, Edelman RR. Fast MRI and its application in obstetrics. Abdom Imaging 1997; 22(6):589–96.

[56] Sidhu RK, Hawkins DF. Prescribing in pregnancy: corticosteroids. Clin Obstet Gynaecol 1981;8(2):383–404.

[57] van der Spuy ZM, Jacobs HS. Management of endocrine disorders in pregnancy: part II. pituitary, ovarian and adrenal disease. Postgrad Med J 1984;60(703):312–20.

[58] Esteban NV, Loughlin T, Yergey AL, et al. Daily cortisol production rate in man determined by stable isotope dilution/mass spectrometry. J Clin Endocrinol Metab 1991;72(1):39–45.

[59] Malchoff CD, Carey RM. Adrenal insufficiency. Curr Ther Endocrinol Metab 1997;6:142–7.

[60] Normington FA, Davies D. Hypertension and oedema complicating pregnancy in Addison's disease. BMJ 1972;2(806):148–9.

[61] James PR, Nelson-Piercy C. Management of hypertension before, during, and after pregnancy. Heart 2004;90(12):1499–504.

[62] Gabbe. Obstetrics: normal and problem pregnancies. 4th edition. New York: Churchhill and Livingston; 2002.

[63] Mulatero P, Stowasser M, Loh KC, et al. Increased diagnosis of primary aldosteronism, including surgically correctable forms, in centers from five continents. J Clin Endocrinol Metab 2004;89(3):1045–50.

[64] Okawa T, Asano K, Hashimoto T, et al. Diagnosis and management of primary aldosteronism in pregnancy: case report and review of the literature. Am J Perinatol 2002;19(1):31–6.

[65] Crane MG, Andes JP, Harris JJ, et al. Primary aldosteronism in pregnancy. Obstet Gynecol 1964;23:200–8.

[66] Wyckoff JA, Seely EW, Hurwitz S, et al. Glucocorticoid-remediable aldosteronism and pregnancy. Hypertension 2000;35(2):668–72.

[67] Brown MA, Wang J, Whitworth JA. The renin-angiotensin-aldosterone system in preeclampsia. Clin Exp Hypertens 1997;19(5–6):713–26.

[68] Wilson M, Morganti AA, Zervoudakis I, et al. Blood pressure, the renin-aldosterone system and sex steroids throughout normal pregnancy. Am J Med 1980;68(1):97–104.

[69] Nielsen AH, Schauser KH, Poulsen K. Current topic: the uteroplacental renin-angiotensin system. Placenta 2000;21(5–6):468–77.

[70] Dorr HG, Heller A, Versmold HT, et al. Longitudinal study of progestins, mineralocorticoids, and glucocorticoids throughout human pregnancy. J Clin Endocrinol Metab 1989; 68(5):863–8.

[71] Lindheimer MD, Katz AI, Nolten WE, et al. Sodium and mineralocorticoids in normal and abnormal pregnancy. Adv Nephrol Necker Hosp 1977;7:33–59.

[72] Boonshaft B, O'Connell JM, Hayes JM, et al. Serum renin activity during normal pregnancy: effect of alterations of posture and sodium intake. J Clin Endocrinol Metab 1968;28(11): 1641–4.

[73] Matsumoto J, Miyake H, Isozaki T, et al. Primary aldosteronism in pregnancy. J Nippon Med Sch 2000;67(4):275–9.

[74] Fujiyama S, Mori Y, Matsubara H, et al. Primary aldosteronism with aldosterone-producing adrenal adenoma in a pregnant woman. Intern Med 1999;38(1):36–9.

[75] Neerhof MG, Shlossman PA, Poll DS, et al. Idiopathic aldosteronism in pregnancy. Obstet Gynecol 1991;78(3 Pt 2):489–91.

[76] Solomon CG, Thiet M, Moore F Jr, et al. Primary hyperaldosteronism in pregnancy: a case report. J Reprod Med 1996;41(4):255–8.

[77] Gordon RD, Fishman LM, Liddle GW. Plasma renin activity and aldosterone secretion in a pregnant woman with primary aldosteronism. J Clin Endocrinol Metab 1967;27(3):385–8.

[78] Aboud E, De Swiet M, Gordon H. Primary aldosteronism in pregnancy: should it be treated surgically? Ir J Med Sci 1995;164(4):279–80.

[79] Baron F, Sprauve ME, Huddleston JF, et al. Diagnosis and surgical treatment of primary aldosteronism in pregnancy: a case report. Obstet Gynecol 1995;86(4 Pt 2):644–5.

[80] Webb JC, Bayliss P. Pregnancy complicated by primary aldosteronism. South Med J 1997; 90(2):243–5.

[81] Hecker A, Hasan SH, Neumann F. Disturbances in sexual differentiation of rat foetuses following spironolactone treatment. Acta Endocrinologica (Copenh) 1980;95(4):540–5.

[82] Deruelle P, Dufour P, Magnenant E, et al. Maternal Bartter's syndrome in pregnancy treated by amiloride. Eur J Obstet Gynecol Reprod Biol 2004;115(1):106–7.

[83] Botchan A, Hauser R, Kupfermine M, et al. Pheochromocytoma in pregnancy: case report and review of the literature. Obstet Gynecol Surv 1995;50(4):321–7.

[84] Lyman DJ. Paroxysmal hypertension, pheochromocytoma, and pregnancy. J Am Board Fam Pract 2002;15(2):153–8.

[85] Cermakova A, Knibb AA, Hoskins C, et al. Post partum phaeochromocytoma. Int J Obstet Anesth 2003;12(4):300–4.

[86] Strachan AN, Claydon P, Caunt JA. Phaeochromocytoma diagnosed during labour. Br J Anaesth 2000;85(4):635–7.

[87] Takai Y, Seki H, Kinoshita K. Pheochromocytoma in pregnancy manifesting hypertensive crisis induced by metoclopramide. Int J Gynaecol Obstet 1997;59(2):133–7.

[88] Harper MA, Murnaghan GA, Kennedy L, et al. Phaeochromocytoma in pregnancy: five cases and a review of the literature. Br J Obstet Gynaecol 1989;96(5):594–606.

[89] Hadden DR. Adrenal disorders of pregnancy. Endocrinol Metab Clin North Am 1995;24(1): 139–51.

[90] Ahn JT, Hibbard JU, Chapa JB. Atypical presentation of pheochromocytoma as part of multiple endocrine neoplasia IIa in pregnancy. Obstet Gynecol 2003;102(5 Pt 2):1202–5.

[91] Peleg D, Munsick RA, Diker D, et al. Distribution of catecholamines between fetal and maternal compartments during human pregnancy with emphasis on L-dopa and dopamine. J Clin Endocrinol Metab 1986;62(5):911–4.

[92] Lenders JW, Pacak K, Eisenhofer G. New advances in the biochemical diagnosis of pheochromocytoma: moving beyond catecholamines. Ann N Y Acad Sci 2002;970:29–40.

[93] Del Giudice A, Bisceglia M, D'Errico M, et al. Extra-adrenal functional paraganglioma (phaeochromocytoma) associated with renal-artery stenosis in a pregnant woman. Nephrol Dial Transplant 1998;13(11):2920–3.

[94] Ilias I, Pacak K. Current approaches and recommended algorithm for the diagnostic localization of pheochromocytoma. J Clin Endocrinol Metab 2004;89(2):479–91.

[95] Devoe LD, O'Dell BE, Castillo RA, et al. Metastatic pheochromocytoma in pregnancy and fetal biophysical assessment after maternal administration of alpha-adrenergic, beta-adrenergic, and dopamine antagonists. Obstet Gynecol 1986;68(Suppl 3):S15–8.

[96] Forest MG. Recent advances in the diagnosis and management of congenital adrenal hyperplasia due to 21-hydroxylase deficiency. Hum Reprod Update 2004;10(6):469–85.

[97] New MI, Carlson A, Obeid J, et al. Prenatal diagnosis for congenital adrenal hyperplasia in 532 pregnancies. J Clin Endocrinol Metab 2001;86(12):5651–7.

[98] Meyer-Bahlburg HF, Dolezal C, Baker SW, et al. Cognitive and motor development of children with and without congenital adrenal hyperplasia after early-prenatal dexamethasone. J Clin Endocrinol Metab 2004;89(2):610–4.

[99] Clayton PE, Miller WL, Oberfield SE, et al. Consensus statement on 21-hydroxylase deficiency from the European Society for Paediatric Endocrinology and the Lawson Wilkins Pediatric Endocrine Society. Horm Res 2002;58(4):188–95.

ELSEVIER
SAUNDERS

Endocrinol Metab Clin N Am
35 (2006) 21–51

ENDOCRINOLOGY
AND METABOLISM
CLINICS
OF NORTH AMERICA

Calcium and Bone Disorders During Pregnancy and Lactation

Christopher S. Kovacs, MD[a],*,
Ghada El-Hajj Fuleihan, MD, MPH[b],*

[a]Health Sciences Centre, St. John's, NL, Canada
[b]Calcium Metabolism and Osteoporosis Program,
American University of Beirut–Medical Center, Riad El Solh, Beirut, Lebanon

Mineral metabolism in the mother must adapt to the demand created by the fetus and placenta, which together draw calcium and other minerals from the maternal circulation to mineralize the developing fetal skeleton. Similarly, mineral metabolism must adapt in the lactating woman to supply sufficient calcium to milk and the suckling neonate. Potential adaptations include increased intake of mineral, increased efficiency of intestinal absorption of mineral, mobilization of mineral from the skeleton, and increased renal conservation of mineral. Despite a similar magnitude of calcium demand by pregnant and lactating women, the adjustments made in each of these reproductive periods differ significantly (Fig. 1). These hormone-mediated adjustments normally satisfy the needs of the fetus and infant with short-term depletions of maternal skeletal calcium content, but without long-term consequences to the maternal skeleton. In states of maternal malnutrition and vitamin D deficiency, however, the depletion of skeletal mineral content may be proportionately more severe and may be accompanied by increased skeletal fragility.

This article reviews present understanding of the adaptations in mineral metabolism that occur during pregnancy and lactation and how these adaptations affect the presentation, diagnosis, and management of disorders of calcium and bone metabolism. Animal data are cited to fill in the gaps where

* Corresponding authors. Basic Medical Sciences, Health Sciences Centre, 300 Prince Philip Drive, St. John's, NL, A1B 3V6 Canada (C.S. Kovacs); Calcium Metabolism and Osteoporosis Program, American University of Beirut–Medical Center, P.O. Box 11-0236, Riad El Solh 4407 2020, Beirut, Lebanon (G.E.-H. Fuleihan).
E-mail addresses: ckovacs@mun.ca (C.S. Kovacs); gf01@aub.edu.lb (G.E.-H. Fuleihan).

0889-8529/06/$ - see front matter © 2005 Elsevier Inc. All rights reserved.
doi:10.1016/j.ecl.2005.09.004
endo.theclinics.com

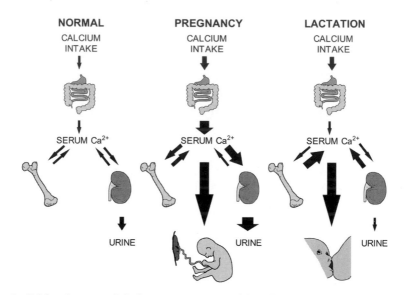

Fig. 1. Calcium homeostasis in human pregnancy and lactation compared with normal. The thickness of arrows indicates a relative increase or decrease with respect to the normal and non-pregnant state. (*Adapted from* Kovacs CS, Kronenberg HM. Maternal-fetal calcium and bone metabolism during pregnancy, puerperium and lactation. Endocr Rev 1997;18:832–72. © 1997 The Endocrine Society; with permission.)

human data are unavailable. The reader also is referred to several other comprehensive reviews on the subject [1–3].

Adaptations during pregnancy

The developing fetal skeleton accretes about 30 g of calcium by term and about 80% of it during the third trimester. This demand for calcium is largely met by a doubling of maternal intestinal calcium absorption, mediated by 1,25-dihydroxyvitamin D_3 (1,25(OH)$_2$$D_3$), or calcitriol, and possibly by other factors.

Mineral ions and calcitropic hormones

Normal pregnancy results in altered levels of calcium and the calcitropic hormones as schematically depicted in Fig. 2 [1]. The ionized calcium (the physiologically important fraction of calcium) remains constant throughout pregnancy. In contrast, the total serum calcium (sum of the ionized, complexed, and albumin-bound fractions of calcium in the circulation) decreases in pregnancy secondary to a decline in serum albumin. In clinical practice, the total serum calcium is more commonly measured than the ionized calcium. The commonly observed decrease in total serum calcium should

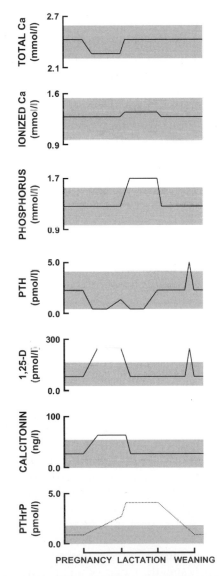

Fig. 2. Longitudinal changes in calcium, phosphorus, and calcitropic hormone levels that occur during pregnancy and lactation. Normal adult ranges are indicated by the shaded areas. The progression in PTHrP levels is depicted by a dashed line to reflect that the data are less complete; the implied comparisons of PTHrP levels in late pregnancy and lactation are uncertain extrapolations because no reports followed patients serially. In both situations, PTHrP levels are elevated. (*Adapted from* Kovacs CS, Kronenberg HM. Maternal-fetal calcium and bone metabolism during pregnancy, puerperium and lactation. Endocr Rev 1997;18:832–72. © 1997 The Endocrine Society; with permission.)

not be mistaken for evidence of "physiologic hyperparathyroidism of pregnancy," an erroneous concept that has persisted in some modern texts [4,5]. The decline in total serum calcium is an unimportant artifact of a nonphysiologic measurement; the ionized calcium is the relevant measurement and always should be assayed if there is any doubt about the true value of the serum calcium during pregnancy (or at any time). Serum phosphorus levels also are normal during pregnancy.

As observed by longitudinal measurements during pregnancy with modern two-site "intact" immunoradiometric assays (IRMA), serum parathyroid hormone (PTH) decreases to the low-normal range (ie, 10–30% of the mean nonpregnant value) during the first trimester, then increases steadily to the mid-normal range by term [6–10]. As judged by the "intact" serum PTH level, the parathyroids are modestly suppressed beginning early in the first trimester and return to apparently normal function by the end of pregnancy. First-generation PTH assays in the 1970s and 1980s were insensitive and measured multiple, biologically inactive fragments of PTH; a few studies with these assays had detected higher levels of PTH during pregnancy in humans. Those early studies of PTH in pregnancy, combined with the observation that total serum calcium decreases during pregnancy, reinforced the erroneous concept that secondary hyperparathyroidism occurs during pregnancy. Modern "intact" assays have made it clear that in well-nourished women, ionized calcium is normal throughout pregnancy, and that PTH is suppressed during early pregnancy. "Bio-intact" PTH assays have been developed that detect true full-length PTH [11]; the levels are likely similar to levels obtained with the more widely used "intact" PTH assays, but no study has examined this. In contrast to the normal suppression of PTH during pregnancy, there is evidence that PTH may increase above normal in late pregnancy in women from Malay, who have very low intakes of calcium [12].

Total $1,25(OH)_2D_3$ levels double early in pregnancy and maintain this increase until term; free $1,25(OH)_2D_3$ levels are increased from the third trimester and possibly earlier. The increase in $1,25(OH)_2D_3$ may be largely independent of changes in PTH because PTH levels typically are decreasing at the time of the increase in $1,25(OH)_2D_3$. The maternal kidneys likely account for most, if not all, of the increase in $1,25(OH)_2D_3$ during pregnancy, although the decidua, placenta, and fetal kidneys may contribute a small amount. The relative contribution of the maternal kidneys is based on several lines of evidence [1], including the report of an anephric woman on hemodialysis who had low $1,25(OH)_2D_3$ levels before and during a pregnancy [13]. The renal 1α-hydroxylase may be upregulated in response to factors such as PTH-related protein (PTHrP), estradiol, prolactin, and placental lactogen (evidence from animal studies is reviewed by Kovacs and Kronenberg [1]).

Serum calcitonin levels also increase during pregnancy, with the C cells of the thyroid, breast, and placenta possibly contributing to the circulating level of calcitonin. It has been postulated that calcitonin protects the maternal skeleton from excessive resorption of calcium, but this hypothesis is unproved.

No human studies have addressed the question, although studies in genetically engineered mice have shown that the absence of calcitonin does not impair the ability of mice to increase skeletal mineral content during pregnancy [14].

PTHrP levels are increased during late pregnancy, as determined by assays that detect PTHrP fragments encompassing amino acids 1 through 86. Because PTHrP is produced by many tissues in the mother and fetus (including the placenta, amnion, decidua, umbilical cord, fetal parathyroids, and breast), it is unclear which sources contribute to the increase detected in the maternal circulation. PTHrP may contribute to the elevations in $1,25(OH)_2D_3$ and the suppression of PTH that are noted during pregnancy, although there is evidence that PTHrP may not be as potent as PTH in stimulating the renal 1α-hydroxylase in vivo [15]. PTHrP has other roles during pregnancy, including the regulation of placental calcium transport in the fetus [1,16]. PTHrP also may have a role in protecting the maternal skeleton during pregnancy because the carboxyl-terminal portion of PTHrP ("osteostatin") has been shown to inhibit osteoclastic bone resorption [17].

Pregnancy induces significant changes in the levels of other hormones, including the sex steroids, prolactin, placental lactogen, and insulin-like growth factor type 1. Each of these may have direct or indirect effects on calcium and bone metabolism during pregnancy, but these issues have not been explored.

Intestinal absorption of calcium

Several clinical studies have shown that intestinal absorption of calcium is doubled during pregnancy from 12 weeks of gestation (the earliest time point studied); this seems to be a major maternal adaptation to meet the fetal need for calcium [1]. This increase may be the result of a $1,25(OH)_2D_3$-mediated increase in intestinal calbindin$_{9K}$-D and other proteins. Based on evidence from limited animal studies [1], prolactin and placental lactogen (and possibly other factors) also may mediate part of the increase in intestinal calcium absorption. The increased absorption of calcium early in pregnancy may allow the maternal skeleton to store calcium in advance of the peak fetal demands that occur later in pregnancy.

Renal handling of calcium

The 24-hour urine calcium excretion is increased by 12 weeks of gestation (the earliest time point studied), and the amount excreted may exceed the normal range [1]. Because fasting urine calcium values are normal or low, the increase in 24-hour urine calcium likely reflects the increased intestinal absorption of calcium (absorptive hypercalciuria). The elevated calcitonin levels of pregnancy also may promote renal calcium excretion.

Skeletal calcium metabolism

Animal models indicate that histomorphometric parameters of bone turnover are increased during pregnancy, which could be interpreted to mean that mineral is mobilized from the maternal skeleton to contribute to the fetal skeleton [18]. Serial measurements of bone mineral density by dual x-ray absorptiometry (DXA) in several strains of normal mice have shown, however, that bone mineral content increases by 5% to 10% during pregnancy [14,19], and the increased bone turnover of pregnancy might reflect (at least in rodents) an anabolic or bone formative state, as opposed to a net bone resorptive state. As noted later in the lactation section, a net loss of bone mineral content occurs during lactation in humans and rodents. An increase in bone mineral content during pregnancy might serve to protect the maternal skeleton against excessive demineralization and fragility during lactation.

Comparable histomorphometric data are not available for human pregnancy. In one study [20], 15 women who electively terminated a pregnancy in the first trimester (8–10 weeks) had bone biopsy evidence of increased bone resorption, including increased resorption surface, increased numbers of resorption cavities, and decreased osteoid. These findings were not present in biopsy specimens obtained from nonpregnant controls or in biopsy specimens obtained at term from 13 women who had elective cesarean sections.

Most human studies of skeletal calcium metabolism in pregnancy have examined changes in "bone markers," that is, serum indices that reflect bone formation and serum or urine indices that reflect bone resorption. These studies have been fraught with numerous confounding variables that cloud the interpretation of the results, including the lack of prepregnancy baseline values; effects of hemodilution in pregnancy on serum markers; increased glomerular filtration rate (GFR) and renal clearance; altered creatinine excretion; placental, uterine, and fetal contributions to the markers; degradation and clearance by the placenta; and lack of diurnally timed or fasted specimens. Given these limitations, many studies have reported that urinary markers of bone resorption (24-hour collection) are increased from early pregnancy to mid-pregnancy (including deoxypyridinoline, pyridinoline, and hydroxyproline). Conversely, serum markers of bone formation (generally not corrected for hemodilution or increased GFR) often decrease from prepregnancy or nonpregnant values in early pregnancy or mid-pregnancy, increasing to normal or greater before term (including osteocalcin, procollagen I carboxypeptides and bone-specific alkaline phosphatase). It is conceivable that the bone formation markers are artifactually lowered by normal hemodilution and increased renal clearance of pregnancy, obscuring any real increase in the level of the markers. One study that adjusted for the confounding effects of hemodilution and altered GFR showed that osteocalcin production was not reduced in pregnancy [21]. Total alkaline phosphatase increases early in pregnancy largely because of contributions from the placental fraction and is not a useful marker of bone formation in pregnancy.

Based on the scant bone biopsy data and the measurements of bone markers (with the aforementioned confounding factors), one cautiously may conclude that bone turnover is increased in human pregnancy from 10 weeks of gestation. There is comparatively little maternal-fetal calcium transfer occurring at this stage of pregnancy compared with the peak rate of calcium transfer in the third trimester. One might have anticipated that markers of bone turnover would increase particularly in the third trimester; however, no further increase was seen at that time.

Changes in skeletal calcium content have been assessed in humans through the use of sequential bone density studies during pregnancy. Because of concerns about fetal radiation exposure, few such studies have been done. Such studies are confounded by changes in body composition and weight during normal pregnancy, which can lead to artifactual changes in bone density. Using single-photon or dual-photon absorptiometry (SPA/DPA), several prospective studies did not find a significant change in cortical or trabecular bone density during pregnancy [1]. Several more recent studies have used DXA before conception (range 1–8 months prior, but not always stated) and after delivery (range 1 6 weeks postpartum) [21–27]. Most studies involved 16 or fewer subjects. One study found no change in lumbar spine bone density measurements obtained preconception and within 1 to 2 weeks postdelivery [23], whereas the other studies reported decreases of 4% to 5% in lumbar spine bone density with the postpartum measurement taken 1 to 6 weeks postdelivery. The puerperium is associated with bone density losses of 1% to 3% per month in women who lactate (see lactation section), and it is important that the postpartum measurement be done as soon as possible after delivery. Other longitudinal studies have found a progressive decrease during pregnancy in indices thought to correlate with bone mineral density, as determined by ultrasound measurements at a peripheral site, the os calcis [28]. Although the longitudinal studies with SPA/DPA suggested no change in trabecular or cortical bone density during pregnancy, the subsequent evidence from preconception and postdelivery DXA measurements and peripheral ultrasound measurements suggests that there may be a small net loss of maternal bone mineral content during normal human pregnancy. None of all the aforementioned studies could address the question as to whether skeletal calcium content increases early in pregnancy in advance of the third trimester, as has been observed in normal mice. Further studies, with larger numbers of patients, are needed to clarify the extent of bone loss during pregnancy.

It seems certain that any acute changes in bone metabolism during pregnancy do not normally cause long-term changes in skeletal calcium content or strength. Numerous studies of osteoporotic or osteopenic women have failed to find a significant association of parity with bone density or fracture risk [1,29]; however, a few studies of women with extremely low calcium or vitamin D intake found that pregnancy may compromise skeletal strength and density (see later). Although most clinical studies could not separate out the effects of parity from the effects of lactation, it may be reasonable to conclude that if parity has any effect on bone density or fracture risk, it normally must be only a modest effect. A more recent study of twins indicated that there may be a small protective effect of parity and lactation on maintaining bone mineral content [30].

Adaptations during lactation

About 280 to 400 mg of calcium is lost through breast milk daily, with losses of 1000 mg or more in women who are nursing twins. A temporary demineralization of the skeleton seems to be the main mechanism by which lactating women meet these calcium requirements. This demineralization does not seem to be mediated by PTH or calcitriol, but may be mediated by PTHrP in the setting of a decrease in estrogen levels.

Mineral ions and calcitropic hormones

The normal lactational changes in maternal calcium, phosphorus, and calcitropic hormone levels are schematically depicted in Fig. 2 [1]. The mean ionized calcium level of exclusively lactating women is increased, although it remains within the normal range. Serum phosphorus levels also are higher during lactation, and the level may exceed the normal range. Because reabsorption of phosphorus by the kidneys seems to be increased, the increased serum phosphorus levels may reflect the combined effects of the increased flux of phosphorus into the blood from diet and from skeletal resorption in the setting of decreased renal phosphorus excretion.

"Intact" PTH, as determined by a two-site IRMA assay, has been found to be reduced 50% or more in lactating women during the first several months. It increases to normal at weaning, but may rise above normal after weaning (levels of bio-intact PTH have not been reported yet during lactation). In contrast to the high $1,25(OH)_2D_3$ levels of pregnancy, maternal free and bound $1,25(OH)_2D_3$ levels decrease to normal within days of parturition and remain there throughout lactation.

PTHrP levels are significantly higher in lactating women and mice than in nonlactating controls, as measured by two-site IRMA assays. The source of PTHrP seems be the breast or mammary tissue because PTHrP has been detected in milk at concentrations exceeding 10,000 times the level found in the blood of patients with hypercalcemia of malignancy or normal human controls. A small increase in the maternal level of PTHrP can be shown after suckling [31]. Blood levels of PTHrP were reduced in lactating mice that had the PTHrP gene ablated only from mammary tissue compared with normal lactating mice [32]. PTHrP seems to play several roles within the breast, as indicated by studies in animals that suggest PTHrP may regulate mammary development and blood flow. The calcium-sensing receptor is expressed in the breast during lactation, where it regulates PTHrP production and the calcium and water content of the milk (Fig. 3) [33].

PTHrP plays a key role during lactation in regulating the demineralization of the skeleton. In response to suckling [31] and in response to signaling from the calcium-sensing receptor expressed by lactating mammary tissue (see Fig. 3) [33], PTHrP reaches the maternal circulation from mammary

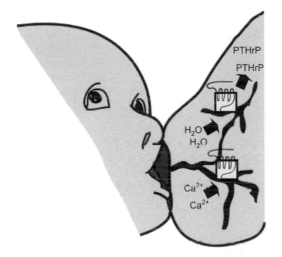

Fig. 3. The calcium receptor (represented schematically) is expressed in mammary tissue during lactation (but not pregnancy), wherein it has several key functions as elucidated from studies in mice [33]. The calcium receptor monitors the systemic concentration of calcium to control PTHrP synthesis and the supply of calcium to the breast. An increase in systemic calcium or the administration of a calcimimetic inhibited PTHrP, whereas a decrease in systemic calcium stimulated PTHrP. The calcium receptor also directly regulates the calcium and fluid composition of milk. The administration of calcium or a calcimimetic stimulated the transport of calcium into the breast, and the administration of a calcimimetic enhanced the entry of water into the milk, making it less viscous. (*From* Kovacs CS. Calcium and bone metabolism during pregnancy and lactation. J Mammary Gland Biol Neoplasia 2005;10(2):105–18. © 2005 Springer Science and Business Media BV; with permission.)

tissue and stimulates resorption of calcium from the maternal skeleton, renal tubular reabsorption of calcium, and (indirectly) suppression of PTH (Fig. 4). In a sense, the breast becomes an accessory parathyroid gland during lactation, but the "hyperparathyroidism" of lactation is increased secretion of PTHrP, not PTH. The strongest evidence in support of this model comes from the study of mice in which the PTHrP gene was ablated at the onset of lactation, but only within mammary tissue [32]. The lactational decrease in bone mineral content was significantly blunted in the absence of mammary gland production of PTHrP. Other evidence for the central role of PTHrP in lactation comes from humans, in that PTHrP levels correlate negatively with PTH levels and positively with the ionized calcium levels of lactating women [31,34], and that higher PTHrP levels correlate with greater losses of bone mineral density during lactation in humans [35]. Observations in aparathyroid women provide evidence of the impact of PTHrP in calcium homeostasis during lactation (see later).

Calcitonin levels are elevated in the first 6 weeks of lactation. Studies in mice lacking the gene that encodes calcitonin indicate that calcitonin may modulate the rate of skeletal resorption during lactation. Calcitonin-null mice lost more than 50% of skeletal mineral content during 3 weeks of

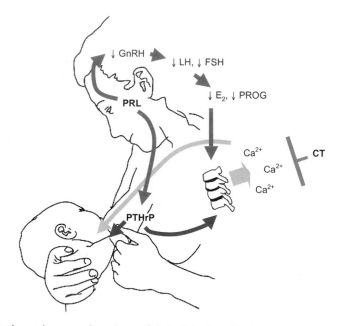

Fig. 4. The breast is a central regulator of skeletal demineralization during lactation. Suckling induces release of prolactin. Suckling and prolactin inhibit the hypothalamic gonadotropin-releasing hormone (GnRH) pulse center, which suppresses the gonadotropins (luteinizing hormone [LH], follicle-stimulating hormone [FSH]), leading to low levels of the ovarian sex steroids (estradiol and progesterone). PTHrP production and release from the breast is controlled by several factors, including suckling, prolactin, and the calcium receptor. PTHrP enters the bloodstream and combines with systemically low estradiol levels to upregulate bone resorption markedly. Increased bone resorption releases calcium and phosphate into the bloodstream, which reach the breast ducts and are actively pumped into the breast milk. PTHrP also passes into the milk at high concentrations, but whether PTHrP plays a role in regulating calcium physiology of the neonate is unknown. Calcitonin (CT) may inhibit skeletal responsiveness to PTHrP and low estradiol. (*From* Kovacs CS. Calcium and bone metabolism during pregnancy and lactation. J Mammary Gland Biol Neoplasia 2005;10(2):105–18. © 2005 Springer Science and Business Media BV; with permission.)

lactation, approximately twice that of normal littermate sisters [14,36]. The calcitonin-depleted mice still regained all of the lost mineral content after weaning, which indicates that although calcitonin is needed in the short-term to prevent severe losses of mineral content and potential skeletal fragility, calcitonin is not required in the long-term because the skeletal losses of mineral are restored anyway. The human equivalent of absence of calcitonin might explain some cases of osteoporosis of lactation (see later).

Intestinal absorption of calcium

Intestinal calcium absorption decreases to the nonpregnant rate from the increased rate of pregnancy. This decrease in absorption corresponds to the decrease in $1,25(OH)_2D_3$ levels to normal.

Renal handling of calcium

In humans, the GFR decreases during lactation, and the renal excretion of calcium typically is reduced to very low levels. This situation suggests that tubular reabsorption of calcium must be increased, to account for reduced calcium excretion in the setting of increased serum calcium.

Skeletal calcium metabolism

Histomorphometric data from animals consistently show increased bone turnover during lactation, with losses of 30% of bone mineral achieved during 2 to 3 weeks of normal lactation in the rat [1], whereas a similar amount is lost in the lactating mouse within 21 days [19]. The loss is greatest in the trabecular bone of rats and mice. Comparative histomorphometric data are lacking for humans, and in place of that, serum markers of bone formation and urinary markers of bone resorption have been assessed in numerous cross-sectional and prospective studies of lactation. Some confounding factors discussed with respect to pregnancy apply to the use of these markers in lactating women. During lactation, GFR is reduced, and the intravascular volume is more contracted. Urinary markers of bone resorption (24-hour collection) increase two to three times above normal during lactation and are higher than the levels attained in the third trimester. Serum markers of bone formation (not adjusted for hemoconcentration or reduced GFR) are generally high during lactation and increase over the levels attained during the third trimester. Total alkaline phosphatase declines immediately postpartum owing to loss of the placental fraction, but still may remain above normal because of the elevation in the bone-specific fraction. Despite the confounding variables, these findings suggest that bone turnover is significantly increased during lactation.

In women, serial measurements of bone density during lactation (by SPA, DPA, or DXA) have shown a decline of 3% to 10% in bone mineral content after 2 to 6 months of lactation at trabecular sites (lumbar spine, hip, femur and distal radius), with smaller losses at cortical sites [1,29,37]. The peak rate of loss is 1% to 3% per month, far exceeding the rate of 1% to 3% per year that can occur in women with postmenopausal osteoporosis, who are considered to be losing bone rapidly. Loss of bone mineral from the maternal skeleton seems to be a normal consequence of lactation and may not be preventable by increasing the calcium intake above the recommended dietary allowance. Several studies have shown that calcium supplementation does not reduce significantly the amount of bone lost during lactation [38–41]. The lactational decrease in bone mineral density correlates with the amount of calcium lost in the breast milk [42].

The mechanisms controlling the rapid loss of skeletal calcium content are not fully understood. The reduced estrogen levels of lactation are important, but are unlikely to be the sole explanation. To estimate the effects of estrogen deficiency during lactation, it is worth noting the alterations in calcium and bone metabolism that occur in reproductive-age women who have estrogen deficiency induced by gonadotropin-releasing hormone agonist therapy for endometriosis and other conditions. Six months of acute estrogen deficiency induced by gonadotropin-releasing hormone agonist therapy leads to 1% to 4% losses in trabecular (but not cortical) bone density, increased urinary calcium excretion, and suppression of $1,25(OH)_2D_3$ and PTH levels [1]. During lactation, women are not as estrogen deficient, but they lose more bone mineral density (at trabecular and cortical sites), have normal (as opposed to low) $1,25(OH)_2D_3$ levels, and have reduced (as opposed to increased) urinary calcium excretion. The difference between isolated estrogen deficiency and lactation may be due to the effects of other factors (eg, PTHrP) that add to the effects of estrogen withdrawal in lactation (Fig. 5). The relative influences of estrogen deficiency and PTHrP have been partially discerned in normal mice, in which it has been shown that treatment with pharmacologic doses of estrogen blunted, but did not abolish, the normal demineralization that occurs during lactation [43].

The bone density losses of lactation are substantially reversed during weaning at a rate of 0.5% to 2% per month [1,29,40]. The mechanism for this restoration of bone density is uncertain and largely unexplored, but preliminary evidence from animal models suggests that PTH, calcitriol, calcitonin, and estrogen may not be required to achieve that restoration. In the long-term, the consequences of lactation-induced depletion of bone mineral seem clinically unimportant in most women. Most epidemiologic studies of premenopausal

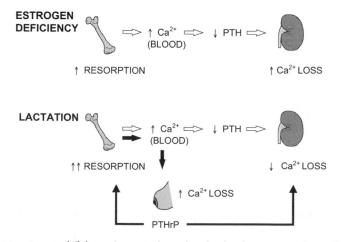

Fig. 5. Acute estrogen deficiency (eg, gonadotropin-releasing hormone analogue therapy) increases skeletal resorption and raises the blood calcium; PTH is suppressed, and renal calcium losses are increased. During lactation, the combined effects of PTHrP (secreted by the breast) and estrogen deficiency increase skeletal resorption, reduce renal calcium losses, and raise the blood calcium, but calcium is directed into the breast milk. (*From* Kovacs CS, Kronenberg HM. Maternal-fetal calcium and bone metabolism during pregnancy, puerperium and lactation. Endocr Rev 1997;18:832–72. © 1997 The Endocrine Society; with permission.)

and postmenopausal women have found no adverse effect of a history of lactation on peak bone mass, bone density, or hip fracture risk [1,29].

Disorders of bone and mineral metabolism during pregnancy and lactation

As previously discussed, pregnancy is a state of hyperabsorptive hypercalciuria, characterized by high levels of calcitriol, increasing levels of PTHrP, suppressed PTH levels, stable serum ionized calcium levels, and enhanced urinary calcium excretion (see Fig. 2). Lactation is characterized by further increments in PTHrP levels, whereas calcitriol levels return to normal. The estimated daily increase in calcium requirements (0.3 g/d) to meet the fetal demands for bone mineralization and the maternal requirements for milk synthesis are largely through enhanced intestinal calcium absorption during pregnancy and through maternal bone resorption during lactation [42]. Disorders of bone and mineral homeostasis that occur in the nonpregnant state may manifest differently during pregnancy and lactation as a result of the differing hormonal changes that occur in these two distinct reproductive intervals.

Primary hyperparathyroidism

Primary hyperparathyroidism occurs rarely during pregnancy; the true incidence is unknown because hyperparathyroidism may remain asymptomatic and go undiagnosed in uncomplicated pregnancies. In the general population, the estimated incidence of hyperparathyroidism increased from 16/100,000 before 1974 (before routine automated screening) to a peak of 112/100,000 years later, then subsequently declined to 4/100,000 [44]. Most subjects were older than age 45 years [44]. The incidence of hyperparathyroidism in women of childbearing age in an older series was estimated to be approximately 8/100,000 per year [45]. Approximately 150 cases have been reported in the English literature to date [46,47]. Two studies retrospectively evaluated 850 parathyroidectomies during the period 1960–1991 and 750 parathyroidectomies during 1975–1996 and revealed that parathyroidectomies during pregnancies accounted for 1.4% and 0.8% of total surgeries [46,48]. The diagnosis may be obscured by the normal pregnancy-induced changes that decrease the total serum calcium and suppress PTH; finding the ionized calcium to be increased and the PTH to be detectable would indicate primary hyperparathyroidism in most cases.

Hyperparathyroidism in a pregnant patient can mean considerable morbidity for the mother and the fetus. Complications have been reported in 67% of mothers and 80% of fetuses and neonates [49], complications that are in large part due to maternal hypercalcemia. The histopathologic distribution in hyperparathyroidism of pregnancy is comparable to that reported in large series spanning all age groups [50]. A series of 100 cases of hyperparathyroidism diagnosed during pregnancy or postdelivery revealed adenomas in 89%, hyperplasia in 9%, and carcinoma in 2% [46].

Manifestations and complications in pregnant women

In a report of 45 pregnant women with hyperparathyroidism, 38% complained of nausea, vomiting, or abdominal pain; 24% reported renal colic; 22% had muscular weakness; 22% manifested mental symptoms; and 11% complained of skeletal pain or fatigue; only 20% were asymptomatic [51]. Other clinical manifestations included hyperemesis gravidarum, weight loss, seizure, or other symptoms mimicking preeclampsia [46,48]. Many of the aforementioned symptoms are nonspecific and could have been due to the pregnancy itself. Objective findings included the following: 24% had nephrolithiasis or nephrocalcinosis, 16% had urinary tract infections, 13% had bone disease on radiograph, and 11% had pancreatitis [51]. In another large series of 63 cases, 38% had evidence of bone disease, 54% had evidence of renal disease, and 30% had evidence of both [52]. The high prevalence of stone disease may be explained by pregnancy-induced hyperabsorptive hypercalciuria that augments the hypercalciuria that otherwise would occur secondary to hyperparathyroidism itself. The prevalence of pancreatitis complicating hyperparathyroidism varied among reports (range 6–13%) [51,53–55] and usually occurred during the second or third trimester [56]. In a series of 75 cases, pancreatitis was the presenting illness in 5 cases, 2 of which had concomitant hypercalcemic crisis [55]. Of the few other cases of acute parathyroid crisis reported during pregnancy [53,57], one became clinically apparent 3 days postpartum followed by rapid deterioration, pancreatitis, respiratory failure, shock, and unsuccessful resuscitation [57]. The patient had been hypercalcemic at 16 weeks of gestation, but was asymptomatic at that time, leading the authors to suggest that the increased fetal need for calcium may have protected the mother from severe hypercalcemia before delivery [57]. Susceptibility to fractures owing to hyperparathyroidism during pregnancy is uncommon. Bilateral femoral neck fractures and rib fractures have been reported in two cases of severe hyperparathyroidism diagnosed during pregnancy, wherein PTH levels were 20-fold above the upper limit of normal, and in one case, the hyperparathyroidism was due to parathyroid carcinoma [58,59].

Complications in Fetuses

The most frequent serious complications in fetuses include stillbirth, miscarriage, and neonatal tetany. The percentage of affected pregnancies terminating in stillbirth, neonatal death, and neonatal tetany declined over the decades from 13% to 2%, from 8% to 2%, and from 38% to 15% [52]. Perinatal death occurred in 25% to 30% of neonates, whereas neonatal complications were noted in 50%, with tetany being at the forefront in infants born to untreated mothers [46,60–62]. Neonatal tetany is a common presentation of unrecognized hyperparathyroidism during pregnancy. The pathophysiology of the hypocalcemia and tetany is the suppression of fetal parathyroid function from maternal hypercalcemia, which becomes clinically evident when the maternal calcium flow is interrupted at birth [63].

Although the neonatal hypocalcemia and hypoparathyroidism are usually transient, resolving with treatment within 3 to 5 months [52], it has been reported to occur initially as late as 2.5 months postpartum [64] and may be permanent [52,61,65]. Bottle-fed infants were more likely to develop hypocalcemia than breastfed ones because of the higher phosphate-to-calcium ratio in cow's milk compared with breast milk [52].

Management of the mother and neonate

Parathyroidectomy performed during pregnancy prevents fetal and neonatal morbidities. The first successful parathyroidectomy during pregnancy was performed by Petit and Clark in 1947 [66]. A review comparing the outcomes of 109 mothers with hyperparathyroidism during pregnancy who were treated medically ($n = 70$) or surgically ($n = 39$) revealed that neonates of mothers with untreated hypercalcemia run a greater risk of complications [46]. In patients treated medically, there were 53% neonatal complications and 16% neonatal deaths, as opposed to a 12.5% incidence of neonatal complications and 2.5% neonatal deaths in patients who underwent parathyroidectomy [46]. Parathyroidectomy is best performed during the second trimester, after completion of organogenesis in the fetus and to avoid the poor outcomes of surgery during the third trimester [51,52,54,62]. In one series, premature labor with neonatal death occurred in four of seven third-trimester surgeries [54]. Parathyroidectomy in the third trimester is warranted, however, when the risks outweigh the benefits, and the procedure has been performed successfully in such cases [47,67].

Treatment options for hyperparathyroidism in pregnancy are influenced by the symptoms and severity of disease and gestational age. Optimal management requires a multidisciplinary approach; surgery should be performed only by an experienced parathyroid surgeon. Symptomatic and severe disease should be treated surgically, preferably in the second trimester, whereas mild asymptomatic disease diagnosed in the third trimester may continue to be observed until after delivery. A consensus for other cases is missing, however. Medical treatment includes adequate hydration and correction of electrolyte abnormalities [49]. Pharmacologic agents to treat hypercalcemia have not been studied adequately in pregnancy. Calcitonin, a pregnancy category B medication of the US Food and Drug Administration, does not cross the placenta and has been used safely in pregnancy [49]. Oral phosphate, a pregnancy category C medication, has been used in pregnancy; its most common side effects are diarrhea and hypokalemia. It should be avoided in patients with renal failure or high serum phosphate because of the risk of soft tissue calcifications [49]. Bisphosphonates and mithramycin are contraindicated because of their adverse effects on fetal development; bisphosphonates in particular may interfere with normal endochondral bone development. High-dose magnesium has been suggested as a therapeutic alternative for hyperparathyroidism in pregnancy, although its effectiveness is uncertain. This divalent cation decreases serum PTH and calcium levels by activating the calcium-sensing receptor, and at the same time it treats premature labor associated with hypercalcemia [68,69]. Experience with any of the aforementioned pharmacologic therapies is limited to individual case reports [49]; consequently, no medical therapy can be claimed to be better than any other. Medical therapy should be coupled with maternal surveillance and the monitoring of serum calcium and electrolytes and the initiation of antenatal testing with serial fetal ultrasound starting at 28 weeks of gestation. Parathyroidectomy is recommended postpartum in cases that were followed medically during pregnancy. Lactation is not contraindicated in women with untreated hyperparathyroidism, but worsening of hypercalcemia and accelerated skeletal losses may be anticipated because of the combined effects of PTHrP and hyperparathyroidism to stimulate bone resorption.

Neonatal hypoparathyroidism secondary to maternal hyperparathyroidism is usually transient (see earlier) and is treated with calcium supplementation and calcitriol. These neonates also should be fed milk formulas high in calcium and low in phosphate to minimize the risk of hypocalcemia. The prevalence and severity of complications from hyperparathyroidism in mothers and neonates have and will continue to decrease over time, owing to increased surveillance, earlier intervention, and improved surgical and anesthetic technology [52,60,61].

Familial benign hypocalciuric hypercalcemia

Familial benign hypocalciuric hypercalcemia (FBHH) is an autosomal dominant disorder that is caused by inactivating mutations in the calcium-sensing receptor that cause hypercalcemia and hypocalciuria [70,71]. In contrast to patients with hyperparathyroidism, patients with FBHH do not experience bone demineralization or nephrolithiasis. FBHH has been reported in pregnancy with no clinical sequelae in the mother [72]. As anticipated, maternal hypercalcemia has caused suppression of PTH synthesis in the fetus, however, and subsequent hypocalcemia and tetany in the neonate [72,73]. The treatment of neonates is similar to that of children born to mothers with hyperparathyroidism (see earlier).

The calcium-sensing receptor is expressed in the epithelial ducts of breast tissue and has been shown to modulate the production of PTHrP and the transport of calcium into milk in a mouse model [33]. Activating mutations of this receptor in women with FBHH theoretically could enhance the degree of skeletal demineralization during lactation and the calcium content of milk, but this has not been studied.

Hypoparathyroidism

Patients usually are known to have hypoparathyroidism or aparathyroidism before pregnancy, and the therapeutic dilemma revolves around adjustment of the treatment, which may vary widely. In 1966, O'Leary et al [74] reported two cases of hypoparathyroidism treated with high doses of calcium and vitamin D wherein the mothers gave birth to healthy infants after uncomplicated pregnancies. Despite physiologic increments in endogenous calcitriol levels during pregnancy, several studies since have documented increased requirements for exogenous calcium and calcitriol therapy as pregnancy progressed in patients with hypoparathyroidism [75–78]. Conversely, in numerous other case reports, women with hypoparathyroidism have been reported to require less calcium and vitamin D supplementation during pregnancy [1]. Potential explanations for requiring less supplementation during pregnancy include pregnancy-induced increments in calcitriol from placental sources, the potential effect of PTHrP in the maternal circulation to stimulate the renal 1α-hydroxylase, and other pregnancy-related factors (eg, prolactin or placental lactogen) that may stimulate the renal 1α-hydroxylase or enhance intestinal calcium absorption independently of calcitriol. The last-mentioned has been reported exclusively in animal models [1]. In some case reports, it seems that the normal, artifactual decrease in total serum calcium during pregnancy was the parameter that led to treatment with increased calcium and calcitriol supplementation. Although few cases report measurements of ionized calcium, several do mention that the increments in vitamin D were due to maternal symptoms of hypocalcemia or tetany.

Consequently, there is no established therapeutic regimen for the treatment of hypoparathyroidism during pregnancy, but numerous principles exist that help to guide treatment decisions. Calcitriol levels normally increase during pregnancy and contribute (at least in part) to the enhanced intestinal calcium absorption of pregnancy; most women should receive an increase in the dosage of calcitriol at least initially. The total serum calcium is less informative, and the ionized calcium should be monitored in these patients. Undertreatment results in maternal hypocalcemia; increases the risk of premature labor and of neonatal secondary hyperparathyroidism; and may lead to neonatal skeletal demineralization, subperiosteal bone resorption, and osteitis fibrosa cystica [79]. Conversely, overtreatment may lead to maternal hypercalcemia and neonatal hypoparathyroidism and raises the potential concerns of teratogenicity that has been shown using older vitamin D preparations [80,81]. The active forms of vitamin D, such as calcitriol and 1α-calcidiol, have the advantages of a shorter half-life and lower risk of toxicity. A study reported the outcome of pregnancy in 10 women treated with calcitriol at doses of 0.25 μg/d to 3.25 μg/d [75]. In 8 of 10 pregnancies, healthy infants were delivered. In two cases, serious adverse events occurred, including premature closure of the frontal fontanelle and stillbirth, but the causative role of calcitriol could not be established [75]. Details regarding nine additional cases of hypoparathyroidism and vitamin D–resistant rickets were provided in the same publication and confirmed the lack of toxicity or teratogenicity from vitamin D supplementation during pregnancy [75].

In contrast to the conflicting literature on the effects of pregnancy on hypoparathyroidism, calcium and vitamin D or calcitriol requirements in hypoparathyroid patients have been shown consistently to decrease during lactation [77,78], such that the patients become hypercalcemic unless the supplements are reduced substantially or discontinued. The decreased requirement for calcium and calcitriol occurs at a time when circulating PTHrP levels are high in the maternal circulation of these hypoparathyroid women [76,82,83]. PTHrP may stimulate endogenous calcitriol formation; in one patient, the calcitriol level initially declined below the lower limit of normal when calcium and calcitriol were discontinued, but thereafter the calcitriol level remained in the lower half of the normal range as lactation proceeded [82]. PTHrP also facilitates maternal bone resorption in the presence of postpartum estrogen deficiency. The aforementioned activity may explain why lactation can eliminate temporarily the requirement for supplemental calcium and calcitriol in hypoparathyroid women.

The management of hypoparathyroidism during pregnancy and lactation is challenging. The use of calcium supplementation with calcitriol is recommended, along with monitoring of symptoms of hypocalcemia and of serum ionized calcium levels (not the total serum calcium) to titrate the calcitriol dose as pregnancy progresses. In general, the requirements in calcitriol vary during the second half of pregnancy, but are expected to decrease during lactation.

Pseudohypoparathyroidism

In case reports of pseudohypoparathyroidism, a state characterized by inherited resistance to PTH, patients have hypocalcemia, hypophosphatemia, and high PTH levels. Such patients have been reported to become normocalcemic during pregnancy without ingesting therapeutic amounts of calcium and vitamin D [84]. The mechanism by which pseudohypoparathyroidism is improved in pregnancy is unclear. It may include increased placental secretion of calcitriol, wherein levels have been reported to double or triple in two case reports during the second and third trimesters [84].

The impact of lactation on calcium metabolism in pseudohypoparathyroidism is less well documented. These patients do not have skeletal resistance to PTH, and it is possible that calcium and vitamin D requirements may decrease secondary to enhanced skeletal resorption owing to the combined effects of endogenous high PTH levels, increasing PTHrP release from the breast, and lactation-induced estrogen deficiency. Women with pseudohypoparathyroidism might be expected to lose more bone density than normal during lactation, but this has not been studied.

Osteoporosis associated with pregnancy and lactation

Osteoporosis associated with pregnancy and lactation has been recognized for more than 5 decades [85] and usually presents during late pregnancy or early postpartum [85–88]. It is still debatable whether pregnancy and lactation are causal or accidentally associated with the condition. It is equally unclear whether these osteoporotic fractures reflect architectural deterioration of a previously abnormal skeleton or whether pregnancy and lactation themselves account in large part for the bone loss and fragility fractures, situations that may be compounded by low calcium intake and vitamin D deficiency. As reviewed previously, skeletal demineralization normally occurs during lactation as a consequence of the actions of mammary gland–derived PTHrP in the setting of low estradiol levels and is not preventable by increased calcium intake; osteoporotic fractures may occur in some women during lactation when the demineralization is excessive or the skeleton is unable to tolerate the normal lactational losses of mineral. PTHrP levels were high in one case of lactational osteoporosis and were found to remain elevated for months after weaning [89]. One study, which followed 13 women with pregnancy-associated osteoporosis for 8 years, showed that bone mineral density at the spine and hip increased significantly, leading the investigators to conclude that a large part of the bone loss had been related to the pregnancy itself [86]. Conversely, a high prevalence of fractures in 35 subjects presenting with pregnancy-associated osteoporosis raised the possibility of a genetic factor [90]. The recognition that absence of endogenous calcitonin in mice more than doubles the lactational losses raises the consideration that some women might have a genetic deficiency in calcitonin, its receptor, or some other factor [14,36]. Because bone density is not normally measured in premenopausal women, the bone density before pregnancy or at the end of lactation is usually unknown, and the debate regarding the relative contribution of pregnancy or lactation-associated bone changes versus preexisting abnormalities in the skeleton will continue.

Clinical features

Patients present at a mean age of 27 to 28 years, usually in the setting of a first pregnancy, and no clear association with parity has been found [86–88]. In more than 60% of cases, patients complain of back pain in the lower thoracic or lumbar area, pain that can be quite debilitating secondary to vertebral collapse [86–88]. In such cases, the pain usually improves spontaneously over weeks, but in a few the severe pain may persist for several years [87]. Others present with hip pain, otherwise known as transient osteoporosis of the hip, as part of a syndrome of monarticular or polyarticular pain over other lower extremity joints, including the ankles, which is accentuated with the use of the joint [86–88,91]. Of the more than 200 cases of transient osteoporosis of the hip that have been reported, one third occurred in women in their third trimester of pregnancy or in the early postpartum period [91–93]. The differential diagnosis of this condition includes inflammatory joint disorders, avascular necrosis of the hip, bone marrow edema, and reflex sympathetic dystrophy. In contrast to the last-mentioned condition, patients with transient regional osteoporosis of the hip lack a history of trauma and the typical physical findings of muscle spasm and skin changes

[92]. In contrast to vertebral osteoporosis, recurrences in transient regional osteoporosis of the hip have been described in 40% of total cases, but no series has described this syndrome exclusively in pregnant women [91].

Pathogenesis and laboratory findings

The pathogenesis of pregnancy-associated osteoporosis (presenting with vertebral compression fractures) and transient osteoporosis of the hip differs. In a few cases of the former, secondary causes of bone loss could be identified, including anorexia nervosa, hyperparathyroidism, osteogenesis imperfecta, and corticosteroid or heparin therapy [87,88,90]. One report described pregnancy-associated osteoporosis after oocyte donation in a woman with ovarian failure [94]. Serum calcium and phosphate levels were normal, and no consistent abnormalities in the calciotropic hormones were reported [87,88]. Bone biopsy specimens obtained in some cases have confirmed the diagnosis of osteoporosis, and no osteomalacia was found [87,88]. Bone density tended to be low when measured [86,88]. In a series of 24 patients, the mean Z-score was -1.98 (± 1.5, $n = 15$) at the lumbar spine and -1.48 (± 1.5, $n = 15$) at the total hip [88]. In transient osteoporosis of the hip, radiographs or MRI revealed reduced bone density and increased water content of the marrow cavity [91].

Diagnostic studies and therapeutic interventions

Patients should be screened for secondary causes of bone loss, a large proportion of which may be treatable. Most cases improve symptomatically within a few weeks with conservative measures [87,91]. Myriad pharmacologic agents have been used in individual cases, including calcium, vitamin D, testosterone, estrogen, calcitonin, and bisphosphonates, with increments in bone mineral density reaching 27% at the spine and 7% at the hip in patient case treated with alendronate for 6 months [87]. Because these are usually reports on individual cases and lack controls, the efficacy of such interventions is unproved, and the interventions are not warranted.

In severe cases of osteoporosis, it may be prudent to discourage breast-feeding, the rationale being that the skeleton may not be able to tolerate the normal demineralization that lactation would induce. Patients should be cautioned against carrying heavy weights to avoid additional stress on the spine, and the use of a supportive corset may be helpful. Patients should be reassured that substantial increments in bone mineral density will occur over time [86], and that the condition in cases of vertebral collapse is unlikely to recur. In cases of transient osteoporosis of the hip, patients usually do well with conservative measures, including bed rest. Symptoms and radiograph abnormalities resolve within a few months of their onset [91], but may recur, in contrast to cases with vertebral fracture symptoms, which usually do not recur.

Disturbances in bone and mineral metabolism from the administration of magnesium sulfate during pregnancy

The administration of intravenous magnesium sulfate for 24 to 72 hours is one of the mainstay therapies for the treatment of preterm labor and for the treatment of preeclampsia and eclampsia. Its effect is mediated by action on the myoneural junction. In vitro at high doses, magnesium suppresses PTH levels, similarly to other divalent and trivalent cations, albeit with a lower potency than calcium. This effect now is recognized to occur through the calcium-sensing receptor, a receptor heavily expressed in the parathyroid glands and kidneys [70,95]. Long-term tocolytic therapy using magnesium sulfate generally has been considered safe [96], although few reports have raised concerns about its safety to mothers and neonates.

Maternal complications

Hypocalcemia has been described in several cases in which the women received magnesium to suppress premature labor [97–99]. In a study of seven such cases, a loading dose of 6 g of intravenous magnesium sulfate followed by a maintenance dose of 2 g/h resulted in a rapid increase in the mean serum magnesium level from 2 mg/dL to 6 mg/dL within 1 hour, coupled with an almost concomitant decline in the serum PTH levels, which only partially recovered in 3 hours despite substantial decrements in total and ionized serum calcium levels below the lower limit of normal [98]. A similar pattern for maternal and neonatal profiles was noted in a study of 15 women treated with magnesium sulfate [99]. A Medline literature search for articles published in English in the period 1966–2002 on magnesium sulfate and hypocalcemia revealed four cases of maternal symptomatic hypocalcemia, with serum calcium levels reaching 5.3 mg/dL in one case. Two mothers had a positive Chvostek and Trousseau sign or tetany; three of these cases were noted to have concomitant low PTH levels [100].

Although the short-term administration of magnesium sulfate may lower maternal serum calcium through an effect on PTH secretion, long-term administration for 2 to 3 weeks was associated with increments in serum PTH levels, possibly as an appropriate adaptive mechanism to prolonged hypocalcemia. It has been suggested that urinary loss of calcium may be a major pathophysiologic mechanism for the hypocalcemia and in such instances may result in ultimate impairment of bone mineralization [101]. In a study of 20 subjects given intravenous magnesium sulfate for premature labor, serum magnesium and phosphorus levels increased, serum calcium levels decreased concomitantly with an increase in serum PTH, and substantial increments in urinary magnesium and calcium were noted, reaching mean levels two to three times the upper limit of normal [101]. Prolonged magnesium administration for several weeks also has been associated with maternal forearm bone loss prospectively, osteoporosis by bone mineral density, and bilateral calcaneal stress fractures postpartum [101–103].

Neonatal complications

Administration of intravenous magnesium to mothers before delivery increased neonatal serum magnesium and decreased PTH levels, whereas the effect on neonatal total and ionized calcium levels varied [97,99]. Studies evaluating the impact of neonatal hypermagnesemia on neonatal outcomes have yielded conflicting results [97,104–106]. Respiratory depression and hypotonia were reported in 16 cases of neonatal hypermagnesemia [106]. A follow-up study of 35 infants born to toxemic mothers treated with magnesium sulfate for 2 to 4 days suggested that neonates whose mothers had received prolonged administration may be more likely to manifest respiratory depression [105]. Cord blood and neonatal serum magnesium levels were of little diagnostic value to the clinical picture except in cases of severe hypermagnesemia [105,107], confirming the general observation that circulating serum magnesium levels do not reflect intracellular and total body magnesium stores. Conversely, a study of 118 infants born to mothers who had received intramuscular magnesium in doses of 10 to 95 g concluded that the neonatal death rate was lower than that of the total newborn population [104]. Respiratory depression, hypotonia, and need for intubation were not evaluated in that report, however [104]. Neonatal bone abnormalities have been reported with long-term use of magnesium sulfate. The first report by Lamm et al [108] described a congenital form of rickets manifested by defective ossification of bone and enamel in the teeth of the offspring of mothers who had received magnesium sulfate during pregnancy. Several cases of abnormal mineralization of metaphyses since have been reported in neonates born to mothers who received prolonged intravenous magnesium and had high serum magnesium levels [109–111]. The proposed mechanism for defective mineralization of bones involves the inhibition of calcification of osteoid in which calcium-binding sites are occupied by magnesium [109,110].

Some of these conflicting findings regarding neonatal morbidity from maternal administration of magnesium sulfate may be explained by the route and duration of magnesium sulfate administration, by the variability in the ranges of cord magnesium levels reached, and by the gestational age of the neonates. Postdelivery, there was a delay in normalization of the serum magnesium level for a few days resulting from the limitation of magnesium excretion by the newborn's immature kidneys [97].

Management issues

There are no guidelines for the monitoring of pregnant women receiving magnesium sulfate. Neonates born to mothers receiving long-term magnesium sulfate and experiencing severe hypermagnesemia (> 7 mg/dL) are more likely to have hypotonia, respiratory depression, and bone abnormalities [97,105,107,111]. Subjects receiving such therapy for periods exceeding 1 or 2 days should be monitored carefully, with the measurement of maternal serum calcium and magnesium levels, coupled with monitoring the fetal movement. Symptomatic neonates can be managed by maintaining ventilation for 24 to 48 hours and providing intravenous fluids for electrolyte balance for a few days, after which marked clinical improvement is usually noted [105]. Intravenous calcium to antagonize the central nervous system depression and peripheral neuromuscular blockade has been used, with careful monitoring of the heart rate [105].

Low calcium intake

There are limited data that low calcium intake in the mother may adversely affect fetal mineral accretion and maternal bone mineral metabolism [112]. In women with low dietary calcium intake, there are differing results as to whether or not calcium supplementation during pregnancy improved maternal or neonatal bone density [3]. There is short-term evidence that maternal turnover was reduced when 1.2 g of calcium was given for 20 days to 31 Mexican women with a mean calcium intake of 1 g during weeks 25 to 30 of gestation [113]. In a double-blind study conducted in 256 pregnant women, 2 g of calcium supplementation improved bone mineral content in infants of supplemented mothers who were in the lowest quintile of calcium intake [114].

During lactation, there is no firm evidence that low calcium intake leads to impaired breast milk quality or accentuates maternal bone loss [115]. Even in women with very low calcium intakes, the same amount of mineral was lost during lactation from the skeleton compared with women who had supplemented calcium intakes, and the breast milk calcium content was unaffected by calcium intake or vitamin D status [116–118]. Conversely, because high calcium intakes do not affect the degree of skeletal demineralization that occurs during lactation [38–41], it is unlikely that increasing calcium supplementation above normal would affect skeletal demineralization.

In general, the physiologic changes in calcium and bone metabolism that usually occur during pregnancy and lactation are likely to be sufficient for fetal bone growth and breast milk production in women with reasonably sufficient calcium intake [115]. The inclusion of calcium supplementation for pregnant women with low calcium intake could be defended, however, and is strengthened further by the possible link between low calcium intake, preeclampsia, and increased blood pressure in the offspring [112]. Increased calcium intake also is recommended in adolescent mothers to meet the need of reproduction and maternal bone growth [115]. There is evidence that the skeleton of an undernourished adolescent recovers fully from lactational losses, but there is some concern that peak bone mass might not be attained subsequently [119].

Vitamin D deficiency

In humans and in animal models, vitamin D deficiency or the absence of the vitamin D receptor can lead to adverse neonatal outcomes, including neonatal rickets, craniotabes, decreased wrist ossification centers, and impaired tooth enamel formation [120]. These features generally are not present at birth, but appear postnatally as intestinal calcium absorption becomes vitamin D dependent. Although vitamin D supplementation of pregnant mothers at risk for vitamin D deficiency improved neonatal serum calcium concentrations and resulted in a trend for greater height and length in the offspring [112], a Cochrane review of 232 women in two trials reported conflicting results [121]. Although there is no evidence to indicate a beneficial effect of vitamin D supplementation during pregnancy above the amounts needed to prevent vitamin D deficiency, optimal levels for vitamin D supplementation are unclear [122]. An arbitrary daily recommended intake has been set at 400 IU/d, but likely needs revision upward [123]. Recommendations for vitamin D supplementation either for women of childbearing age or for lactating women were not mentioned in the new US dietary guidelines issued in 2005 [124].

Scientific data pertaining to vitamin D supplementation during lactation are even scarcer than data on vitamin D supplementation during pregnancy. An arbitrary daily recommended intake has been set at 400 IU/d, but may be insufficient [123]. Whether vitamin D deficiency impairs the ability to restore maternal skeleton postweaning is unclear [1]. Lactating mothers supplemented with 1000 IU to 2000 IU of vitamin D for 15 weeks experienced increments in circulating maternal 25-hydroxyvitamin D_3 levels of 16 ng/mL to 23 ng/mL [122]. It has been suggested that vitamin D supplementation of lactating mothers would improve vitamin D nutrition in the mother and the breastfeeding infant; this has not been shown yet, but is currently under investigation [122]. Breastfed infants of vitamin D–deficient mothers should receive vitamin D supplementation to avoid nutritional rickets [125]. There is low penetrance of vitamin D into breast milk, and it is more efficient to give the vitamin D supplement directly to the infant, although supplementing the mother with high doses has been shown to work [126].

Hypercalcemia of malignancy

Hypercalcemia of malignancy, an extremely rare occurrence, has been reported in two cases—one in metastatic breast cancer and the other in renal cell carcinoma [127,128]. In both reports, the disease was rapidly progressive and resulted in premature delivery at 29 and 32 weeks of gestation and maternal demise within 4 months postpartum. On the first day postdelivery, both infants were hypercalcemic, and one subsequently developed hypocalcemia from transient hypoparathyroidism. Intravenous pamidronate was used shortly before delivery in one case with normalization of maternal serum calcium within 5 days of pamidronate administration [128]. Treatment in such cases includes adequate aggressive hydration with close monitoring, furosemide, and possibly calcitonin. Because bisphosphonates cross the placenta, their use should be reserved for life-threatening situations.

Neonatal hypoparathyroidism from maternal therapy with radioactive iodine

Inadvertent maternal therapy with radioactive iodine during pregnancy may result in neonatal hypoparathyroidism, similar to what has been reported in adults treated with high-dose radioactive iodine. A mother was reported to have received 103 mCi of iodine-131 (^{131}I) for thyroid carcinoma at 10 weeks of gestation when she was unaware of her pregnancy. Her neonate experienced occasional episodes of stiffening and turning blue during the first 2 months that accelerated and led to a hospital admission for respiratory distress, tonic-clonic seizures, and ultimate tracheostomy [129]. The infant was found be hypocalcemic, with documented hypoparathyroidism and severe hypothyroidism. The infant was discharged after 1 month of hospitalization with a tracheostomy and ongoing treatment with calcium, dihydrotachysterol, and thyroid hormone. It is likely that the fetal thyroid gland accumulated sufficient amounts of ^{131}I to result in destruction of fetal thyroid and parathyroid tissue from the emitted β particles [129].

Summary

Studies of pregnant women indicate that the fetal calcium demand is met largely by intestinal calcium absorption, which from early pregnancy onward more than doubles. The studies of biochemical markers of bone turnover, DXA, and ultrasound are inconclusive, but suggest that the maternal skeleton also contributes calcium to the developing fetus. In contrast, during lactation, skeletal calcium resorption is the dominant mechanism by which calcium is supplied to the breast milk; renal calcium conservation is also apparent. Lactation produces an obligatory skeletal calcium loss regardless of maternal calcium intake, but the calcium is completely restored to the skeleton after weaning through mechanisms that are not understood. The adaptations during pregnancy and lactation lead to novel presentations and management issues for known disorders of calcium and bone metabolism, such as primary hyperparathyroidism, hypoparathyroidism, and vitamin D deficiency. Finally, although some women experience fragility fractures as a consequence of pregnancy or lactation, in most women the changes in calcium and bone metabolism during pregnancy and lactation are normal and without adverse consequences in the long-term.

References

[1] Kovacs CS, Kronenberg HM. Maternal-fetal calcium and bone metabolism during pregnancy, puerperium and lactation. Endocr Rev 1997;18:832–72.

[2] Kovacs CS. Calcium and bone metabolism in pregnancy and lactation. J Clin Endocrinol Metab 2001;86:2344–8.

[3] Prentice A. Pregnancy and lactation. In: Glorieux FH, Petifor JM, Jüppner H, editors. Pediatric bone: biology and diseases. New York: Academic Press; 2003. p. 249–69.

[4] Chesney RW, Specker BL, McKay CP. Mineral metabolism during pregnancy and lactation. In: Coe FL, Favus MJ, editors. Disorders of bone and mineral metabolism. 2nd edition. Philadelphia: Lippincott, Williams & Wilkins; 2002. p. 347–59.

[5] Taylor RN, Lebovic DI. The endocrinology of pregnancy. In: Greenspan FS, Gardner DG, editors. Basic and clinical endocrinology. 7th edition. New York: Lange Medical Books/McGraw-Hill; 2004. p. 637–57.

[6] Dahlman T, Sjoberg HE, Bucht E. Calcium homeostasis in normal pregnancy and puerperium: a longitudinal study. Acta Obstet Gynecol Scand 1994;73:393–8.

[7] Gallacher SJ, Fraser WD, Owens OJ, et al. Changes in calciotrophic hormones and biochemical markers of bone turnover in normal human pregnancy. Eur J Endocrinol 1994; 131:369–74.

[8] Cross NA, Hillman LS, Allen SH, et al. Calcium homeostasis and bone metabolism during pregnancy, lactation, and postweaning: a longitudinal study. Am J Clin Nutr 1995;61: 514–23.

[9] Rasmussen N, Frolich A, Hornnes PJ, Hegedus L. Serum ionized calcium and intact parathyroid hormone levels during pregnancy and postpartum. Br J Obstet Gynaecol 1990;97: 857–9.

[10] Seki K, Makimura N, Mitsui C, et al. Calcium-regulating hormones and osteocalcin levels during pregnancy: a longitudinal study. Am J Obstet Gynecol 1991;164:1248–52.

[11] Gao P, D'Amour P. Evolution of the parathyroid hormone (PTH) assay—importance of circulating PTH immunoheterogeneity and of its regulation. Clin Lab 2005;51: 21–9.

[12] Singh HJ, Mohammad NH, Nila A. Serum calcium and parathormone during normal pregnancy in Malay women. J Matern Fetal Med 1999;8:95–100.

[13] Turner M, Barre PE, Benjamin A, et al. Does the maternal kidney contribute to the increased circulating 1,25-dihydroxyvitamin D concentrations during pregnancy? Miner Electrolyte Metab 1988;14:246–52.

[14] Woodrow JP, Noseworthy CS, Fudge NJ, et al. Calcitonin/calcitonin gene-related peptide protect the maternal skeleton from excessive resorption during lactation [abstract]. J Bone Miner Res 2003;18(Suppl 2):S37.

[15] Horwitz MJ, Tedesco MB, Sereika SM, et al. Direct comparison of sustained infusion of human parathyroid hormone-related protein-(1–36). J Clin Endocrinol Metab 2003;88: 1603–9.

[16] Kovacs CS, Lanske B, Hunzelman JL, et al. Parathyroid hormone-related peptide (PTHrP) regulates fetal-placental calcium transport through a receptor distinct from the PTH/PTHrP receptor. Proc Natl Acad Sci U S A 1996;93:15233–8.

[17] Cornish J, Callon KE, Nicholson GC, Reid IR. Parathyroid hormone-related protein-(107–139) inhibits bone resorption in vivo. Endocrinology 1997;138:1299–304.

[18] Marie PJ, Cancela L, Le Boulch N, Miravet L. Bone changes due to pregnancy and lactation: influence of vitamin D status. Am J Physiol 1986;251:E400–6.

[19] Sharpe CJ, Fudge NJ, Kovacs CS. A rapid 35% flux in bone mass occurs during pregnancy and lactation cycles in mice [abstract]. International Bone and Mineral Society Meeting, Osaka, Japan, June 3–7, 2003. Bone 2003;32(Suppl):S227.

[20] Purdie DW, Aaron JE, Selby PL. Bone histology and mineral homeostasis in human pregnancy. Br J Obstet Gynaecol 1988;95:849–54.

[21] Naylor KE, Iqbal P, Fledelius C, et al. The effect of pregnancy on bone density and bone turnover. J Bone Miner Res 2000;15:129–37.

[22] Black AJ, Topping J, Durham B, et al. A detailed assessment of alterations in bone turnover, calcium homeostasis, and bone density in normal pregnancy. J Bone Miner Res 2000;15:557–63.

[23] Ritchie LD, Fung EB, Halloran BP, et al. A longitudinal study of calcium homeostasis during human pregnancy and lactation and after resumption of menses. Am J Clin Nutr 1998; 67:693–701.

[24] Ulrich U, Miller PB, Eyre DR, et al. Bone remodeling and bone mineral density during pregnancy. Arch Gynecol Obstet 2003;268:309–16.

[25] Kaur M, Pearson D, Godber I, et al. Longitudinal changes in bone mineral density during normal pregnancy. Bone 2003;32:449–54.

[26] Gambacciani M, Spinetti A, Gallo R, et al. Ultrasonographic bone characteristics during normal pregnancy: longitudinal and cross-sectional evaluation. Am J Obstet Gynecol 1995;173:890–3.

[27] Pearson D, Kaur M, San P, et al. Recovery of pregnancy mediated bone loss during lactation. Bone 2004;34:570–8.

[28] To WW, Wong MW, Leung TW. Relationship between bone mineral density changes in pregnancy and maternal and pregnancy characteristics: a longitudinal study. Acta Obstet Gynecol Scand 2003;82:820–7.

[29] Sowers M. Pregnancy and lactation as risk factors for subsequent bone loss and osteoporosis. J Bone Miner Res 1996;11:1052–60.

[30] Paton LM, Alexander JL, Nowson CA, et al. Pregnancy and lactation have no long-term deleterious effect on measures of bone mineral in healthy women: a twin study. Am J Clin Nutr 2003;77:707–14.

[31] Dobnig H, Kainer F, Stepan V, et al. Elevated parathyroid hormone-related peptide levels after human gestation: relationship to changes in bone and mineral metabolism. J Clin Endocrinol Metab 1995;80:3699–707.

[32] VanHouten JN, Dann P, Stewart AF, et al. Mammary-specific deletion of parathyroid hormone-related protein preserves bone mass during lactation. J Clin Invest 2003;112:1429–36.

[33] VanHouten J, Dann P, McGeoch G, et al. The calcium-sensing receptor regulates mammary gland parathyroid hormone-related protein production and calcium transport. J Clin Invest 2004;113:598–608.

[34] Kovacs CS, Chik CL. Hyperprolactinemia caused by lactation and pituitary adenomas is associated with altered serum calcium, phosphate, parathyroid hormone (PTH), and PTH-related peptide levels. J Clin Endocrinol Metab 1995;80:3036–42.

[35] Sowers MF, Hollis DW, Shapiro B, et al. Elevated parathyroid hormone-related peptide associated with lactation and bone density loss. JAMA 1996;276:549–54.

[36] Woodrow JP, Hoff AO, Gagel RF, Kovacs CS. Calcitonin treatment rescues calcitonin-null mice from excessive bone resorption during lactation [abstract]. J Bone Miner Res 2004; 19(Suppl):SA518.

[37] Laskey MA, Prentice A. Effect of pregnancy on recovery of lactational bone loss [letter]. Lancet 1997;349:1518–9.

[38] Cross NA, Hillman LS, Allen SH, Krause GF. Changes in bone mineral density and markers of bone remodeling during lactation and postweaning in women consuming high amounts of calcium. J Bone Miner Res 1995;10:1312–20.

[39] Kalkwarf HJ, Specker BL, Bianchi DC, Ranz J, Ho M. The effect of calcium supplementation on bone density during lactation and after weaning. N Engl J Med 1997;337:523–8.

[40] Polatti F, Capuzzo E, Viazzo F, et al. Bone mineral changes during and after lactation. Obstet Gynecol 1999;94:52–6.

[41] Kolthoff N, Eiken P, Kristensen B, Nielsen SP. Bone mineral changes during pregnancy and lactation: a longitudinal cohort study. Clin.Sci (Colch) 1998;94:405–12.

[42] Laskey MA, Prentice A, Hanratty LA, et al. Bone changes after 3 mo of lactation: influence of calcium intake, breast-milk output, and vitamin D-receptor genotype. Am J Clin Nutr 1998;67:685–92.

[43] VanHouten JN, Wysolmerski JJ. Low estrogen and high parathyroid hormone-related peptide levels contribute to accelerated bone resorption and bone loss in lactating mice. Endocrinology 2003;144:5521–9.

[44] Wermers RA, Khosla S, Atkinson EJ, et al. The rise and fall of primary hyperparathyroidism: a population-based study in Rochester, Minnesota, 1965–1992. Ann Intern Med 1997; 126:433–40.

[45] Heath H, Hodgson SF, Kennedy MA. Primary hyperparathyroidism: incidence, morbidity, and potential economic impact in a community. N Engl J Med 1980;302: 189–93.

[46] Kelly TR. Primary hyperparathyroidism during pregnancy. Surgery 1991;110:1028–34.

[47] Haenel LC, Mayfield RK. Primary hyperparathyroidism in a twin pregnancy and review of fetal/maternal calcium homeostasis. Am J Med Sci 2000;319:191–4.

[48] Kort KC, Schiller HJ, Numann PJ. Hyperparathyroidism and pregnancy. Am J Surg 1999; 177:66–8.

[49] Schnatz PF, Curry SL. Primary hyperparathyroidism in pregnancy: evidence-based management. Obstet Gynecol Surv 2002;57:365–76.

[50] El-Hajj Fuleihan G. Pathogenesis and etiology of primary hyperparathyroidism. In: Rose BD, editor. UpToDate 13.1. Wellesley (MA): UpToDate; 2005.

[51] Kristoffersson A, Dahlgren S, Lithner F, Jarhult J. Primary hyperparathyroidism in pregnancy. Surgery 1985;97:326–30.

[52] Shangold MM, Dor N, Welt SI, et al. Hyperparathyroidism and pregnancy: a review. Obstet Gynecol Surv 1982;37:217–28.

[53] Clark D, Seeds JW, Cefalo RC. Hyperparathyroid crisis and pregnancy. Am J Obstet Gynecol 1981;140:840–2.

[54] Carella MJ, Gossain VV. Hyperparathyroidism and pregnancy: case report and review. J Gen Intern Med 1992;7:448–53.

[55] Croom RD, Thomas CG. Primary hyperparathyroidism during pregnancy. Surgery 1984; 96:1109–18.

[56] Inabnet WB, Baldwin D, Daniel RO, Staren ED. Hyperparathyroidism and pancreatitis during pregnancy. Surgery 1996;119:710–3.

[57] Matthias GS, Helliwell TR, Williams A. Postpartum hyperparathyroid crisis: case report. Br J Obstet Gynaecol 1987;94:807–10.

[58] Negishi H, Kobayashi M, Nishida R, et al. Primary hyperparathyroidism and simultaneous bilateral fracture of the femoral neck during pregnancy. J Trauma 2002;52:367–9.

[59] Hess HM, Dickson J, Fox HE. Hyperfunctioning parathyroid carcinoma presenting as acute pancreatitis in pregnancy. J Reprod Med 1980;25:83–7.

[60] Wagner G, Transhol L, Melchior JC. Hyperparathyroidism and pregnancy. Acta Endocrinol (Copenh) 1964;47:549–64.

[61] Ludwig GD. Hyperparathyroidism in relation to pregnancy. N Engl J Med 1962;267: 637–42.

[62] Delmonico FL, Neer RM, Cosimi AB, et al. Hyperparathyroidism during pregnancy. Am J Surg 1976;131:328–37.

[63] Kaplan EL, Burrington JD, Klementschitsch P, et al. Primary hyperparathyroidism, pregnancy, and neonatal hypocalcemia. Surgery 1984;96:717–22.

[64] Ip P. Neonatal convulsion revealing maternal hyperparathyroidism: an unusual case of late neonatal hypoparathyroidism. Arch Gynecol Obstet 2003;268:227–9.

[65] Bruce J, Strong JA. Maternal hyperparathyroidism and parathyroid deficiency in the child, with account of effect of parathyroidectomy on renal function, and of attempt to transplant part of tumor. QJM 1955;24:307–19.

[66] Petit D, Clark R. Hyperparathyroidism and pregnancy. Am J Surg 1947;74:860–4.

[67] Schnatz PF. Surgical treatment of primary hyperparathyroidism during the third trimester. Obstet Gynecol 2002;99(5 Pt 2):961–3.

[68] Rajala B, Abbasi RA, Hutchinson HT, Taylor T. Acute pancreatitis and primary hyperparathyroidism in pregnancy: treatment of hypercalcemia with magnesium sulfate. Obstet Gynecol 1987;70(3 Pt 2):460–2.

[69] Dahan M, Chang RJ. Pancreatitis secondary to hyperparathyroidism during pregnancy. Obstet Gynecol 2001;98(5 Pt 2):923–5.

[70] Brown EM, Pollak M, Seidman CE, et al. Calcium-ion-sensing cell-surface receptors. N Engl J Med 1995;333:234–40.

[71] El-Hajj Fuleihan G, Heath HH. Familial benign hypocalciuric hypercalcemia and neonatal severe hyperparathyroidism. In: Bilezikian JP, Marcus R, Levine MA, editors. The parathyroids: basic and clinical concepts. 2nd edition. New York: Academic Press; 1994. p. 607–23.

[72] Powell BR, Buist NR. Late presenting, prolonged hypocalcemia in an infant of a woman with hypocalciuric hypercalcemia. Clin Pediatr (Phila) 1990;29:241–3.

[73] Thomas BR, Bennett JD. Symptomatic hypocalcemia and hypoparathyroidism in two infants of mothers with hyperparathyroidism and familial benign hypercalcemia. J Perinatol 1995;15:23–6.

[74] O'Leary JA, Klainer LM, Neuwirth RS. The management of hypoparathyroidism in pregnancy. Am J Obstet Gynecol 1966;94:1103–7.

[75] Callies F, Arlt W, Scholz HJ, et al. Management of hypoparathyroidism during pregnancy—report of twelve cases. Eur J Endocrinol 1998;139:284–9.

[76] Caplan RH, Beguin EA. Hypercalcemia in a calcitriol-treated hypoparathyroid woman during lactation. Obstet Gynecol 1990;76:485–9.

[77] Salle BL, Berthezene F, Glorieux FH, et al. Hypoparathyroidism during pregnancy: treatment with calcitriol. J Clin Endocrinol Metab 1981;52:810–3.

[78] Sadeghi-Nejad A, Wolfsdorf JI, Senior B. Hypoparathyroidism and pregnancy: treatment with calcitriol. JAMA 1980;243:254–5.

[79] Landing BH, Kamoshita S. Congenital hyperparathyroidism secondary to maternal hypoparathyroidism. J Pediatr 1970;77:842–7.

[80] Taussig HB. Possible injury to the cardiovascular system from vitamin D. Ann Intern Med 1966;65:1195–200.

[81] Friedman WF, Mills LF. The relationship between vitamin D and the craniofacial and dental anomalies of the supravalvular aortic stenosis syndrome. Pediatrics 1969;43:12–8.

[82] Mather KJ, Chik CL, Corenblum B. Maintenance of serum calcium by parathyroid hormone-related peptide during lactation in a hypoparathyroid patient. J Clin Endocrinol Metab 1999;84:424–7.

[83] Shomali ME, Ross DS. Hypercalcemia in a woman with hypoparathyroidism associated with increased parathyroid hormone-related protein during lactation. Endocr Pract 1999;5:198–200.

[84] Breslau NA, Zerwekh JE. Relationship of estrogen and pregnancy to calcium homeostasis in pseudohypoparathyroidism. J Clin Endocrinol Metab 1986;62:45–51.

[85] Nordin BE, Roper A. Postpregnancy osteoporosis: a syndrome? Lancet 1955;1:431–4.

[86] Phillips AJ, Ostlere SJ, Smith R. Pregnancy-associated osteoporosis: does the skeleton recover? Osteoporos Int 2000;11:449–54.

[87] Khovidhunkit W, Epstein S. Osteoporosis in pregnancy. Osteoporos Int 1996;6:345–54.

[88] Smith R, Athanasou NA, Ostlere SJ, Vipond SE. Pregnancy-associated osteoporosis. QJM 1995;88:865–78.

[89] Reid IR, Wattie DJ, Evans MC, Budayr AA. Post-pregnancy osteoporosis associated with hypercalcaemia. Clin Endocrinol (Oxf) 1992;37:298–303.

[90] Dunne F, Walters B, Marshall T, Heath DA. Pregnancy associated osteoporosis. Clin Endocrinol (Oxf) 1993;39:487–90.

[91] Lakhanpal S, Ginsburg WW, Luthra HS, Hunder GG. Transient regional osteoporosis: a study of 56 cases and review of the literature. Ann Intern Med 1987;106:444–50.

[92] Arayssi TK, Tawbi HA, Usta IM, Hourani MH. Calcitonin in the treatment of transient osteoporosis of the hip. Semin Arthritis Rheum 2003;32:388–97.

[93] Curtiss PH Jr, Kincaid WE. Transitory demineralization of the hip in pregnancy: a report of three cases. J Bone Joint Surg Am 1959;41:1327–33.

[94] Khastgir G, Studd JW, King H, et al. Changes in bone density and biochemical markers of bone turnover in pregnancy-associated osteoporosis. Br J Obstet Gynaecol 1996;103:716–8.

[95] Brown EM, El Hajj Fuleihan G, Chen CJ, Kifor O. A comparison of the effects of divalent and trivalent cations on parathyroid hormone release, 3',5'-cyclic-adenosine

monophosphate accumulation, and the levels of inositol phosphates in bovine parathyroid cells. Endocrinology 1990;127:1064–71.

[96] Wilkins IA, Goldberg JD, Phillips RN, et al. Long-term use of magnesium sulfate as a tocolytic agent. Obstet Gynecol 1986;67(3 Suppl):38S–40S.

[97] Donovan EF, Tsang RC, Steichen JJ, et al. Neonatal hypermagnesemia: effect on parathyroid hormone and calcium homeostasis. J Pediatr 1980;96:305–10.

[98] Cholst IN, Steinberg SF, Tropper PJ, et al. The influence of hypermagnesemia on serum calcium and parathyroid hormone levels in human subjects. N Engl J Med 1984;310: 1221–5.

[99] Cruikshank DP, Pitkin RM, Reynolds WA, et al. Effects of magnesium sulfate treatment on perinatal calcium metabolism: I. maternal and fetal responses. Am J Obstet Gynecol 1979; 134:243–9.

[100] Koontz SL, Friedman SA, Schwartz ML. Symptomatic hypocalcemia after tocolytic therapy with magnesium sulfate and nifedipine. Am J Obstet Gynecol 2004;190:1773–6.

[101] Smith LG Jr, Burns PA, Schanler RJ. Calcium homeostasis in pregnant women receiving long-term magnesium sulfate therapy for preterm labor. Am J Obstet Gynecol 1992;167: 45–51.

[102] Hung JW, Tsai MY, Yang BY, Chen JF. Maternal osteoporosis after prolonged magnesium sulfate tocolysis therapy: a case report. Arch Phys Med Rehabil 2005;86:146–9.

[103] Levav AL, Chan L, Wapner RJ. Long-term magnesium sulfate tocolysis and maternal osteoporosis in a triplet pregnancy: a case report. Am J Perinatol 1998;15:43–6.

[104] Stone SR, Pritchard JA. Effect of maternally administered magnesium sulfate on the neonate. Obstet Gynecol 1970;35:574–7.

[105] Lipsitz PJ. The clinical and biochemical effects of excess magnesium in the newborn. Pediatrics 1971;47:501–9.

[106] Lipsitz PJ, English IC. Hypermagnesemia in the newborn infant. Pediatrics 1967;40: 856–62.

[107] Savory J, Monif GR. Serum calcium levels in cord sera of the progeny of mothers treated with magnesium sulfate for toxemia of pregnancy. Am J Obstet Gynecol 1971; 110:556–9.

[108] Lamm CI, Norton KI, Murphy RJ, et al. Congenital rickets associated with magnesium sulfate infusion for tocolysis. J Pediatr 1988;113:1078–82.

[109] Santi MD, Henry GW, Douglas GL. Magnesium sulfate treatment of preterm labor as a cause of abnormal neonatal bone mineralization. J Pediatr Orthop 1994;14:249–53.

[110] Cumming WA, Thomas VJ. Hypermagnesemia: a cause of abnormal metaphyses in the neonate. AJR Am J Roentgenol 1989;152:1071–2.

[111] Malaeb SN, Rassi AI, Haddad MC, et al. Bone mineralization in newborns whose mothers received magnesium sulphate for tocolysis of premature labour. Pediatr Radiol 2004;34: 384–6.

[112] Prentice A. Micronutrients and the bone mineral content of the mother, fetus and newborn. J Nutr 2003;133(Suppl 2):1693S–9S.

[113] Janakiraman V, Ettinger A, Mercado-Garcia A, et al. Calcium supplements and bone resorption in pregnancy: a randomized crossover trial. Am J Prev Med 2003;24:260–4.

[114] Koo WW, Walters JC, Esterlitz J, et al. Maternal calcium supplementation and fetal bone mineralization. Obstet Gynecol 1999;94:577–82.

[115] Prentice A. Calcium in pregnancy and lactation. Annu Rev Nutr 2000;20:249–72.

[116] Prentice A, Jarjou LM, Cole TJ, et al. Calcium requirements of lactating Gambian mothers: effects of a calcium supplement on breast-milk calcium concentration, maternal bone mineral content, and urinary calcium excretion. Am J Clin Nutr 1995;62:58–67.

[117] Prentice A, Jarjou LM, Stirling DM, et al. Biochemical markers of calcium and bone metabolism during 18 months of lactation in Gambian women accustomed to a low calcium intake and in those consuming a calcium supplement. J Clin Endocrinol Metab 1998;83: 1059–66.

[118] Prentice A, Yan L, Jarjou LM, et al. Vitamin D status does not influence the breast-milk calcium concentration of lactating mothers accustomed to a low calcium intake. Acta Paediatr 1997;86:1006–8.

[119] Bezerra FF, Mendonca LM, Lobato EC, et al. Bone mass is recovered from lactation to postweaning in adolescent mothers with low calcium intakes. Am J Clin Nutr 2004;80: 1322–6.

[120] Specker B. Vitamin D requirements during pregnancy. Am J Clin Nutr 2004;80(Suppl): 1740S–7S.

[121] Mahomed K, Gulmezoglu AM. Vitamin D supplementation in pregnancy. Cochrane Database Syst Rev 2000;2:CD000228.

[122] Hollis BW, Wagner CL. Assessment of dietary vitamin D requirements during pregnancy and lactation. Am J Clin Nutr 2004;79:717–26.

[123] Hollis BW. Circulating 25-hydroxyvitamin D levels indicative of vitamin D sufficiency: implications for establishing a new effective dietary intake recommendation for vitamin D. J Nutr 2005;135:317–22.

[124] Department of Health and Human Services and the Department of Agriculture. Dietary guidelines for Americans 2005. Executive summary. January 12, 2005. Available at: http://www.health.gov/dietaryguidelines/dga2005/document/html/executivesummary.htm. Accessed April 25, 2005.

[125] Thomson K, Morley R, Grover SR, Zacharin MR. Postnatal evaluation of vitamin D and bone health in women who were vitamin D-deficient in pregnancy, and in their infants. Med J Aust 2004;181:486–8.

[126] Hollis BW, Wagner CL. Vitamin D requirements during lactation: high-dose maternal supplementation as therapy to prevent hypovitaminosis D for both the mother and the nursing infant. Am J Clin Nutr 2004;80(Suppl):1752S–8S.

[127] Usta IM, Chammas M, Khalil AM. Renal cell carcinoma with hypercalcemia complicating a pregnancy: case report and review of the literature. Eur J Gynaecol Oncol 1998;19:584–7.

[128] Illidge TM, Hussey M, Godden CW. Malignant hypercalcaemia in pregnancy and antenatal administration of intravenous pamidronate. Clin Oncol (R Coll Radiol) 1996;8:257–8.

[129] Richards GE, Brewer ED, Conley SB, Saldana LR. Combined hypothyroidism and hypoparathyroidism in an infant after maternal ^{131}I administration. J Pediatr 1981;99:141–3.

ELSEVIER
SAUNDERS

Endocrinol Metab Clin N Am
35 (2006) 53–78

ENDOCRINOLOGY
AND METABOLISM
CLINICS
OF NORTH AMERICA

Management of Gestational Diabetes: Pharmacologic Treatment Options and Glycemic Control

Oded Langer, MD, PhD*

*Department of Obstetrics and Gynecology, St. Luke's–Roosevelt Hospital Center,
University Hospital of Columbia University, New York, NY, USA*

Diabetes mellitus is one of the most common medical complications of pregnancy; gestational diabetes mellitus (GDM) accounts for approximately 90% to 95% of all cases. GDM is defined as carbohydrate intolerance of variable severity with onset or first recognition during pregnancy. The definition is applicable regardless of whether insulin is used to treat the disease or if the condition persists after pregnancy. It does not exclude the possibility that unrecognized glucose intolerance may have antedated the pregnancy [1]. In the United States, approximately 135,000 to 200,000 women are diagnosed annually with GDM. Approximately 9% to 12% of undiagnosed type 2 diabetes is included in the GDM population. The overall increase in obesity including women of reproductive age parallels the increase in GDM and type 2 diabetes [2].

Pregnancy is characterized by hyperinsulinemia and insulin resistance in response to the diabetogenic effects of normal carbohydrate metabolism [3]. During the first trimester and early in the second trimester, increased insulin sensitivity occurs secondary to the relatively higher levels of estrogen. In contrast, in the late second and early third trimesters, there is increased insulin resistance and reduced sensitivity to insulin action. A variety of hormones—placental lactogen, leptin, progesterone, prolactin, cortisol and adiponectin—are instrumental in these changes.

GDM and type 2 diabetes share impaired insulin secretion and insulin resistance. Insulin resistance results in decreased glucose uptake in skeletal

* Department of Obstetrics and Gynecology, St. Luke's–Roosevelt Hospital Center, University Hospital of Columbia University, 1000 Tenth Avenue, Suite 10A, New York, NY 10019.

   E-mail address: odlanger@chpnet.org

0889-8529/06/$ - see front matter © 2005 Elsevier Inc. All rights reserved.
doi:10.1016/j.ecl.2005.09.007   *endo.theclinics.com*

muscles, white adipose tissue, and liver and suppression of hepatic glucose production. The risk factors associated with type 2 diabetes and GDM are comparable (eg, obesity, ethnicity, family history). β-Cell adaptation to insulin resistance is impaired in women with GDM and may be a universal response to insulin resistance because it is found in many ethnic groups. Women with a history of GDM are at an increased risk for subsequent development of type 2 diabetes (50%–80%). Type 2 diabetes and GDM arguably may be the same disease with different names [4–6].

Adverse perinatal outcome

Maternal hyperglycemia with resultant fetal hyperinsulinemia is central to the pathophysiology of diabetic complications in pregnancy. The infants of GDM women are at a 3 to 8 fold increased risk for stillbirth and aberrant fetal growth (macrosomia and growth restriction) and metabolic (eg, hypoglycemia and hypocalcemia), hematologic (eg, bilirubinemia and polycythemia), and respiratory complications that increase neonatal intensive care unit admission rates and birth trauma (eg, shoulder dystocia) [7,8].

Congenital anomalies and spontaneous abortions are more serious complications in pregestational diabetes than in GDM. Because of the relatively high rate of undiagnosed type 2 diabetic women in the GDM population (10%), a concerted effort should be made to rule out the presence of congenital malformations. Approximately 50% of all pregnancies are unplanned and do not have the advantages of preconception care. GDM in most cases is diagnosed between 20 and 30 weeks of gestation (after the organogenesis period), decreasing the rate of congenital malformations in this population is difficult to achieve [9–12]. In these cases, the main role of the obstetrician is early diagnosis in lieu of prevention. In addition, these patients and their fetuses are exposed to long-term complications, such as obesity in adolescence and later in life [13,14], higher rates of diabetes and potential intellectual impairment of the infant [15,16].

Achieving a normal glucose profile in pregnancy

Good glycemic control achieved with intensified therapy prevents microvascular and macrovascular complications [17] and improves pregnancy outcome and the overall quality of life [18]. The glucose profiles of normal pregnant women without diabetes are based on studies with small sample sizes, conducted for a single day during the third trimester in a hospital environment under strict dietary limitations [19,20]. One study [21] reported a gradual increase in mean blood glucose in the third trimester, whereas another study [22] measured continuous blood glucose in obese and nonobese nondiabetic women. The results of both studies imply that currently recommended normoglycemia criteria as targets for glycemic control in women with diabetes do not target the actual normal levels in pregnancies of non-diabetic women (Table 1) [1,23,24].

Optimizing clinical outcome for various diabetic complications in pregnancy occurs at different levels of blood glucose. A decreased rate of congenital anomalies was observed when the postprandial threshold was less than 140 mg/dL or the preprandial threshold was less than 120 mg/dL [25–28]. In contrast, a mean blood glucose of less than 100 mg/dL to 110 mg/dL was associated with fewer large-for-gestational-age (LGA) or macrosomic newborns [10,18,29–31]. This association suggests that there are clinical thresholds for optimizing pregnancy rather than an absolute number for normoglycemia that in many cases is unobtainable. Because macrosomia and fetal hyperinsulinemia are the central complications in GDM, the targeted threshold needs to be mean blood glucose of 90 mg/dL to 100 mg/dL and postprandial blood glucose of 110 mg/dL to 120 mg/dL.

Intensified therapy in pregnancy

It is well established that the level of metabolic control in nonpregnant patients with pregestational diabetes influences the incidence and development of retinopathy, nephropathy, and neuropathy. The levels of glycemia achieved in studies on nonpregnant subjects (DCCT, UKPDS) [17,32] were significantly higher, however, than the targeted levels of glycemia during pregnancy.

Managing women with either pregestational diabetes or GDM using intensified therapy helps to establish adequate glycemic control. Such intensive therapy involves using memory-based self-monitoring blood glucose,

Table 1
Recommended therapeutic thresholds for pregnant and nonpregnant subjects compared with the glycemic profile in nondiabetic pregnant women

Criteria[a]	Therapeutic objective studies [Ref.]				Glycemic profile in nondiabetics (first author [Ref.])	
	DCCT [17][b]	ACOG [23]	ADA [24]	4th Int'l [1]	Parretti [21]	Yogev [22]
Fasting (mg/dL)	70–120	60–90	< 105	< 95	55–60 ± 5	75 ± 12
Premeal (mg/dL)	70–120	60–105	—	—	NA	78 ± 11
Postmeal (mg/dL)						
1 h	—	< 130–140	< 155	< 140	98–105 ± 5	97.0 ± 11
2 h	—	< 120	< 130	< 120	85–95 ± 6	105 ± 13
90–120 min	< 180	—	—	—	—	—
2 AM–6 AM (mg/dL)	> 65	60–90	—	—	60–65 ± 5	68.3 ± 10
Mean (mg/dL)	NA	100	—	—	74.7 ± 5.2	84.0 ± 18

Abbreviation: NA, not available.
[a] To convert glucose values from mg/dL to mM/L, multiply by 0.056.
[b] Data for the nonpregnant state.

multiple injections of insulin or its equivalent, diet, and an interdisciplinary team effort. Regardless of the treatment strategy, the purpose of intensified therapy is to achieve the targeted level of glycemic control that diminishes the rate of hypoglycemia and ketosis and maximizes perinatal outcome. Although there is ample evidence associating glycemic control and the occurrence of maternal/fetal complications, association does not prove cause and effect. It does provide the rationale for glucose control, however.

In a prospective study involving 1145 intensified therapy and 1316 conventional therapy GDM patients, the author observed that intensified therapy resulted in a pregnancy outcome comparable to that in the general population [18]. Independent of the type of diabetes and the treatment modality employed, capillary self-monitoring blood glucose accurately quantifies blood glucose, providing sufficient data to make suitable adjustments in the timing and dose of insulin. Diabetic patients seem to accept the self-monitoring blood glucose technique readily, which provides a sense of empowerment and involves patients in the efforts to improve pregnancy outcome. These performance measures seem comparable for all ethnic groups [33–35]. When the pregnancy outcome of conventional therapy patients was compared with that of untreated GDM patients, there were similar rates of adverse outcome. This finding suggests the inability of conventional therapy to maintain targeted levels of glycemic control.

In a pilot randomized study in 1997, Garner and coworkers [36] studied the effect of strict glycemic control and tertiary care versus routine obstetric care in the management of women with normal fasting glucose levels (diet-controlled GDM). Among 300 GDM women studied, there were no differences in mean birth weight, macrosomia, or birth trauma. The mode of delivery also was similar between the two groups, whereas the treatment group did have lower preprandial and postprandial glucose levels during the third trimester.

This feasibility study reveals several areas of concern. The rate of macrosomia was 19% in the untreated group and 16% in the treated group. These macrosomia rates are 40% to 80% above the baseline rate reported in Canada for nondiabetic populations and raise the question of the quality of glycemic control in this study. The women in the control arm could have been self-treating by modifying their own diet on the basis of self-education. Ideally the control group should be unaware that they have GDM and should be blinded to their oral glucose tolerance test results. It is possible that the women in the control group received feedback from knowing the results of home glucose monitoring, with resultant behavioral changes. Ten percent of the untreated control group who tested their blood glucose levels 1 day each week were removed from the study and treated for hyperglycemia. Finally, the authors stated that there is "… no difference in maternal or fetal outcomes; the sample size was not large enough to allow any conclusions or recommendations on the effect of treatment versus no treatment in gestational diabetes mellitus" [36]. Nonetheless, regardless of the limitations of sample size, they chose to conclude that "… The study suggests that intensive treatment of GDM may have little effect on birth weight, birth trauma, operative delivery, or neonatal metabolic disorders" [36].

Treatment modalities in gestational diabetes

The introduction of new pharmacologic alternatives for treatment (insulin analogues and oral antidiabetic agents) and their use in pregnancy make it worthwhile to consider proven and potential benefits during gestation. Although treatment modalities for achieving targeted levels of glycemic control in type 1 diabetes, type 2 diabetes, and GDM differ, diet, exercise, insulin, and oral antidiabetic drugs are the chief means of reducing blood glucose concentrations. In pregnant women with type 2 diabetes, oral antidiabetic drugs have not been tested adequately in terms of whether targeted glycemic levels can be achieved.

Diet and exercise: modalities that enhance glucose control

Diet is the mainstay of treatment in GDM whether or not pharmacologic therapy is introduced. Dietary control with a reduction in fat intake and the substitution of complex carbohydrates for refined carbohydrates seeks to achieve and maintain the maternal blood glucose profile essential during gestation. Two current approaches are recommended: decreasing the proportion of carbohydrates to 35% to 40% in a daily regimen of three meals and three to four snacks [1,23,24,37] or lowering the glycemic index so that carbohydrates account for approximately 60% of daily intake. The assignment of daily caloric intake is similar for women with either GDM or pregestational diabetes and is calculated based on prepregnancy body mass index (BMI) [1,23,24]. In general, for normal-weight women (BMI 20–25), 30 kcal/kg should be prescribed; for overweight and obese women (BMI > 25–34), calories should be restricted to 25 kcal/kg; and for morbidly obese women (BMI > 34), calories should be restricted to 20 kcal/kg or less. Caloric restrictions of 30% in obese patients are associated with the same rate of macrosomia as in the general population. When caloric restrictions are applied, free fatty acids and ketone bodies may increase (starvation ketosis), requiring daily assessment of the ketones in the morning urine; if positive, blood assessment needs to be done [38]. A moderate exercise program for pregnant diabetic women who are willing and able may improve postprandial blood glucose levels and insulin sensitivity [24,39]. Some women are less able to exercise owing to issues of socioeconomic limitations, obesity, and multiparity.

Insulin therapy

Types of insulin to manage diabetes in pregnancy

Insulin production has progressed from animal species to human insulin preparations produced with recombinant DNA technology to the current insulin analogues designed primarily to improve pharmacokinetic features for subcutaneous administration. This succession of advances represents almost a century of research [40,41]. When comparing insulin lispro (Humalog) and human insulins, placental transfer, efficacy, and the cost-to-benefit ratio must be considered. Insulin lispro, insulin aspart and human insulin have few differences in receptor binding and metabolic and mitogenic potency, although insulin lispro has slightly increased binding to the insulin-like growth factor-1 receptor [41–43]. Continuous subcutaneous infusion of insulin lispro in nonpregnant subjects with either type 1 diabetes or type 2 diabetes was associated with a decreased frequency of severe hypoglycemic episodes, limited postprandial glucose excursions, and a possible decrease in glycosylated hemoglobin. Insulin lispro provides greater convenience in the timing of administration (analogues administered 15 minutes after start of meal compared with soluble insulin taken 30 minutes before a meal) [41,43]. Currently, data are limited on the efficacy of the drug.

Human insulin is recommended during pregnancy because data using insulin analogues are lacking [24] (only 282 women, mostly type 1 diabetics, treated with insulin lispro and 15 women treated with aspart reported in the literature). Studies on insulin lispro showed an improvement in glycemic control, increased patient satisfaction, and a decrease in hypoglycemic episodes, but scant data on maternal and neonatal outcomes (Table 2). In the nonpregnant state, insulin glargine has been reported to have a theoretical toxicologic effect for the development of mammary, ovarian, and bone tumors and the development of retinopathy. There are currently seven case reports on the use of insulin glargine and no data on the use of detemir in pregnancy [41,43].

Insulin analogues: placental transfer and safety concerns

The association between proliferative retinopathy and type of insulin analogue used in gestation is controversial. In one report, 3 of 10 women, with type 1 or type 2 diabetes who had no evidence of retinopathy before pregnancy developed proliferative retinopathy that required laser therapy during the third trimester while receiving insulin lispro [44]. This observation has been hotly debated (see Table 2) [44–60]. The affected patients had abnormal glycemic levels; it is likely that poor glycemic control, not insulin lispro, led to proliferative retinopathy.

There are anecdotal case reports of congenital anomalies with the use of insulin analogues. The issue of whether insulin lispro and other analogues cross the placenta also is debated. Bauman and Yalow [61] showed that insulin by itself does not cross the placenta, but does so when complexed to insulin antibodies. Menon and coworkers [62] reported that animal and human insulin crossed the placenta in 51 mothers with type 1 diabetes in an amount directly related to the level of the mother's anti-insulin antibodies. In another study, 4 of 19 women with gestational diabetes being treated with insulin lispro received intravenous infusion of the drug during

Table 2
Studies reporting the use of insulin analogs in pregnancy

Study (first author, year [Ref.])	Study design	Type of diabetes	No. of patients treated			DPR	Anomalies	Neonatal outcome	
			L	H	Other			Complications	LGA
Diamond, 1997 [46]	CR	1	2	—		—	2/2	—	—
Jovanovic, 1999 [45]	RCT	GDM	19	23		—	—	—	16%
Kitzmiller, 1999 [44]	Retro	1 and 2	10	—		3/10	—	—	—
Bhattacharyya, 1999 [47]	Retro	1 and 2	16	21		NP	—	—	—
Buchbinder, 2000 [48]	Retro	1	12	42		NP	0/12	—	—
Bhattacharyya, 2001 [49]	Retro	1 and 2, GDM	20	57		—	L: 1/20 H H: 9/57	—	—
Persson, 2002 [50]	RCT	1	16	17		—	—	—	—
Loukovaara, 2003 [51]	Prosp	1	36	33		NP	—	—	—
Durand-Gonzales, 2003 [52]	CR	GDM	1	—		—	—	—	—
Garg, 2003 [53]	Retro	1	25	35		—	L: 2/25 H: 2/35	—	24% Macrosomia > 4000 g
Mecacci, 2003 [54]	RCT	GDM	25	24		—	—	—	—
Carr, 2004 [55]	RCT	Diabetes	9	—		NP	—	—	—
Idama, 2001 [56]	Retro	1	7	—		—	0/7	—	57%
Cypryk, 2004 [57]	Retro	PGDM	25	46		—	—	Hypoglycemia Lispro: 17% Human: 23%	Lispro: 44% Human: 30%
Masson, 2003 [58]	Retro	1	50	26		P (6 cases)	6/76	Hypoglycemia: 41%	35%
Pettitt, 2003 [59]	RCT	GDM	—	—	15[a]	—	—	—	—
Devlin, 2002 [60]	CR	1	—	—	1[b]	—	—	—	—

Abbreviations: CR, case report; DPR, diabetes proliferative retinopathy; H, human; L, lispro; NP, no progression; P, progression; RCT, randomized control trial; Retro, retrospective; —, no data.

[a] Insulin aspart.
[b] Insulin glargine.

labor; insulin lispro was not detected in the umbilical cord blood of the infants [45].

Using an in vitro model in which human placentas were perfused, Challier and coworkers [63] reported evidence of human insulin in the fetal perfusate after infusion into the maternal compartment of the placenta. Boskovic and coworkers [64] evaluated 11 term human placentas obtained from uncomplicated pregnancies immediately after delivery. No placental transfer was detected during perfusion with insulin lispro (100 μU/mL and 200 μU/mL). In contrast, there was a concentration-dependent transfer to the fetal perfusate at insulin lispro levels of 580 μU/mL and higher. Finally, the investigators compared actual maternal serum level and administered doses of insulin lispro. Mothers treated with 50 U of insulin lispro achieved serum concentrations greater than 200 μU/mL with an apparent linear correlation between dose and levels [64]. The investigators did not evaluate placentas of diabetic mothers, however. Placentas generally are affected by the disease, which may influence the perfusion characteristics. One can speculate that even in the presence of lower insulin doses, placental transfer may occur. Although it is unlikely that insulin lispro in therapeutic doses would cross the placenta, the high dose of insulin required in pregnancy, especially in GDM and type 2 diabetes, to achieve established levels of glycemic control needs to be weighed against the potential for placental transfer and adverse outcome for the fetus.

Before using insulin analogues to treat pregnant women, several issues need to be addressed: Can pregnant women achieve targeted levels of glycemic control with the use of insulin lispro? The response is yes; the quality of glycemic control parallels the accepted criteria recommended during pregnancy. Is the quality of glycemic control during pregnancy with the use of insulin lispro comparable to that with the use of regular insulin? Is the incidence of hypoglycemic incidents similar? Six published studies compared the use of insulin lispro and regular insulin in pregnancy. Most of the studies found no significant difference with respect to glycemic control and the incidence of hypoglycemia. Two of the studies were performed on women with GDM with a total of 60 women treated with insulin lispro. In the study by Persson and coworkers [50], there was a lower postprandial glucose concentration after breakfast and a slightly higher rate of hypoglycemia (< 55 mg/dL) in the insulin lispro group. If there is no advantage in using insulin lispro compared with regular insulin, is insulin lispro as safe in pregnancy as regular insulin? Insulin lispro may be more user-friendly with negligible differences in glycemic control and hypoglycemia. These assets cannot currently justify extensive use of the drug, however, before establishing its safety in well-controlled clinical trials.

Which patients should receive pharmacologic therapy?

When diet fails to achieve targeted levels of glycemic control, insulin and antidiabetic agents are validated treatment options. Available guidelines differ regarding the threshold of fasting plasma glucose at which pharmacologic therapy (glyburide or insulin) should be initiated [23,24,65]. Some authors recommend a threshold of fasting plasma glucose 95 mg/dL or greater [1,65] whereas others recommend a threshold of 105 mg/dL or greater [23,24]. Using a fasting plasma glucose threshold of 95 mg/dL or greater decreases the rate of macrosomia and LGA infants [66,67].

Most authorities agree on initiation of drug therapy with elevated postprandial values ($\geq$ 120 mg/dL for 2 hours or $\geq$ 140 mg/dL for 1 hour). Using these standards, approximately 30% to 50% of women with GDM require pharmacologic therapy when diet therapy alone fails to reduce glycemic levels. When patients who qualified for diet therapy were evaluated, only patients who achieved established levels of glycemic control improved insulin secretion and sensitivity. Patients who failed to achieve glycemic control, although exhibiting slightly improved insulin sensitivity, did not achieve the same level of insulin response and sensitivity as nondiabetic women [68]. Studies using continuous blood glucose monitoring have shed new light on the existing controversy whether to test blood glucose at 1 or 2 hours postprandial in pregnant women. The author found that the time from start of meal to the postprandial peak is approximately 80 to 90 minutes depending on the type of diabetes and regardless of level of glycemia. In nondiabetic pregnant women, the peak postprandial value was 110 mg/dL. The association between this physiologic characteristic and pregnancy outcome needs to be evaluated before changing current clinical thresholds [22,69].

Can the fetus provide a marker for pharmacologic initiation?

Three randomized controlled studies addressed the use of fetal abdominal circumference to guide insulin therapy. This approach combined maternal glucose and fetal growth parameters. The studies suggest that some women, despite glucose levels above established targets ($\geq$ 105 mg/dL) may not derive a fetal benefit from intensified therapy [70–72]. In a randomized study with a large sample size, the author found similar results. In the author's study, subjects who did not achieve targeted levels of glycemic control had higher rates of macrosomia and LGA infants, however, regardless of abdominal circumference [73]. The limitation of the use of abdominal circumference at 28 weeks' gestation as a measure for insulin initiation is that it is snapshot information, whereas fetal growth is longitudinal. Most environmental effects (eg, glucose) occur during the third trimester, which is also the time of most fetal growth. A fetus at 28 weeks' gestation in the 40th percentile of growth can double its weight and reach the 85th percentile under the influence of elevated blood glucose. Using the fetus as an additional marker for the decision-making process in initiating pharmacologic therapy is an attractive approach. It should not be used as a single predictor, but in conjunction with GDM severity parameters and level of glycemic control throughout pregnancy

How long is diet therapy maintained before initiating pharmacologic treatment?

Consensus and hard data are lacking regarding how long diet therapy should be maintained before initiating pharmacologic treatment. In a study by the author, 70% of the subjects with initial fasting plasma glucose less than 95 mg/dL achieved targeted levels of glycemia within 2 weeks of dietary management, but no significant improvement occurred thereafter [74]. The failure to initiate insulin therapy in a timely manner may lead to fetal hyperinsulinemia and associated complications. Premature initiation of insulin therapy without knowing whether glycemic control can be achieved with diet alone may cause unnecessary drug treatment. When GDM is diagnosed after 30 to 33 weeks of gestation, and minimal time is available for achieving targeted glycemic control, pharmacologic therapy should be initiated. There is greater flexibility in treatment modalities when GDM is diagnosed early in the third trimester.

Insulin requirements in gestational diabetes

To evaluate the insulin dose required to achieve targeted levels of glycemic control, multiple blood glucose determinations should be performed [18,75]. Insulin requirements may change during GDM. The author observed a biphasic increase in insulin requirements among 57 women with GDM who then had normal oral glucose tolerance tests postpartum [76]. The first phase was characterized by a significant weekly increase until the 30th week of gestation, after which the insulin dose remained unchanged. Insulin requirements for obese subjects in the study were 0.9 U/kg compared with 0.8 U/kg for nonobese patients. There was a significant difference in variability as measured by the coefficient of variation (45% versus 25%; $P < .01$). The total insulin dose required to reach the established level of glycemic control for most patients is 40 U to 90 U (body-weight–dependent). Women with GDM seem to benefit from frequent visits during the 20th to 30th weeks of gestation for insulin adjustment.

In a pregnant diabetic patient, the rationale for insulin therapy is based on mimicking the physiology of insulin secretion. The basal insulin is supplied by the administration of NPH/lente/ultralente insulin at bedtime or before breakfast and at bedtime. The meal-related (glucose excursion) insulin includes the use of insulin lispro before meals (0–15 min) or Regular insulin before meals (30–45 min). This algorithm provides the foundation for the use of intensified therapy (multiple injections daily) versus conventional therapy (one to two injections daily) [77].

The calculation for the insulin dose in GDM women is based on prepregnancy BMI. For nonobese patients, 0.8 U/kg is used and for overweight and obese women, 0.9 to 1 U/kg is used, then current maternal pregnancy weight is multiplied by the amount of insulin. A woman at 28 weeks' gestation currently weighing 85 kg but based on prepregnancy BMI, classified as overweight/obese would require a total calculated insulin dose of

85×1 (unit) $= 85$. The total insulin dose is divided so that two thirds is administered in the morning, which is further split in a ratio of 2:1 (intermediate and rapid-acting), and one third is administered with supper and bedtime in a ratio of 1:1 (rapid-acting and intermediate). The rapid-acting dose is administered with supper, and the intermediate dose is taken before bedtime. If after 3 to 7 days the GDM patient has not achieved the desired level of glycemic control, the total insulin dose should increase by 10% to 20% and thereafter adjusted when needed. The actual total insulin dose in GDM women is 40% higher than the calculated (starting) dose [76]. The decreased insulin sensitivity characterizes pregnancy and in particular GDM patients. As a rule of thumb, before every insulin administration, self-monitoring blood glucose assessment needs to occur.

Oral antidiabetic agents as alternatives to insulin therapy

A variety of oral agents may be alternatives to insulin therapy for women with GDM. Sulfonylureas are insulin secretagogues (eg, glyburide and glipizide). The primary action of glyburide is to increase insulin secretion, decreasing hepatic glucose production with resultant reversal of hyperglycemia and indirect improvement of insulin sensitivity [78] Antidiabetic drug groups include meglitinides (insulin secretagogues, such as the rapid-acting repaglinide, which limit postprandial hyperglycemia), biguanides (eg, metformin, which decreases insulin resistance), α-glucosidase inhibitors (eg, acarbose, which reduces intestinal absorption of starch and glucose), and thiazolidinediones (eg, rosiglitazone and pioglitazone). All have been used successfully in the treatment of nonpregnant patients with type 2 diabetes. Each may be used alone or in combination with other oral agents or insulin.

Most of these drugs have not been studied in pregnancy or only minimally so. The most data regarding safety in pregnancy for oral antidiabetic drugs are with the use of glyburide. To date, 1261 women treated with glyburide have been reported in the literature. For insulin analogues and oral antidiabetic drugs, none of the studies were blinded (Table 3). Many experts and authoritative bodies have recommended using glyburide as an alternative to insulin [65,79–83]. Others have not firmly advocated the use of oral agents in pregnancy and recommend further evaluation [24,84,85]. The use of oral agents is a pragmatic alternative to insulin therapy in pregnancy because of ease of administration and patient satisfaction with a noninvasive treatment. However valid these reasons, the introduction of a new drug is unjustified if improvements in pregnancy outcome and cost-effectiveness are not evaluated definitively.

Is there increased risk for fetal anomalies with the use of oral antidiabetic drugs?

For a drug to be potentially effective and safe in pregnancy, it should not cross the placenta or should not be detrimental to the fetus at concentrations

Table 3
Studies reporting use of oral antidiabetic agents in pregnancy

| Study (first author, year [Ref.]) | Study design | Type of diabetes | No. of patients | | | | Achievement of good control | Neonatal outcome | |
			Glyburide	Regular insulin	Metformin	Other		Complications	LGA
Langer, 2000 [78]	RCT	GDM	201	203			82% and 88%	No difference in metabolic complications, congenital anomalies, and PNM	12% and 13%
Lim, 1997 [93]	Prosp, observ	GDM	33	21			No significant difference	No significant difference in metabolic complications and PNM	No significant difference
Conway, 2004 [94]	Prosp, observ	GDM	75				84%	NA	NA
Kremer, 2004 [95]	Prosp, observ	GDM	73				81%		Macrosomia: 19%
Chmait, 2004 [96]	Prosp, observ	GDM	69				82%	Caesarean section: 36%	Macrosomia: 7%

Gilson, 2002 [97]	Prosp, observ	GDM	22	22	82%	No significant difference in the rate between insulin- and glyburide-treated groups	No significant difference between insulin and glyburide groups
Fines, 2003 [98]	Retro case-control	GDM	40	44	NA	No difference in ponderal index between the groups	Less macrosomia in the glyburide group (5/40 vs 11/44)
Velazques, 2003 [99]	Case series	GDM	31	7	Improved level of glycemic control in the glyburide group: 82%	No hypoglycemic events in the glyburide group	LGA in the glyburide and in the insulin group: 16% and 29%
Pendsey, 2002 [100]	RCT	2	23	Repaglinide: 23	Improved level of glycemic control		
Glueck, 2004 [90]	Prosp, observ	PCOS		42		GDM developed in 7.1% of patients	
Glueck, 2002 [91]	Prosp and retro observ	PCOS	33	w/o metformin: 39		GDM developed in 3% of patients treated with metformin vs 27% w/o treatment	

(continued on next page)

Table 3 (*continued*)

Study (first author, year [Ref.])	Study design	Type of diabetes	No. of patients				Achievement of good control	Neonatal outcome	
			Glyburide	Regular insulin	Metformin	Other		Complications	LGA
Coetzee, 1984 [101]	Retro	2			78			Drug deemed safe in first trimester	
Coetzee, 1986 [102]	Retro	GDM and 2			126			Reduced PNM	
Coetzee, 1979 [103]	Prosp, observ	GDM and 2			60		GDM: 81.4% Type 2 diabetes: 46.2%		
Hellmuth, 2000 [104]	Prosp, observ	GDM		42	50	Sulfonylurea: 68		No significant difference in neonatal morbidity. Higher rate of preeclampsia (32% vs 10%) and PNM (11.6% vs 1.3%) in metformin group	

Study	Design	Type	n	n	Treatment	Outcome	Result
Notelovitz, 1971 [105]	RCT	GDM and 2	25	52	Tolbutamide chlorpropamin: 2 × 52	Using oral hypoglycemic: 80% Using insulin: 36%	No significant difference in PNM, metabolic complications, and congenital anomalies
Yogev, 2004 [106]	Prosp	GDM	25	30	Diet treated: 27	Mean blood glucose similar in all groups	Significantly lower rate of maternal hypoglycemia in glyburide group
Moore, 2005 [107]	RCT	GDM	31	32		Blood glucose similar	Perinatal outcome similar
Ramos, 2005 [108]	Retro	GDM	236	316		Blood glucose similar	Perinatal outcome similar

Abbreviations: NA, not available; Observ, observational; PNM, perinatal mortality; Prosp, prospective; RCT, randomized controltrial; Retro, retrospective; w/o, without.

that are clinically indicated for the mother. Case reports and small retrospective studies in women receiving first-generation sulfonylureas raised concern about congenital anomalies [86,87]. Potential effects on the fetus, mainly hypoglycemia and growth stimulation [87], were reported. A report of increased rates of congenital malformations involved 20 type 2 diabetes patients who had hyperglycemia before conception (hemoglobin $A_{1c} > 8$). It is impossible to determine if the reported rate of anomalies was due to the use of the drug or the preexisting hyperglycemia [86]. In contrast, several studies showed that anomalies in the infants of women who received oral antidiabetic agents were associated with altered maternal glucose metabolism and not the drug [88]. A meta-analysis failed to show an increased risk for fetal anomalies with sulfonylureas [89]. Metformin seems to be unassociated with congenital malformations in patients with polycystic ovary syndrome and reduces the occurrence of GDM and spontaneous abortion (see Table 3) [90–92].

Does glyburide cross the placenta?

The placenta of the diabetic mother is characterized by capillary dilation, relatively immature villous structure, and chronic disturbances in intervillous circulation. The author examined the placentas of nondiabetic and diabetic mothers in vitro and showed that glyburide (glibenclamide) does not cross the human placenta from the maternal to fetal circulation in significant amounts. There was virtually no drug transport even when concentrations three to four times higher than peak therapeutic levels were employed [109–111]. The author also showed that first-generation sulfonylureas diffused across the placenta most freely [109–111]. There is evidence that the qualitative aspects of transfer are comparable between placentas obtained during the first and third trimesters [64,112]. In mothers treated with therapeutic plasma concentrations of glyburide, the drug was undetectable in the cord blood of their neonates [78]. No data exist on the long-term effects on the infant when oral antidiabetic drugs and insulin analogues are used in the mother. Glyburide exhibits less transfer across the placenta compared with other agents, underscoring its potential therapeutic usefulness.

Because glyburide does not cross the placenta, it cannot affect neonatal hypoglycemia or fetal anomalies. In addition, most GDM patients are identified between 24 and 28 weeks' gestation. The fetus is not exposed to the drug during organogenesis. In rare cases of early diagnosis in the first trimester (perhaps type 2) and recognized type 2 diabetes, current data suggest that the use of glyburide or metformin would not increase the rate of anomalies influenced by the level of glycemic control. Although a randomized study would be the ideal model to address this issue, it is highly unlikely that it would be performed for ethical considerations (see Table 3).

Glyburide pharmacology and administration

The pharmacologic mechanism of action of glyburide is to increase insulin secretion, and its secondary effect is to decrease insulin resistance by reducing glucose toxicity. Its onset of action is approximately 4 hours, and duration of action is about 10 hours. After achieving the targeted therapeutic level, the drug covers the basal requirement and the postprandial excursions of glucose. The starting dose is 2.5 mg orally in the morning. If the targeted level of glycemia has not been reached, 2.5 mg is added to the morning dose. If indicated (after 3–7 days), 5 mg is added in the evening. Thereafter, the dose is increased by 5 mg to a total of 20 mg/day. If patients fail to achieve established levels of glycemic control, long-acting insulin can be added to the regimen [78].

The abnormal level of glycemia in GDM can be controlled by monotherapy with glyburide and probably metformin. Can monotherapy with glyburide achieve targeted levels of glycemia required in pregnancy in type 2 patients? Although this issue has not been studied extensively, one can speculate that monotherapy may not be sufficient. Combination therapy with other oral antidiabetic drugs, with proven efficacy and safety, would help subjects achieve established levels of glycemic control. Another alternative is the combination of insulin and glyburide, which would result in a lower dose of insulin compared with the use of monotherapy with insulin.

Glyburide compared with insulin

Several studies evaluated the efficacy of oral antidiabetic agents during pregnancy (see Table 3). Most studies showed that these agents were comparable to insulin in achieving established levels of glycemic control and pregnancy outcome. The author compared glyburide with standard insulin therapy in a randomized controlled trial in 404 GDM women [78]. The primary outcome was the ability to achieve established levels of glycemic control; insulin and glyburide had comparable results. The success in achieving glycemic control with glyburide was reconfirmed by several studies (Tables 3 and 4). Adequate glycemic control was obtained with significantly fewer hypoglycemic episodes in the glyburide group compared with the insulin group [78]. Using a continuous glucose monitoring system that recorded data every 5 minutes for 72 continuous hours with 288 measurements per day, asymptomatic hypoglycemic events (> 30 consecutive minutes of glucose values < 50 mg/dL) occurred in 63% of subjects receiving insulin compared with 28% of subjects receiving glyburide [106].

The insulin-treated patients and glyburide-treated patients achieved comparable results in many variables: cord-serum insulin concentrations, incidence of macrosomia, increased Ponderal index, LGA infants, neonatal metabolic complications (hypoglycemia, polycythemia, and hyperbilirubinemia), respiratory complications, and cesarean delivery [78]. The perinatal outcome in the glyburide and the intensified therapy subjects was comparable (see Table 4).

The author analyzed the association among glyburide dose, GDM severity, and selected maternal and neonatal factors [113]. Glyburide and insulin were equally efficacious for treatment of women with GDM of varying

Table 4
Comparison of selected pregnancy outcomes in conventional versus intensified insulin therapy, glyburide versus insulin, and nondiabetic subjects

Criteria	Therapy comparison [18][a]		Comparison [78]		Nondiabetic [8,18]
	Conventional	Intensified	Glyburide	Insulin	
LGA (%)[b]	20.1	13.1	12.0	13.0	11.9
Macrosomia (%)	13.6	7.1	7.2	4.7	8.1
Ponderal index > 2.85	21.7	13.8	9.0	12.0	22.0
Overall Caesarean section (%)	21.5	15.0	23.0	24.0	13.7
Induction of labor (%)	27	22	33	34	13.0
PET (%)	5.6	5.9	6.0	6.0	7.6
CHTN (%)	6.1	5.8	6.0	9.1	6.2
5-Min Apgar score < 7 (%)	3.2	2.1	3.1	4.2	2.5
Neonatal ICU admission (%)	25.6	6.3	6.0	7.0	4.7
Hypoglycemia (%) < 40 mg/dL	20.0	3.8	9.0	6.0	2.5
Polycythemia (%) > 60%	12.0	0.7	2.0	3.0	1.4
Hyperbilirubinemia (%) > 11 mg/dL	17.5	7.9	6.0	4.0	6.4
Hypocalcemia (%) < 8 mg/dL	4.0	0.3	1.0	1.0	NA
Respiratory complications (%)	6.2	2.3	2.0	3.0	2.1
Shoulder dystocia	1.4	0.4	1.5	1.6	0.5
Perinatal mortality					
Stillbirth	4/1000	1/1000	5/1000	5/1000	4/1000
Neonatal death	2/1000	3/1000	5/1000	5/1000	4.7/1000

Abbreviations: CHTN, chronic hypertension; ICU, intensive care unit; NA, not available; PET, preeclampsia.

[a] Conventional therapy: fasting plasma glucose and 2-h postprandial once weekly, visualized self-monitoring blood glucose 4 times daily; intensified therapy: memory-based self-monitoring blood glucose 7 times daily.

[b] LGA > 90th percentile; macrosomia ≥ 4000 g.

severity when fasting plasma glucose results were between 95 mg/dL and 139 mg/dL. Of patients, 71% required a 10-mg daily dose of glyburide to achieve glycemic control. In all disease severity levels, glyburide and insulin-treated subjects had similar success rates in achieving targeted glucose levels and pregnancy outcomes [113]. Achieving the established level of glycemic control, not the mode of therapy, seems to be the key to improving pregnancy outcome in GDM.

Is glyburide therapy less costly than insulin therapy?

The costs of alternative therapies should be addressed when different medications exhibit similar effectiveness and safety. Goetzel and Wilkins [114] compared the costs of insulin and glyburide and observed that glyburide is considerably less costly (average savings per patient of $166–$200 based on rates in 2000). Glyburide is a cost-effective, patient-friendly, potentially adherence-enhancing therapy that produces perinatal outcome comparable to insulin therapy.

Table 5
Oral antidiabetic drug classification

Drug (trade name)	Mechanism of action	Pregnancy category	Decrease in FPG (mg/dL)	Decrease in hemoglobin A$_{1C}$ (%)	Cross placenta	Excreted in breast milk
Sulfonylureas	Increase insulin secretion		60–70	1.5–2		
Glimepiride (Amaryl)		C			Unknown	Unknown
Glipizide (Glucotrol)		C			Minimal	Unknown
Glipizide-GITS (Glucotrol XL)		—			—	—
Glyburide (DiaBeta, Glynase, Micronase)		B			No	No
Meglitinides	Increase insulin secretion		9–21	0.5–0.8		
Nateglinide (Starlix)		C			Unknown	Unknown
Repaglinide (Prandin)		C			Unknown	Unknown
Biguanide	Decreases hepatic gluconeogenesis; increases insulin sensitivity		59–78	0.9–2		
Metformin (Glucophage)		B			Yes	No
Glitazones	Increase insulin sensitivity; decrease hepatic glucose production		59–80	1.4–2.6		
Pioglitazone (Actos)		C			Unknown	Animals
Rosiglitazone (Avandia)		C			Unknown	Animals

(continued on next page)

Table 5 (*continued*)

Drug (trade name)	Mechanism of action	Pregnancy category	Decrease in FPG (mg/dL)	Decrease in hemoglobin A_{1C} (%)	Cross placenta	Excreted in breast milk
Alpha-glucosidase inhibitors	Slow absorption of carbohydrates in the intestine		20–30	0.5–1		
Acarbose (Precose)		B			Unknown	Animals
Miglitol (Glyset)		B			Unknown	Animals
Insulin			Dose-dependent	Dose-dependent		
Aspart (Novolog)		B			Unknown	No
Lispro (Humalog)		B			Minimal	No
Regular		B			No	No
NPH		B			No	No
Lente		B			No	No
Glargine (Lantus)		C			Unknown	No
Ultralente		B			No	No

Glyburide and lactation

Data are scant on the effect of oral antidiabetic drugs on lactation. Data from two centers, in Canada and in California, suggested that glyburide is not present in the milk of lactating mothers when measured in vivo and in vitro [115].

Summary

Although not universally accepted, the introduction of insulin analogues (mainly insulin lispro, class B), oral antidiabetic agents (mainly glyburide [class B]) (Table 5), and the use of intensified therapy have altered profoundly the management approach in the treatment of diabetes in pregnancy with outcomes comparable to the general population (see Table 4). Insulin lispro is not likely to cross the placenta with the clinically used dose in most type 1 and type 2 diabetic patients. The benefits of this drug are the reduction of nocturnal hypoglycemic episodes and postprandial levels and the ease of patient use. With the establishment of the efficacy for the use of glyburide (and possibly metformin), there is an equally effective alternative to insulin therapy. Glyburide is a cost-effective, patient-friendly, and potentially compliance-enhancing therapy that produces perinatal outcome in GDM pregnancies comparable to traditional insulin therapy. For GDM patients who require pharmacologic therapy, glyburide is the drug of choice, and only patients who fail to achieve glycemic control should begin insulin therapy.

The major obstacles to the creation of evidence-based criteria to guide benefit/risk in pharmacologic therapy in obstetrics is the fear of the potential adverse drug effects on the fetus and the resultant paucity of research. The history of the Food and Drug Administration regulations for prescription drug labeling in pregnancy adds an additional layer of difficulty. The ethical, legal, and medical rhetoric surrounding this dilemma may have exaggerated the potential for fetal harm. There may be greater risk to the fetus in withholding certain medications than in prescribing them. The current evidence-based data for insulin lispro and glyburide support their use in pregnancy. A large-scale multicentric study to evaluate glyburide and insulin analogues would be a practical and enlightening endeavor.

References

[1] Metzger BE, Coustan DR, and the Organizing Committee. Summary and recommendations of the Fourth International Workshop Conference on Gestational Diabetes. Diabetes Care 1998;21(Suppl 2):B161–7.

[2] Mokdad AH, Serdula MK, Dietz WH, et al. The spread of the obesity epidemic in the United States, 1991–1998. JAMA 1999;282:1519–22.

[3] Catalano P, Buchanan TA. Metabolic changes during normal and diabetic pregnancies. In: Reece EA, Coustan DR, Gabbe SG, editors. Diabetes in Women: Adolescence, Pregnancy, and Menopause. Philadelphia: Lippincott, Williams & Wilkins; 2004. p. 129–45.

[4] Pendergrass M, Fazioni E, DeFronzo RA. Non-insulin dependent diabetes mellitus and gestational diabetes mellitus: same disease, another name? Diabetes Rev 1995;3: 584–601.

[5] Buchanan TA, Xiang AH, Peters RK. Response of pancreatic B-cells to improved insulin sensitivity in women at high risk for type 2 diabetes. Diabetes 2000;49:782–8.

[6] Catalano PM, Kirwan JP, Haugel-de Mouzon S, King J. Gestational diabetes and insulin resistance: role in short- and long-term implications for mother and fetus. J Nutr 2003;133: 1674S–83S.

[7] Merlob P, Hod M. Short-term implications: the neonate. In: Hod M, Jovanovic L, Di Renzo GC, et al, editors. Textbook of Diabetes and Pregnancy. London: Martin Dunitz; 2003. p. 289–304.

[8] Langer O, Yogev Y, Most O, et al. Gestational diabetes: the consequences of not treating. Am J Obstet Gynecol 2005;192:989–97.

[9] Simmons D. Persistently poor pregnancy outcomes in IDDM. BMJ 1997;315:263–4.

[10] Langer O, Conway DL. Level of glycemia and perinatal outcome in pregestational diabetes. J Matern Fetal Med 2000;9:35–41.

[11] Dunne FP, Brydon P, Smith T, et al. Pre-conception and diabetes care in insulin dependent diabetes mellitus. QJM 1999;92:175–6.

[12] Janz NK, Herman WH, Becker MP, et al. Diabetes and pregnancy: factors associated with seeking pre-conception care. Diabetes Care 1995;18:157–65.

[13] Silverman BL, Rizzo TA, Cho NH, Metzger BE. Long-term effects of the intrauterine environment. Diabetes 1996;21(Suppl.2):142–9.

[14] Pettitt D, Nelson RG, Saad MF, et al. Diabetes and obesity in the offspring of Pima Indian women with diabetes during pregnancy. Diabetes Care 1993;16:310–4.

[15] Rizzo T, Freinkel N, Metzger B, et al. Correlations between antepartum maternal metabolism and newborn behavior. Am J Obstet Gynecol 1990;163:1458–64.

[16] Rizzo T, Metzger B, Burns W, et al. Correlations between antepartum maternal metabolism and intelligence of offspring. N Engl J Med 1991;325:911–6.

[17] The Diabetes Control and Complications Trial Research Group. The effect of intensified treatment of diabetes on the development and progression of long-term complications in insulin-dependent diabetes mellitus. N Engl J Med 1993;329:977–86.

[18] Langer O, Rodriguez DA, Xenakis EMJ, et al. Intensified versus conventional management of gestational diabetes. Am J Obstet Gynecol 1994;170:1036–47.

[19] Cousins L, Rigg L, Hollingsworth D, et al. The 24-hour excursion and diurnal rhythm of glucose, insulin, and C-peptide in normal pregnancy. Am J Obstet Gynecol 1980;136:483–8.

[20] Phelps RL, Metzger BE, Freinkel N. Carbohydrate metabolism in pregnancy: XVII. diurnal profiles of plasma glucose, insulin, free fatty acids, triglycerides, cholesterol, and individual amino acids in late normal pregnancy. Am J Obstet Gynecol 1981;140:730–6.

[21] Parretti E, Mecacci F, Papini M, et al. Third-trimester maternal glucose levels from diurnal profiles in non-diabetic pregnancies: correlation with sonographic parameters of fetal growth. Diabetes Care 2001;24:1319–23.

[22] Yogev Y, Ben-Haroush A, Chen R, et al. Diurnal glycemic profile in obese and normal weight non-diabetic pregnant women. Am J Obstet Gynecol 2004;191:1655–60.

[23] American College of Obstetricians and Gynecologists. Clinical management guidelines for obstetrician-gynecologists: No. 30. Gestational diabetes. Washington, DC: American College of Obstetricians and Gynecologists; 2001.

[24] American Diabetes Association. Position statement on gestational diabetes mellitus. Diabetes Care 2004;27(Suppl 1):S88–90.

[25] Rosenn B, Miodovnik M, Combs CA, et al. Glycemic thresholds for spontaneous abortion and congenital malformations in insulin-dependent diabetes mellitus. Obstet Gynecol 1994; 84:515–20.

[26] Fuhrman K, Reiher H, Semmler K, et al. Prevention of congenital malformations in infants of insulin-dependent diabetic mothers. Diabetes Care 1983;6:219–24.

[27] Kitzmiller JL, Gavin LA, Gin GD, et al. Preconception care of diabetes: glycemic control prevents congenital anomalies. JAMA 1991;265:731–6.

[28] Pregnancy outcomes in the Diabetes Control and Complications Trial. Am J Obstet Gynecol 1996;174:1343–53.

[29] Langer O. Is normoglycemia the correct threshold to prevent complications in the pregnant diabetic patient? Diabetes Rev 1996;4:2–10.

[30] Drexel H, Bicher A, Sailer S, et al. Prevention of perinatal morbidity by tight metabolic control in gestational diabetes mellitus. Diabetes Care 1988;11:761–8.

[31] Roversi GD, Garguilo M, Nicolini U, et al. Maximal tolerated insulin therapy in gestational diabetes. Diabetes Care 1980;3:479–84.

[32] Prospective Diabetes Study Group UK. Intensive blood glucose control with sulphonylureas or insulin compared with conventional treatment and risk of complications in patients with type 2 diabetes. Lancet 1998;352:837–53.

[33] Langer N, Langer O. Gestational diabetes vs. pre-existing diabetes: comparison of pregnancy mood profiles. Diabetic Educator 2000;26:667–72.

[34] Langer O, Langer N. Is cultural diversity a factor in self-monitoring blood glucose in gestational diabetes? J Assoc Minority Physicians 1995;6:73–7.

[35] Langer N, Langer O. Emotional adjustment to diagnosis and intensified treatment of gestational diabetes. Obstet Gynecol 1994;84:329–34.

[36] Garner P, Okun N, Keely E, et al. A randomized controlled trial of strict glycemic control and tertiary level obstetric care in the management of gestational diabetes: a pilot study. Am J Obstet Gynecol 1997;177:190–5.

[37] Major CA, Henry MJ, De Veciana M, Morgan MA. The effects of carbohydrate restriction in patients with diet-controlled gestational diabetes. Obstet Gynecol 1998;91: 600–4.

[38] Dornhorst A, Nicholls JSD, Probst F, et al. Calorie restriction for treatment of gestational diabetes. Diabetes 1991;404(Suppl 2):161–4.

[39] Artal R. Exercise: the alternative therapeutic intervention for gestational diabetes. Clin Obstet Gynecol 2003;46:479–87.

[40] Owens DR, Zinman B, Bolli GB. Insulins today and beyond. Lancet 2001;358:739–46.

[41] Hirsch I. Insulin analogues. N Engl J Med 2005;352:174–83.

[42] Kurtzhals P, Schaffer L, Sorensen A, et al. Correlations of reception binding and metabolic and mitogen potentials of insulin analogues designed for clinical use. Diabetes 2000;49: 999–1005.

[43] Holleman F, Hoekstra JBL. Insulin lispro. N Engl J Med 1997;337:176–83.

[44] Kitzmiller JL, Main E, Ward B, et al. Insulin lispro and the development of proliferative diabetic retinopathy during pregnancy [letter]. Diabetes Care 1999;22:874–6.

[45] Jovanovic L, Ilic S, Pettitt D, et al. Metabolic and immunologic effects of insulin lispro in gestational diabetes. Diabetes Care 1999;22:1422–7.

[46] Diamond T, Kormas N. Possible adverse fetal effect of insulin lispro [letter]. N Engl J Med 1997;337:1009–10.

[47] Bhattacharyya A, Vice P. Insulin lispro, pregnancy, and retinopathy. Diabetes Care 1999; 22:2101–2.

[48] Buchbinder A, Miodovnik M, McElvy S, et al. Is insulin lispro associated with the development or progression of diabetic retinopathy during pregnancy? Am J Obstet Gynecol 2000;183:1162–5.

[49] Bhattacharyya A, Brown S, Hughes S, Vice P. Insulin lispro and regular insulin in pregnancy. QJM 2001;94:255–60.

[50] Persson B, Swahn ML, Hjertberg R. Insulin lispro therapy in pregnancies complicated by type 1 diabetes mellitus. Diabetes Res Clin Pract 2002;58:115–21.

[51] Loukovaara S, Immonen I, Teramo KA, Kaaja R. Progression of retinopathy during pregnancy in type 1 diabetic women treated with insulin lispro. Diabetes Care 2003;26: 1193–8.

[52] Durand-Gonzalez KN, Guillausseau N, Anciaux ML, et al. Allergy to insulin in a woman with gestational diabetes mellitus: transient efficiency of continuous subcutaneous insulin lispro infusion. Diabetes Metab 2003;29:432–4.

[53] Garg S, Frias JP, Anil S, et al. Insulin lispro therapy in pregnancies complicated by type 1 diabetes: glycemic control and maternal and fetal outcomes. Endocr Pract 2003;9:187–93.

[54] Mecacci F, Carignani L, Cioni R, et al. Maternal metabolic control and perinatal outcome in women with gestational diabetes treated with regular or lispro insulin: comparison with non-diabetic pregnant women. Eur J Obstet Gynaecol Reprod Biol 2003;111:19–24.

[55] Carr K, Idama TO, Masson EA. A randomized controlled trial of insulin lispro given before or after meals in pregnant women with type 1 diabetes—the effect on glycaemic excursion. J Obstet Gynaecol 2004;24:382–6.

[56] Idama TO, Lindow SW, French M. Preliminary experience with the use of insulin lispro in pregnant diabetic women. J Obstet Gynaecol 2001;21:350–1.

[57] Cypryk K, Sobczak M, Pertynska-Marczewska M, et al. Pregnancy complications and peri-natal outcome in diabetic women treated with Humalog (insulin lispro) or regular human insulin during pregnancy. Med Sci Monit 2004;10:129–32.

[58] Masson EA, Patmore JE, Brash PD, et al. Pregnancy outcome in Type 1 diabetes mellitus treated with insulin lispro (Humalog). Diabet Med 2003;20:46–50.

[59] Pettitt DJ, Opsina P, Kolaczynski JW, Jovanovic L. Comparison of an insulin analogue, insulin aspart, and regular human insulin with no insulin gestational diabetes mellitus. Diabetes Care 2003;26:183–6.

[60] Devlin JT, Hothersall L, Wilkins JL. Use of insulin glargine during pregnancy in a type 1 diabetic woman. Diabetes Care 2002;25:1095–6.

[61] Bauman WA, Yalow RS. Transplacental passage of insulin complexed to antibody. Proc Natl Acad Sci U S A 1981;78:4588–90.

[62] Menon RK, Cohen RM, Sperling MA, et al. Transplacental passage of insulin in pregnant women with insulin-dependent diabetes mellitus: its role in fetal macrosomia. N Engl J Med 1990;323:309–15.

[63] Challier JC, Haugel S, Desmaizieres V. Effects of insulin on glucose uptake and metabolism in the human placenta. J Clin Endocrinol Metab 1986;62:803–7.

[64] Boskovic R, Feig DS, Derewlany L, et al. Transfer of insulin lispro across the human placenta. Diabetes Care 2003;26:1390–4.

[65] Reece EA, Homko C, Miodovnik M, Langer O. A consensus report of the diabetes in pregnancy study group of North America Conference. J Matern Fetal Neonat Med 2002;12:362–4.

[66] Langer O. Maternal glycemic criteria for insulin therapy in gestational diabetes mellitus. Diabetes Care 1998;21(Suppl 2):B91–8.

[67] Langer O, Berkus MD, Brustman L, et al. Rationale for insulin management in gestational diabetes mellitus. Diabetes 1991;40(Suppl2):186–90.

[68] Langer O. Management of gestational diabetes. Clin Obstet Gynecol 1999;93:978–82.

[69] Haroush AB, Yogev Y, Langer O, et al. Postprandial glucose profile characteristics in diabetic pregnancies. Am J Obstet Gynecol 2004;2:576–81.

[70] Buchanan TA, Kjos SL, Montoro MN, et al. Use of fetal ultrasound to select metabolic therapy for pregnancies complicated by mild gestational diabetes. Diabetes Care 1994;17:275–83.

[71] Schaefer-Graf U, Kjos S, Fauzan O, et al. A randomized trial evaluating a predominantly fetal growth-based strategy to guide management of gestational diabetes in Caucasian women. Diabetes Care 2004;27:297–302.

[72] Kjos S, Schaefer-Graf U, Sardesi S, et al. A randomized controlled trial using glycemic plus fetal ultrasound parameters versus glycemic parameters to determine insulin therapy in gestational diabetes with fasting hyperglycemia. Diabetes Care 2001;11:1904–10.

[73] Rosenn B, Langer O, Brustman L, et al. It's not just the abdominal circumference: glycemic control still matters [abstract]. American Journal of Obstetrics and Gynecology 2004;189:165.

[74] McFarland MB, Langer O, Conway DL, Berkus M. Dietary therapy for gestational diabetes: how long is long enough? Obstet Gynecol 1999;93:978–82.

[75] Langer O, Mazze RS. Diabetes in pregnancy: evaluating self-monitoring performance and glycemic control with memory-based technology. Am J Obstet Gynecol 1986;155:635–8.

[76] Langer O, Anyaegbunam A, Brustman L, et al. Gestational diabetes: Insulin requirements in pregnancy. Am J Obstet Gynecol 1987;157:669–75.

[77] DeWitt DE, Hirsch IB. Outpatient insulin therapy in type 1 and type 2 diabetes mellitus. JAMA 2003;289:2254–64.

[78] Langer O, Conway DL, Berkus MD, et al. A comparison of glyburide and insulin in women with gestational diabetes mellitus. N Engl J Med 2000;343:1134–8.

[79] Saade G. Gestational diabetes mellitus: a pill or a shot? [editorial] Obstet Gynecol 2005;105: 456–7.

[80] Cefalo RC. A comparison of glyburide and insulin in women with gestational diabetes mellitus. Obstet Gynecol Surv 2001;56:126–7.

[81] Gabbe SG, Graves CR. Management of diabetes mellitus complicating pregnancy. Obstet Gynecol 2003;102:857–68.

[82] Koren G. The use of glyburide in gestational diabetes: An ideal example of "bench to bedside." Pediatr Res 2001;49:734.

[83] Ryan EA. Glyburide was as safe and effective as insulin in gestational diabetes. Evidence Based Medicine 2001;6:79.

[84] Coustan DR. Oral hypoglycemic agents for the Ob/Gyn. Contemp Obstet Gynecol 2001;45–63.

[85] Jovanovic L. The use of oral agents during pregnancy to treat gestational diabetes. Curr Diab Rep 2001;1:69–70.

[86] Piacquadio K, Hollingsworth DR, Murphy H. Effects of in-utero exposure to oral hypoglycemic drugs. Lancet 1991;338:866–9.

[87] Kemball ML, McIver C, Milner RD, et al. Neonatal hypoglycemia in infants of diabetic mothers given sulfonylurea drugs in pregnancy. Arch Dis Child 1970;45:696–701.

[88] Towner D, Kjos SL, Leung B, et al. Congenital malformations in pregnancies complicated by NIDDM. Diabetes Care 1995;18:1446–51.

[89] Gutzin S, Kozer E, Magee L, et al. The safety of oral hypoglycemic agents in the first trimester of pregnancy: a meta-analysis. Can J Clin Pharmacol 2003;10:179–83.

[90] Glueck CJ, Goldenberg N, Wang P, et al. Metformin during pregnancy reduces insulin, insulin resistance, insulin secretion, weight, testosterone and development of gestational diabetes: prospective longitudinal assessment of women with polycystic ovary syndrome from preconception throughout pregnancy. Hum Reprod 2004;19:510–21.

[91] Glueck CJ, Wang P, Kobayashi S, et al. Metformin therapy throughout pregnancy reduces the development of gestational diabetes in women with polycystic ovary syndrome. Fertil Steril 2002;77:520–5.

[92] Jakubowicz DJ, Juorno MJ, Jakubowica S. Effects of metformin on early pregnancy loss in the polycystic ovary syndrome. J Clin Endocrinol Metab 2002;87:524–9.

[93] Lim JM, Tayob Y, O'Brien PM, Shaw RW. A comparison between the pregnancy outcome of women with gestation diabetes treated with glibenclamide and those treated with insulin. Med J Malay 1997;52:377–81.

[94] Conway DL, Gonzales O, Skiver D. Use of glyburide for the treatment of gestational diabetes: the San Antonio experience. J Matern Fetal Neonatal Med 2004;15:51–5.

[95] Kremer CJ, Duff P. Glyburide for the treatment of gestational diabetes. Am J Obstet Gynecol 2004;190:1438–9.

[96] Chmait R, Dinise T, Moore T. Prospective observational study to establish predictors of glyburide success in women with gestational diabetes mellitus. J Perinatol 2004;24(10): 617–22.

[97] Gilson G, Murphy N. Comparison of oral glyburide with insulin for the management of gestational diabetes mellitus in Alaskan native women. Am J Obstet Gynecol 2002;187: S152.

[98] Fines V, Moore T, Castle S. A comparison of glyburide and insulin treatment in gestational diabetes mellitus on infant birth weight and adiposity. Am J Obstet Gynecol 2003;189:S108.

[99] Velazquez MD, Bolnick J, Cloakey D. The use of glyburide in the management of gestational diabetes. Obstet Gynecol 2003;101(Suppl):88S.

[100] Pendsey SP, Sharma RR, Chalkhore SS. Repaglinde: a feasible alternative to insulin in management of gestational diabetes mellitus. Diabetes Res Clin Pract 2002;56(Suppl):S46.

[101] Coetzee EJ, Jackson WP. Oral hypoglycaemics in the first trimester and fetal outcome. S Afr Med J 1984;65:635–7.

[102] Coetzee EJ, Jackson WP. The management of non-insulin-dependent diabetes during pregnancy. Diabetes Res Clin Pract 1985–86;1:281–7.

[103] Coetzee EJ, Jackson WP. Metformin in management of pregnant insulin-independent diabetics. Diabetologia 1979;16:241–5.

[104] Hellmuth E, Damm P, Molsted-Pedersen L. Oral hypoglycaemic agents in 118 diabetic pregnancies. Diabet Med 2001;17:507–11.

[105] Notelovitz M. Sulphonylurea therapy in the treatment of the pregnant diabetic. S Afr Med J 1971;45:226–9.

[106] Yogev Y, Ben-Haroush A, Chen R, et al. Undiagnosed asymptomatic hypoglycemia: diet, insulin, and glyburide for gestational diabetic pregnancy. Obstet Gynecol 2004;104:88–93.

[107] Moore L, Briery C, Martin R, et al. Metformin vs. insulin in A2 diabetics: a randomized clinical trial. Am J Obstet Gynecol 2004;191(Suppl):S8.

[108] Jacobson GF, Ramos GA, Ching JY, et al. Comparison of glyburide and insulin for the management of gestational diabetes in a large managed care organization. Am J Obstet Gynecol 2005;193(1):118–24.

[109] Elliot B, Langer O, Schenker S, Johnson R. Insignificant transfer of glyburide occurs across the human placenta. Am J Obstet Gynecol 1991;165:807–12.

[110] Elliot B, Schenker S, Langer O, et al. Comparative placental transport of oral hypoglycemic agents: a model of human placental drug transfer. Am J Obstet Gynecol 1994;171:653–60.

[111] Elliot B, Langer O, Schussling F. A model of human placental drug transfer. Am J Obstet Gynecol 1997;176:527–30.

[112] Ng WW, Miller RK. Transport of nutrients in the early human placenta: amino acid, creatinine, vitamin B12. Trophoblast Res 1983;1:121–33.

[113] Langer O, Yogev Y, Xenakis EMJ. Insulin and glyburide therapy: dosage, severity level of gestational diabetes and pregnancy outcome. Am J Obstet Gynecol 2004;192:134–9.

[114] Goetzel L, Wilkins I. Glyburide compared to insulin for the treatment of gestational diabetes mellitus: a cost analysis. J Perinatol 2002;22:403–6.

[115] Feig DS, Briggs GG, Kraemer JM, et al. Transfer of glyburide and glipzide into breast milk. Diabetes Care 2005;28:1851–5.

ENDOCRINOLOGY
AND METABOLISM
CLINICS
OF NORTH AMERICA

ELSEVIER
SAUNDERS

Endocrinol Metab Clin N Am
35 (2006) 79–97

Successful Pregnancy in Women with Type 1 Diabetes: From Preconception Through Postpartum Care

Lois Jovanovic, MD[a,b,c,*], Yuichiro Nakai, MD[d]

[a]Keck School of Medicine, University of Southern California at Los Angeles,
Los Angeles, CA, USA
[b]University of California at Santa Barbara, Santa Barbara, CA, USA
[c]Sansum Diabetes Research Institute, Santa Barbara, CA, USA
[d]Department of Medicine, University of California Davis Health Systems,
Sacramento, CA, USA

Using 2002 birth data [1], it is estimated that diabetes affects an estimated 8% of the more than 4 million pregnancies that come to term annually in the United States. Identifying women who require aggressive monitoring and treatment of their diabetes to minimize both maternal and fetal complications during and after pregnancy is a significant challenge for physicians and the health system because almost 75% of pregnancy-related diabetes occurs in women with gestational diabetes or undiagnosed type 2 diabetes.

Conversely, although type 1 diabetes is estimated to account for only 1% to 2% of the pregnancies complicated by diabetes (~ 6000 births in the United States annually), screening is not an issue because the diagnosis of type 1 diabetes is generally well established in a woman's preconception years. As recently as the 1980s, type 1 diabetes and pregnancy were a deadly combination for mothers and especially for fetuses, with rates of fetal perinatal mortality as high as 25% to 30% [2]. Advances over the past 2 decades in home glucose monitoring and insulin administration have provided the technology needed to not only allow women to successfully survive pregnancy but also to decrease the risks of diabetic fetopathy to those of the nondiabetic population [3,4].

Pregnancy in diabetic women is associated with an increase in risk to both the fetus and the mother. Early in the pregnancy there is an emergency

---

* Corresponding author. Sansum Diabetes Research Institute, 2219 Bath Street, Santa Barbara, CA 93105.
E-mail address: ljovanovic@sansum.org (L. Jovanovic).

doi:10.1016/j.ecl.2005.09.008

to normalize the blood glucose to prevent congenital anomalies and spontaneous abortions. As the pregnancy progresses, the mother is at an increased
risk for syncope, hypoglycemia, or diabetic ketoacidosis, all of which need
emergency attention. Later in the pregnancy, she is at risk for accelerated
retinopathy, with the risk of blindness, pregnancy-induced hypertension
and preeclampsia-eclampsia, urinary tract infections, including pyelonephri-
tis, and polyhydramnios. The greatest concern is the increased risk of sudden death in utero for the fetus. All of these dreaded complications can
be obviated or at least minimized with careful planning of the pregnancy
and attention to glucose control.

The additional risks of pregnancy for mothers with type 1 diabetes and
their babies place the emphasis of optimizing maternal and fetal health of
these pregnancies and the focus of this article on (1) appropriate preconception counseling and management goals; (2) optimizing glycemic monitoring
and intensifying insulin therapy during the metabolically dynamic process of
pregnancy; (3) appropriately evaluating women and their fetuses for complications of both diabetes and intensive diabetes therapy during pregnancy;
and (4) peripartum and postpartum glycemic control.

Congenital anomalies

There is an increased prevalence of congenital anomalies and spontaneous abortions in diabetic women who are in poor glycemic control during
the period of fetal organogenesis, which is nearly complete at 7 weeks post-
conception [5]. Thus, a woman may not even know she is pregnant at this
time. For this reason, prepregnancy counseling and planning are essential
in women of childbearing age who have diabetes. Because organogenesis
is complete so early in the fetus' development, if a woman presents to her
health care team and announces that she has missed her period by only
a few days, if the blood glucose levels are normalized immediately [6–10],
there is still is a chance to prevent cardiac anomalies by swiftly normalizing
the glucose levels (although the neural tube defects are probably already set
by the time the period is missed).

Women with type 2 diabetes are less likely to have preconception care
and counseling, often because the diabetes has not yet been diagnosed,
and thus, they are at even greater risk of bearing a birth-defective child.
In one study [11], 40% of women with type 1 diabetes but only 14% with
type 2 diabetes received preconception care.

Another problem for some women with type 2 diabetes is gaining access
to adequate medical care before and after conception. Nowhere is this more
evident than in Hispanic women, in whom the higher prevalence of obesity,
type 2 and gestational diabetes, and increased fertility rates place them at
higher risk for maternal and neonatal complications [12–14]. Pima Indian
women are also at increased risk; they have a 19-fold higher incidence of

type 2 diabetes compared with the general United States population, with an age-adjusted prevalence rate approximately eight times higher [15,16].

A measurement of glycosylated hemoglobin A_{1c} (HbA_{1c}) can, in early pregnancy, estimate the level of glycemic control during the period of fetal organogenesis. There are two important observations in this regard: first, HbA_{1c} values early in pregnancy are correlated with the rates of spontaneous abortion and major congenital malformations [17–19]. Although most studies have been performed in women with type 1 diabetes, the same risk of hyperglycemia applies to those with type 2 diabetes [20,21]; and second, normalizing blood glucose concentrations before and early in the pregnancy can reduce the risks of spontaneous abortion and congenital malformations nearly to that of the general population [22,23].

One report compared 110 women who were 6 to 30 weeks pregnant at the time of referral with 84 women who were recruited before conception and then put on a daily glucose-monitoring regimen [19]. The mean blood glucose concentration was between 60 and 140 mg/dL (3.3 mmol/L and 7.8 mmol/L) in 50% of the latter group of women. The incidence of anomalies was 1.2% in the women recruited before conception versus 10.9% in those first seen during pregnancy. Very similar findings were noted in another study: 1.4% versus 10.4% incidence of congenital abnormalities [23]. Major congenital malformations, which either require surgical correction or significantly affect the health of the child, are more common in infants of diabetic mothers (13% versus 2% in infants of nondiabetic mothers) [24].

The increased rate of spontaneous abortion in poorly controlled diabetic women is believed to be secondary to hyperglycemia, maternal vascular disease, including uteroplacental insufficiency, and possibly immunologic factors [25]. In addition, animal studies suggest that hyperglycemia regulates the expression of an apoptosis (programmed cell death) regulatory gene as early as the preimplantation blastocyst stage, resulting in increased DNA fragmentation [26]. These findings emphasize the importance of glycemic control at the earliest stages of conception.

Ideally, if a diabetic woman plans her pregnancy there is time to create algorithms of care that are individualized, and a woman can be given choices. When a diabetic woman presents in her first few weeks of pregnancy, there is no time for individualization; rather, rigid protocols must substituted urgently to provide optimal control within 24 to 48 hours.

Deleterious effects of strict glycemic control

Despite the clear benefits to the fetus of strict glycemic control, there is a hazard of hypoglycemia. Major complications of hypoglycemia can usually be prevented with careful monitoring and education of the mother [7,23,27]. Very strict glycemic control (mean blood glucose $\leq$ 56 mg/dL) may be deleterious to the fetus and should be avoided. In one study, the most common cause of maternal mortality was related to hypoglycemia [28].

Retinopathy

There are three reported situations in which the rapid normalization of blood glucose level increases the risk for the deterioration of diabetic retinopathy: puberty [29], pregnancy [30], and insulin-like growth factor (IGF)-1 treatment [31]. If two of these events occur in the same patient, the risk for retinopathy progression is potentiated [30,32]. All three situations are associated with increased serum concentrations of growth-promoting factors. It is hypothesized that when the blood glucose level is rapidly decreased, there is increased retinal extravasation of serum proteins. If there is a concomitant increase in the concentration of serum growth-promoting factors, a predisposed retina may deteriorate [33–35].

Pregnancy per se is the condition most frequently reported in which the rapid normalization of blood glucose is associated with retinal deterioration [7,32, 34–36]. Normal pregnancy is associated with a high concentration of many growth-promoting factors [36–38]. Hill and colleagues [33] have reported that a potent mitogenic and angiogenic factor normally absent from the adult circulation becomes detectable by 14 weeks of gestation and is maximal at 22 to 32 weeks of gestation. A placental growth hormone variant had been found to increase throughout pregnancy, along with the human somatomammotropin prolactin [36]. Maternal IGF-1 production has also been shown to increase significantly above nonpregnant levels [37]. It is well known that diabetes mellitus is associated with perturbations of growth hormone IGF-1 in cases of poor metabolic control [38].

If treatment with lispro insulin, a short-acting insulin analog, allows for increasing the rate whereby the hyperglycemic state is normalized, then lispro insulin may play a role in causing the rapid deterioration of retinopathy. It is unlikely, in the few case reports of rapid deterioration of retinopathy in patients taking lispro insulin, that deterioration was caused by the IGF-1 activity of this insulin, because pregnancy alone has such elevated IGF-1 levels.

Human insulin binds to the IGF-1 receptor with an affinity of 0.1% to 0.2% of the affinity of IGF-1. A comparison of lispro and human insulin was made to determine the relative IGF-1 receptor binding affinity in human placental membranes, skeletal muscle, smooth muscle cells, and mammary epithelial cells. Lispro had a slightly higher affinity for the human placental membranes compared with human insulin. No other differences were observed in any other cell lines. Despite the suggested increased affinity, it should be noted that the absolute affinity for the IGF-1 receptor is extremely low for both lispro and human insulin. Concentrations more that 1000 times above normal physiologic range are needed to reach a receptor binding affinity of 50%. IGF-1 is a much larger protein chain than insulin, and there is a 49% homology between human insulin and IGF-1. The reversal of the Asx28 and Asx29 amino aids in lispro increases this homology to 51% because of the analogous position in the IGF-1 molecule. It has been shown that insulin lispro has the same affinity for the IGF-1 receptor as human insulin and that the dissociation kinetics of insulin lispro on the insulin receptor are identical to those of insulin, indicating that insulin lispro should have no excess mitogenic effect through the IGF-1 or insulin receptor [39,40].

Phelps and colleagues [32] have clearly shown that the deterioration of retinopathy correlated significantly with the levels of plasma glucose at entry and with the magnitude of improvement in glycemia during the first 6 to 14 weeks after entry, although the 13 patients with no retinopathy at baseline did not progress to proliferative retinopathy. However, one of the women developed moderate hemorrhages, exudates, and intraretinal microaneurysms. Of their 20 patients with an initial background of retinopathy, two patients progressed to proliferative retinopathy. Laatikainen and colleagues [41] confirmed that the decrease in hemoglobin HbA_{1c} levels was the most rapid in the two patients with the worst progression. They concluded that a rapid near-normalization of glycemic control during pregnancy can accelerate the progression of retinopathy in poorly controlled diabetic patients. The Diabetes in Early Pregnancy (DIEP) study [42] reported the results of 155 type 1 diabetic women who underwent retinal angiography in the first few weeks of gestation and then at term (within 1 week before delivery). In the 140 patients who did not have proliferative retinopathy at baseline, the progression of retinopathy was seen in 10.3%, 21.1%, 18.8%, and 54.8% of patients with no retinopathy, microaneurysms only, mild nonproliferative retinopathy, and moderate to severe nonproliferative retinopathy at baseline, respectively. Proliferative retinopathy developed in 6.3% of patients with mild and 29% of patients with moderate to severe baseline retinopathy. The elevated glycosylated hemoglobin at baseline and the magnitude of improvement of glucose control through week 14 were associated with a higher risk of progression of retinopathy (the adjusted odds ratio [OR] for progression in those with a glycohemoglobin level ≥ 6 standard deviations [SD] above the control mean versus those < 2 SD was 2.7; 95% confidence interval [CI], 1.1%–7.2%; $P = 0.039$). Independent of retinal status, the DIEP study also reported that the duration of diabetes increased the risk of progression such that after 6 years' duration of diabetes the OR was 3.0 (95% CI, 0.5%–17.4%); after 11 to 15 years, the OR was 9.7 (95% CI, 1.9%–49.0%); and after more than 16 years, the OR was 15.0 (95% CI, 3.0%–74.5%); however, hyperglycemia was a stronger risk factor. Additional evidence has been reported by the Diabetes Control and Complications Trial [30]. For women in the conventional care group who became pregnant and thus had immediate intensification of glucose control (n = 135), the retinal status worsened in 47% of the patients, and the OR for progression by the second trimester was 2.6, compared with diabetic women in the conventional group who did not become pregnant.

There is one case report in the literature, which clearly shows that the combination of pregnancy and rapid normalization of severe hyperglycemia is sufficient to explode a previously normal retina. Hagay and colleagues [43] reported a case of a woman with no previously documented hyperglycemia who presented at 8 weeks of gestation with an HbA_{1c} level of 16% and whose ophthalmic examination was reported to be completely normal. She was treated with intensive insulin therapy, and at 12 weeks, her HbA_{1c} level was 5.9%. By the second trimester, she had severe bilateral proliferative diabetic retinopathy that required treatment by photocoagulation.

Based on the above literature review, clearly the five risk factors, which emerge for the prediction of those pregnant diabetic women who will progress to proliferative retinopathy, are baseline evidence of some retinopathy, elevated HbA_{1c} levels at conception, rapid normalization of blood glucose, duration of diabetes for greater than 6 years, and proteinuria.

Because the use of the rapid-acting insulin analogs facilitates the rapid normalization of blood glucose levels [44,45], their use may play a role in the progression of retinopathy, and the clinician must be aware of the retinal status and obtain consultation with a retinal specialist when rapid normalization of blood glucose is undertaken. The literature shows clearly the danger in quickly normalizing blood glucose, regardless of the type of insulin used, in pregnant women with a long duration of diabetes and elevated HbA_{1c} levels in the first trimester, proteinuria, and perhaps type of diabetes.

The schedule of busy clinics may decrease the ability to completely examine the retinae. Mild background retinopathy may be missed, even in the best of settings. Any retinopathy increases the risk, especially if the blood glucose level is elevated. Rather than recommending angiography to all women before each pregnancy is planned, in the case of no retinopathy seen on retinal examination, it is prudent to improve the glucose control slowly. These case reports reinforce the need to intensify preconception care programs to allow the luxury of slowly normalizing the blood glucose and plan the pregnancy only after blood glucose levels have been stabilized within the normal ranges for at least 6 months [42].

When a patient who is already pregnant presents with high glycosylated hemoglobin levels, regardless of the retinal status, she needs to have an ophthalmology consultation on the first day of admission. As the glucose normalization protocol is being initiated, a retinal specialist needs to be on the team, be vigilant, and treat with laser therapy if the retina deteriorates.

Thyroid disease

Type 1 diabetes is associated commonly with other autoimmune endocrine disorders. Thyroid autoantibodies occur more frequently in these patients than in the normal population [46]. Furthermore, an increased prevalence of subclinical hypothyroidism has been reported in pregnant diabetic women [46–49]. Several studies have found a wide range (10%–25%) in the prevalence of postpartum thyroid dysfunction in type 1 diabetic patients [50]. In a report by Haddow and colleagues [51], there is the suggestion that screening pregnant women for hypothyroidism by measuring thyrotropin may be worthwhile and that treating women with serum thyrotropin concentrations at or above the 98th percentile could lead to "an increase of approximately 4 points in IQ scores in their children." Because there is an increased risk of gestational hypothyroidism in diabetic women, all diabetic pregnant women should be screened for hypothyroidism early in their pregnancy and treated immediately if hypothyroidism is documented [51]. Notably, Graves' disease is not more common in type 1 diabetic women than in the general population [46].

Diabetic ketoacidosis

Diabetic ketoacidosis, a complication associated with a high mortality rate in the fetus, may occur. In addition, ketonemia during pregnancy has been associated with decreased intelligence in offspring [52–54], but in these reports there is no mention of an association with fetal malformations. In early pregnancy, ketonuria sometimes occurs in women who are limiting their caloric intake because of nutritional recommendations [55]. Ketonuria resulting from caloric restriction has been shown subsequently not to be associated with decreased intelligence in the offspring, unless it is also associated with severe hyperglycemia (blood glucose levels > 180 mg/dL). Thus, women with moderate to large ketonuria associated with hyperglycemia should immediately alert their physician. Also, if a type 1 diabetic woman is using an insulin infusion pump [53], even short periods of interruption in the infusion may result in ketoacidosis caused by the increased metabolic rate in pregnancy. Thus, many centers are recommending the use of an additional injection of neutral protamine Hagedorn (NPH) insulin at bedtime, in a volume that is 0.1 times the patient's weight in kg, for an appropriate adjustment in the overnight basal metabolism [27,55].

Pregnancy-induced hypertension

Normal first trimester blood pressure is less than 120/80 mmHg [56]. Fetal complications from maternal hypertension include intrauterine growth retardation and fetal demise. The only antihypertensive mediations that have been proven to be safe over the past two generations are methyldopa and hydralazine. When additional medication is needed to maintain normotension, the use of labetolol has been recommended, along with the judicious use of calcium channel blockers and even diuretics. Nifedipine has also been reported to be safe when added after the first trimester. The use of angiotensin converting enzyme (ACE) inhibitors in pregnancy have been associated with congenital anomalies, specifically renal agenesis or renal failure, and thus, they are absolutely contraindicated in pregnancy [57]. However, Hod and colleagues [57] have shown that when ACE inhibitors are used before conception, they decrease the degree of proteinuria, and when they are discontinued at the time of conception, the decreased proteinuria is sustained throughout pregnancy, with an improved maternal and fetal outcome. Although the management of elevated blood pressure in a diabetic pregnant woman is an urgent priority, the means to achieve these goals are limited in pregnancy.

Diabetic nephropathy

Diabetic nephropathy, when not associated with hypertension, does not have an impact on fetal outcome unless the kidney function is more than 50% impaired. Normal creatinine clearance is increased in pregnancy because of the increased metabolic rate and the increased cardiac output by the 10th to 12th week of gestation. Thus, a depression of the creatinine clearance below 50 mL/min is associated with increased fetal loss. Proteinuria greater than 250 mg/dL in the first trimester has been associated with nephrotic syndrome by the third trimester, requiring bed rest and in some cases replacement of protein losses with parenteral supplementation of albumin [25]. Maternal anasarca is not associated with fetal hypdrops, as long as the maternal nutrition includes enough protein for fetal growth [55].

Monitoring glycemic control during pregnancy

The development of accurate, fast, and portable glucose reflectance meters provides patients with the technology to self-assess glycemic control and initiate diabetes management changes numerous times daily, with a goal of normoglycemia. To effectively use newer insulin analogs and dosing strategies to their fullest potential, both the physician and the pregnant patient must understand the techniques, goals, and potential pitfalls of intensifying not only self-monitored blood glucose testing (SMBG) but also HbA_{1c} monitoring and urine ketone testing as well.

The consideration of glycemic goals in the pregnant diabetic woman must take into account the normal glucose ranges in nondiabetic pregnant women. Recently reexamined with the use of continuous glucose monitoring systems, mean fasting glucose values have been shown to range from 61 mg/dL to 75 mg/dL [58–60], decreasing over the course of gestation [59]. In diabetic and nondiabetic pregnancies, maximal postprandial glucose excursions occur between 60 and 90 minutes after meal ingestion and correlate more closely with 1-hour than 2-hour postprandial measurements [60–62]. The mean peak 1-hour postprandial glycemic excursions have been shown to range from 97 to 120.9 mg/dL in nondiabetic women, with negative 3-hour, 100-g oral glucose tolerance tests performed at 24 to 28 weeks gestation, depending on whether the patients passed or failed their 1-hour, 50-g oral glucose challenge test [58]. For diabetic women, fasting and preprandial SMBG must be monitored with treatment goals that are lower than those that are used outside of pregnancy, to goals of 60 to 90 mg/dL. Understanding these nondiabetic pregnancy, normal glucose ranges provides additional support to the previous observation that the macrosomia risk increases with increasing maximal postprandial hyperglycemia $\geq$ 120 mg/dL [4]. While striving to achieve normoglycemia in a type 1 diabetic woman's pregnancy, fasting, pre-prandial, and 1-hour postprandial SMBG testing [4,63] must be carried out to dose insulin safely yet meet the fasting-preprandial glucose goals of 60 mg/dL to 90 mg/dL and 1-hour postprandial glucose goals of 100 mg/dL to 120 mg/dL [64].

Because of the high frequency of SMBG testing required in pregnancy, the use of alternative site SMBG testing is appealing, but the dynamically changing blood glucose concentrations after eating may be identified at finger sites before they are detected at forearm or thigh sites [65]. Because no studies have evaluated the use of blood glucose values from alternative sites in pregnancy, alternative site SMBG testing must be discouraged. The eventual availability of real-time continuous glucose monitoring sensors holds the promise of not only significantly reducing the number of finger-stick blood glucose assessments but also raising the awareness of glycemic excursions [66,67], which can occur commonly, particularly in women with type 1 diabetes, between SMBG measurements. At the time of this writing, no such system is available currently for commercial use.

Glycosylated hemoglobin testing

Until real-time continuous glucose monitoring systems are in routine clinical use to accurately assess 24-hour glycemia, frequent HbA_{1c} monitoring will remain valuable as an assessment of blood glucose excursions occurring at non-SMBG time points. Whereas the HbA_{1c} testing frequency in a nonpregnant population is commonly timed to assess a new steady state of glycemic control, during the compressed time frame of pregnancy (in which 2 weeks represents 5% of a normal gestation), the need to recognize and treat worsening glycemic control as promptly as possible can be facilitated by examining HbA_{1c} changes because they reflect trends in glycemic control. Because clinically and statistically significant differences in HbA_{1c} can be detected at 2-week intervals [68,69], HbA_{1c} assessment every 2 weeks during gestation is recommended.

Nondiabetic pregnant women evaluated by continuous glucose monitoring systems maintain mean blood glucose levels of or less than 100 mg/dL [60], and treating diabetic pregnant women to this mean glucose goal significantly decreases perinatal mortality [70]. Knowing that a mean blood glucose goal of 100 mg/dL correlates with an HbA_{1c} goal of 5% [71], discordant SMBG and HbA_{1c} results should prompt investigation because poor control, undetected by the patient's current SMBG routine, is assumed. Additionally, when using HbA_{1c} measurement as an indicator of glycemic control during pregnancy, it is important to establish a normal HbA_{1c} range, created to reflect the fact that the mean blood glucose levels of nondiabetic pregnant women are approximately 20% lower than in the nonpregnant state [72,73].

Urinary ketone testing

In the nonpregnant state, home urine ketone assessments can be performed in times of hyperglycemia (blood glucose concentration > 180 mg/dL) to assess for evidence of diabetic ketoacidosis. Although many clinicians still use urinary ketone monitoring in pregnancy to ensure maternal nutrition, there are several reasons that this is of limited value when the maternal blood glucose concentration is less than 180 mg/dL in an otherwise uncomplicated diabetic pregnancy. Urinary ketones are frequently positive, without positive serum ketones or acidosis caused by extremely efficient renal ketone clearance [73,74], and are frequently found in urine specimens from nondiabetic pregnant women [75]. Rat models of pregnancy affected by diabetes have demonstrated embryonic malformations in vitro when exposed to markedly elevated ketones [76], but prospective human studies have not found correlations between ketonemia and fetal malformation or pregnancy loss [53]. In a separate study [52], the presence of ketonuria was not correlated with an impaired intellectual growth of the offspring when the maternal blood glucose was controlled adequately. As long as adequate maternal nutrition, reflected by appropriate maternal weight gain, is maintained and the pregnant woman is not ill or hyperglycemic, routine morning urinary ketone testing is of limited value. Additional insulin should be prescribed based on evidence of hyperglycemia, not evidence of ketonuria. Furthermore, increasing carbohydrate intake for the sole purpose of preventing positive urine ketones can result in overfeeding and worsening glycemic control, potentially increasing the risk of macrosomia.

Treatment

There are several components to the treatment of diabetes in pregnant women, the administration of insulin, exercise, and diet.

Insulin doses

The starting insulin dose is calculated to be 0.7 U/kg/d, divided into three to four injections of short- and intermediate-acting insulin. Thecapillary glucose needs to be measured before and 1 hour after each meal, at bedtime, and at 3 AM to assure that there is around-the-clock glucose control. Each day the insulin is adjusted based on the blood glucose measurements such that the optimal dose of insulin is derived on a daily basis. Only human insulin should be used in pregnant women. Most women with type 1 diabetes require at least three injections per day [41,45,48]. A two-injection regimen can cause nocturnal hypoglycemia if the evening meal dose of intermediate-acting insulin peaks during the middle of the night [27].

Total daily insulin requirements typically rise during gestation. This is caused primarily by the effects of human placental lactogen, which has somatotropic properties. The average insulin requirement in pregnant women with type 1 diabetes rises from 0.7 U/kg/d in the first trimester, often increasing to 0.8 U/kg/d for weeks 18 to 26, 0.9 U/kg/d for weeks 26 to 36, and 1.0 U/kg/d for weeks 36 to term. Massively obese women may need initial doses of 1.5 U/kg/d to 2.0 U/kg/d to overcome the combined insulin resistance of pregnancy and obesity [54]. Declining insulin requirements may occur at 9 to 12 weeks of gestation and again at 38 to 40 weeks of gestation [27]. These changes in insulin requirement are thought to be caused by the luteal-placental shift in progesterone seen in the late first trimester and to the onset of labor, with increased glucose use that occurs when uterine contractions commence.

The total daily dose is divided such that 50% is given as a basal dose, using an insulin infusion pump or NPH insulin, divided into two to three daily injections spaced 8 to 12 hours apart. The meal-related dose then is the other 50% of the insulin requirement. Recent reports have shown that insulin lispro is safe in pregnancies complicated by type 1 diabetes [77]. However, the studies using insulin aspart and the long-acting insulin analogs detemir and glargine have not yet been published.

Some clinicians have recommended using insulin pumps to achieve optimal glycemic control during pregnancy [78,79]. Most pregnant women require at least three infusion rates in a 24-hour period, in particular a low-dose basal from 12 midnight to 4 AM, an increased rate in the early morning hours, from 4 AM to 10 AM, to counteract the increased release of the anti-insulin hormones cortisol and growth hormone, and an intermediate basal during the rest of the day, from 10 AM to 12 midnight. A protocol for calculating infusion rates has been described elsewhere [80].

Role of exercise

Gestational diabetes differs from a pregnancy in type 1 diabetes because the former is a disorder primarily of impaired glucose clearance. As a result, therapies that overcome peripheral resistance to insulin, such as exercise, are preferable to insulin. In comparison, in women with type 1 diabetes who are already taking insulin, the benefits of exercise are not so clear. Exercise can contribute to the "brittleness" of diabetes, with the risk of exercise-induced hypoglycemia. Women who exercised before pregnancy can usually continue under the supervision of their obstetrician. However, exercise is not recommended in women who are deconditioned and did not exercise before pregnancy [80].

Diet

The optimal diet takes into account caloric intake, carbohydrate content, and the distribution of meals throughout the day. The appropriate caloric intake depends on the pregravid weight, with the following general recommendations:

- ~30 kcal/kg/d if the woman is at her ideal body weight
- ~24 kcal/kg/d if the woman ≥ 20% to 50% above ideal body weight
- 12–18 kcal/kg/d if the woman is > 50% above ideal body weight
- 36–40 kcal/kg/d if the woman is > 10% below ideal body weight

The recommended distribution of calories is 40% to 50% carbohydrate, 20% protein, and 30% to 40% fat. Many physicians find that maintaining glycemic control requires a diet in which carbohydrate accounts for no more than 40% of calories [3,54]. Postprandial blood glucose values depend largely on the carbohydrate content of the meal, and it is the postprandial blood glucose concentration that has the most important role in macrosomia [4,63].

Most programs recommend three meals and three snacks per day. An acceptable caloric distribution would be 10% of calories at breakfast, 30% at both lunch and dinner, and 30% as snacks. A daily supplement of ferrous sulfate and folate is also recommended.

Fetal surveillance

The high perinatal mortality once associated with a diabetic pregnancy has decreased significantly, largely caused by improved glycemic control [81]. In the past, unexplained fetal death occurred in 10% to 30% of type 1 diabetic pregnancies, typically after the 36th week of gestation in women with poor glycemic control, associated with macrosomia, hydramnios, pre-eclampsia, and vascular disease. Fetal surveillance, therefore, is of utmost importance in optimizing a good outcome for both mother and fetus, especially in the perilous third trimester. Ultrasonography is the most useful tool for the assessment of the fetus. It can be used to (1) estimate gestational age; (2) screen for structural anomalies; (3) evaluate growth; (4) assess amniotic fluid volume; and (5) determine fetal status dynamically through Doppler and biophysical studies.

Ultrasonographic estimates of gestational age are most accurate if they are performed in early pregnancy. The gestational age, determined by a crown–rump length measured in the first trimester, will be accurate within 5 days. Ultrasonographic estimates of gestational age are not reliable after the 28th week and cannot be used to determine the estimated date of delivery [82].

Macrosomia is more apparent in some fetal structures, such as the liver and abdomen. As a result, ultrasonographic estimates that use the fetal abdominal circumference to calculate fetal weight may not be as accurate as in normal fetuses in which growth is proportional. Macrosomia is usually defined as fetal weight greater than 4.0 kg to 4.5 kg or birth weight above the 90th percentile for gestational age [83–85]. Macrosomic fetuses are at an increased risk for a prolonged second stage of labor, shoulder dystocia, operative delivery, and perinatal death [83].

Macrosomia occurs in approximately 88% of fetuses in whom the abdominal circumference and estimated fetal weight both exceed the 90th percentile [61,85]. The biparietal diameter and head circumference appear to be less predictive of macrosomia. Undiagnosed macrosomia may lead to birth trauma if vaginal delivery ensues. Before the onset of labor, an assessment of the fetal size is paramount.

In contrast to macrosomia, intrauterine growth retardation (usually defined as birth weight below the 10th percentile for gestational age) is uncommon in diabetic pregnancies. It is associated with uteroplacental insufficiency and occurs primarily in pregnancies complicated by diabetic vasculopathy or preeclampsia [25].

Ultrasonography is essential for the evaluation of congenital anomalies. A structural ultrasonogram can detect both neural tube defects and major cardiac defects by this time. Infants of diabetic mothers are at an increased risk for neural tube defects, which occur in approximately 2% of diabetic pregnancies (versus 0.1%–0.2% in the general population) [86]. Other congenital anomalies that occur with higher frequency in infants of diabetic mothers include anencephaly, microcephaly, caudal regression syndrome, and genitourinary and gastrointestinal anomalies. Congenital heart disease is also common, including a specific type of hypertrophic cardiomyopathy, atrial and ventricular septal defects, transposition of the great vessels, and coarctation of the aorta. Hydramnios can occur because of increased amniotic fluid osmolality and polyuria secondary to fetal hyperglycemia [87]. Ultrasonography is performed in the third trimester for the assessment of growth and development and the presence of macrosomia.

Maternal diabetes alone does not increase the risk for chromosomal abnormalities such as Down syndrome. As a result, the indications for invasive testing, such as amniocentesis and chorionic villous sampling, are the same as in the general population.

Guidelines for antepartum surveillance vary and usually depend on the clinical situation and the discretion of the physician. In women who have diet-controlled gestational diabetes, fetal surveillance is not initiated usually until 40 weeks' gestation, because these women are at very low risk for complications. More rigorous monitoring is recommended for women who have additional indications for closer fetal surveillance. Most centers defer testing until the 35th week of gestation if there is excellent glycemic control, but testing is started much earlier in women who have poor control, nephropathy, or hypertension. In these women, antepartum testing is begun at 26 to 28 weeks, when fetal survival is likely if delivery were to occur. Antepartum fetal testing should be performed twice per week. Doppler umbilical artery velocimetry has shown increased placental resistance in women with vasculopathy and poor glycemic control, which increase the risk of intrauterine growth retardation and preeclampsia [82,88].

Labor and delivery

Maternal hyperglycemia is the major cause of neonatal hypoglycemia. As a result, the peripartum maintenance of maternal euglycemia is essential. The following general recommendations can be made: insulin is still required before active labor and can be given subcutaneously or by intravenous infusion, with a goal of maintaining blood glucose concentrations between 70 mg/dL and 90 mg/dL. One method of insulin infusion consists of the intravenous administration of 15 U of regular insulin in 150 mL of normal saline at a rate of 1 U/h to 3 U/h. Normal saline may be sufficient to maintain euglycemia when labor is anticipated. As the mother enters active labor, insulin resistance decreases rapidly (because expulsion of the fetoplacental unit leads to the cessation of production of somatomammotropin, which has a short half-life), and insulin requirements drop to zero. Thus, continuing insulin therapy is likely to lead to hypoglycemia. To prevent hypoglycemia, glucose should be infused at a rate of 2.5 mg/kg/min should be given [89]. Capillary blood glucose should be measured hourly. The glucose infusion should be doubled for the next hour if the blood glucose value is less than 60 mg/dL. On the other hand, values of 120 mg/dL or more require the administration of regular insulin subcutaneously or intravenously until the blood glucose value falls to 70 mg/dL to 90 mg/dL. At this time, the insulin dose is titrated to maintain normoglycemia while glucose is infused at a rate of 2.5 mg/kg/min. Bolus doses of glucose should not be given because they can raise maternal blood glucose concentrations and increase the risk of neonatal hypoglycemia, fetal hypoxia, and fetal or neonatal acidosis. If a cesarean section is planned, the bedtime NPH insulin dose may be given on the morning of surgery and every 8 hours thereafter if surgery is delayed [90].

Postpartum

Insulin requirements drop sharply after delivery, and the new mother may not require insulin for 24 to 72 hours. Insulin requirements should be recalculated at this time, at approximately 0.6 U/kg/d, based on postpartum weight. Postpartum caloric requirements are approximately 25 kcal/kg/d and somewhat higher (27 kcal/kg/d) in lactating women.

Glycemic control is somewhat more erratic in lactating diabetic women, with more frequent episodes of hypoglycemia. Because the risk of life-threatening hypoglycemia is increased in the immediate postpartum period, especially if a woman is lactating, preventing postpartum hypoglycemia is the primary goal. Hypoglycemia occurring in the middle of the night can be prevented if the NPH dose before bed is deleted and regular insulin is given instead at 3 AM in low doses, after the mother has finished nursing the infant [91].

Summary

Although the successful outcome rate of pregnancies complicated by diabetes is now approaching the rate seen in a normal healthy pregnant population, this improvement is realized only when careful attention is paid to the metabolic, hemodynamic, and vascular perturbations associated with the changes of pregnancy. The diabetic woman must not only pay attention to her nutrition but also blunt momentary swings in her blood glucose by taking frequent blood glucose determinations and perfectly calculated doses of insulin. In addition, she must be under constant surveillance for a host of other complications of pregnancy, such as hypertension, retinopathy, infection, acidosis, thyroid dysfunction, nephropathy, and sudden death in utero. Any or all of these problems become medical emergencies if left untreated. Thus, rigorous vigilance to sustain normoglycemia, normotension, retinal health, normal thyroid function, renal health, and fetal well-being are all paramount in the management of pregnancies complicated by diabetes.

References

[1] Martin JA, Hamilton BE, Sutton PD, et al. Births: final data for 2002. Natl Vital Stat Rep 2003;52:1.
[2] Perinatal mortality and congenital malformations in infants born to women with insulin-dependent diabetes mellitus: United States, Canada, and Europe, 1940–1988. MMWR Morb Mortal Wkly Rep 1990;39:363.
[3] Jovanovic L, Druzin M, Peterson CM. Effect of euglycemia on the outcome of pregnancy in insulin-dependent diabetic women as compared with normal control subjects. Am J Med 1981;71:921.
[4] Jovanovic L, Peterson CM, Reed GF, et al, for the National Institute of Child Health and Human Development–Diabetes in Early Pregnancy Study. Maternal postprandial glucose levels and infant birth weight: the Diabetes in Early Pregnancy Study. Am J Obstet Gynecol 1991;164:103.
[5] Mills JL, Baker L, Goldman A. Malformations in infants of diabetic mothers occur before the seventh gestational week: implications for treatment. Diabetes 1979;23:292.
[6] Mills JL, Knopp RH, Simpson JL, et al. Lack of relation of increased malformation roles in infants of diabetic mothers to glycemic control during organogenesis. N Engl J Med 1988; 318:671.
[7] Kitzmiller JL, Gavin LA, Gin GD, et al. Preconception care of diabetes: glycemic control prevents congenital anomalies. JAMA 1991;265:731.
[8] Mills JL, Simpson JL, Driscoll SG, et al, for the National Institutes of Child Health and Human Development—Diabetes in Early Pregnancy Study: Incidence of spontaneous abortion among normal women and insulin dependent diabetic women whose pregnancies were identified within 21 days of conception. N Engl J Med 1988;319:1617.

 [9] Miller E, Hare JW, Cloherty JP, et al. Elevated maternal hemoglobin A1C in early pregnancy and major congenital anomalies in infants of diabetic mothers. N Engl J Med 1981;304(22): 1331–4.

[10] Fuhrmann K, Ruher H, Semmler K, et al. Prevention of congenital malformations in infants of insulin dependent diabetic mothers. Diabetes Care 1983;6:219.

[11] Janz NK, Herman WH, Becker MP, et al. Diabetes and pregnancy: factors associated with seeking pre-conception care. Diabetes Care 1995;18(2):157–65.

[12] Forsbach G, Contreras-Soto JJ, Fong G. Prevalence of gestational diabetes and macrosomic infants in Mexican population. Diabetes Care 1988;11:235.

[13] Hollingsworth DR, Vaucher Y, Yamamoto TR. Diabetes in pregnancy in Mexican Americans. Diabetes Care 1991;14:695.

[14] Mestman JH. Outcome of diabetes screening in pregnancy and perinatal morbidity in infants of mothers with mild impairment in glucose tolerance. Diabetes Care 1980;3:447.

[15] Knowler WC, Bennett PH, Hamman RF. Diabetes incidence and prevalence in Pima Indians: a 19-fold greater incidence than in Rochester, Minnesota. Am J Epidemiol 1978;108: 497.

[16] Knowler WC, Pettit DJ, Saad MF. Diabetes mellitus in Pima Indians: incidence, risk factors, and pathogenesis. Diabet Metab Rev 1990;6:1.

[17] Damm P, Molsted-Pederson L. Significant decrease in congenital malformations in newborn infants of an unselected population of diabetic women. Am J Obstet Gynecol 1989;161:1163.

[18] Greene MF, Hare JW, Cloherty JP, et al. First trimester hemoglobin A1C and risk for major malformation and spontaneous abortion in diabetic pregnancy. Teratology 1989;39:225.

[19] Ylinen K, Aula P, Stenman UH, et al. Risk of minor and major fetal malformations in diabetics with high haemoglobin A1C values in early pregnancy. BMJ 1984;289(6441):345–6.

[20] Becerra JE, Khoury MJ, Cordero JF. Diabetes mellitus during pregnancy and risks for specific birth defects: a population-based case-control study. Pediatrics 1990;85:1.

[21] Towner D, Kjos SL, Leung B. Congenital malformations in pregnancies complicated by NIDDM. Diabetes Care 1995;18:1446.

[22] Fuhrmann K, Reiher H, Semmler K, et al. The effect of intensified conventional insulin therapy before and during pregnancy on the malformation rate in offspring of diabetic mothers. Exp Clin Endocrinol 1984;83:173.

[23] Steel JM, Johnstone FD, Hepburn DA, et al. Can prepregnancy care of diabetic women reduce the risk of abnormal babies? BMJ 1990;301:1070.

[24] Cousins L. Etiology and prevention of congenital anomalies among infants of overt diabetic women. Clin Obstet Gynecol 1991;34:481.

[25] Kitzmiller JL, Watt N, Driscoll SG. Decidual arteriopathy in hypertension and diabetes in pregnancy and immunofluorescent studies. Am J Obstet Gynecol 1981;141:773.

[26] Moley KH, Chi MM, Knudson CM, et al. Hyperglycemia induces apoptosis in preimplantation embryos through cell death effector pathways. Nat Med 1998;4:1421.

[27] Jovanovic L, Mills Jl, Knopp RH, et al, for the National Institute of Child Health and Human Development-Diabetes in Early Pregnancy Study Group. Declining insulin requirement in the late first trimester of diabetic pregnancy. Diabetes Care 2001;24:1130–6.

[28] Leinonen PJ, Hiilesmaa VK, Kaaja RJ, et al. Maternal mortality in type 1 diabetes. Diabetes Care 2001;24:1501–2.

[29] Daneman D, Drash AL, Lobes LA. Progressive retinopathy with improved control in diabetic dwarfism (Mauriac's syndrome). Diabetes Care 1981;4:360–4.

[30] Lachin J, Clearly P, Molitch M, et al, for the DCCT Research Group. Pregnancy increases the risk of complication in the DCCT. Diabetes 1998;47(Suppl 1):S1091.

[31] Van Ballegooie E, Hooymans JMM, Timerman Z. Rapid deterioration of diabetic retinopathy during treatment with continuous subcutaneous insulin infusion. Diabetes Care 1984;7: 236–41.

[32] Phelps RL, Sakol L, Metzger BE, et al. Changes in diabetic retinopathy during pregnancy: correlations with regulation of hyperglycemia. Arch Ophthalmol 1986;104:1806–10.

[33] Hill DJ, Clemmons DR, Riley SC, et al. Immunohistochemical localization of insulin like growth factors and IGF binding proteins-1,-2, and -3 in human placenta and fetal membranes. Placenta 1993;14:1–12.

[34] Larinkari J, Laatikainen L, Ranta T. Metabolic control and serum hormone levels in relationship to retinopathy in diabetic pregnancy. Diabetologia 1982;22:327–31.

[35] Merimee TJ, Zapf J, Froesch ER. Insulin-like growth factors: studies in diabetics with and without retinopathy. N Engl J Med 1983;309:527–31.

[36] MacLeod JN, Worsley I, Ray Y, et al. Human growth hormone variant is a biologically active somatogen and lactogen. Endocrinology 1991;128:1298–302.

[37] Gluckman PD. The endocrine regulation of fetal growth in late gestation: the role of insulin-like growth factors. T J Clin Endocinol Metab 1995;80:1047–50.

[38] Holly JMP, Amiel SA, Sandhu RR, et al. The role of growth hormone in diabetes mellitus. J Endocrinol 1988;118:353–64.

[39] DiMarchi RD, Chance RE, Long HB, et al. Preparation of an insulin with improved pharmacokinetics relative to human insulin through consideration of structural homology with insulin-like growth factor-1. Horm Res 1994;41(Suppl 2):S93–6.

[40] Llewelyn J, Slieker LJ, Zimmermann JL. Pre-clinical studies on insulin lispro. Drugs Today (Barc) 1998;34(Suppl C):C11–21.

[41] Laatikainen L, Teramo K, Hieta-Heikurainen H, et al. A controlled study of he influence of continuous subcutaneous insulin infusion treatment on diabetic retinopathy during pregnancy. Acta Medica Scandinavica 1987;221:367–76.

[42] Chew EY, Mills JL, Metzger BE, et al, for the National Institute of Child Health and Human Development-Diabetes in Early Pregnancy Study. Metabolic control and progression of retinopathy: The Diabetes In Early Pregnancy Study. Diabetes Care 1995;18:631–7.

[43] Hagay ZJ, Schachter M, Pollack A, et al. Case report: development of proliferative retinopathy in a gestational diabetes patient following rapid metabolic control. Eur J Obstet Gynecol Reprod Biol 1994;57:211–3.

[44] Anderson JH, Brunelle RL, Koivisto VA. Reduction of postprandial hyperglycemia and frequency of hypoglycemia in IDDM patients on insulin-analog treatment. Diabetes 1997;46: 265–70.

[45] Jovanovic L, Ilic S, Pettitt DJ, et al. The metabolic and immunologic effects of insulin lispro in gestational diabetes. Diabetes Care 1999;22:1422–7.

[46] Betterle C, Zanette F, Pedini B, et al. Clinical and subclinical organ-specific autoimmune manifestations in Type 1 (insulin-dependent) diabetic patients and their first-degree relatives. Diabetologia 1989;26:431–6.

[47] Bech K, Hoier-Madsen M, Feldt-Rasmussen U, et al. Thyroid function and autoimmune manifestations in insulin-dependent diabetes mellitus during and after pregnancy. Acta Endocrinol (Copenh) 1991;124:534–9.

[48] Jovanovic L, Peterson CM. De novo clinical hypothyroidism in pregnancies complicated by type 1 diabetes, subclinical hypothyroidism, and proteinuria: a new syndrome. Am J Obstet Gynecol 1988;159:442–6.

[49] Alvarez-Marfany M, Roman SH, Drexler Aj, et al. Long-term prospective study of postpartum thyroid dysfunction in women with insulin dependent diabetes mellitus. J Clin Endocrinol Metab 1994;79:10–6.

[50] Gerstein HC. Incidence of postpartum thyroid dysfunction in patients with type I diabetes mellitus. Ann Intern Med 1993;118:419–23.

[51] Haddow JE, Palomaki GE, Allan WC, et al. Maternal thyroid deficiency during pregnancy and subsequent neuropsychological development of the child. N Engl J Med 1999;341: 549–55.

[52] Rizzo T, Metzger BE, Nurns WJ. Correlations between antepartum maternal metabolism and intelligence of offspring. N Engl J Med 1991;325:911.

[53] Jovanovic L, Metzger BE, Knopp RH, et al. The Diabetes in Early Pregnancy Study: beta-hydroxybutyrate levels in type 1 diabetic pregnancy compared with normal pregnancy.

NICHD-Diabetes in Early Pregnancy Study Group (DIEP). National Institute of Child Health and Development. Diabetes Care 1998;21(11):1978–84.

[54] Jovanovic L, Peterson CM. Sweet success, but an acid aftertaste [editorial]? N Engl J Med 1991;325:959–60.

[55] Jovanovic L, Peterson CM. Dietary manipulation as a primary treatment strategy for pregnancies complicated by diabetes. J Am Coll Nutr 1990;9:320.

[56] Peterson CM, Jovanovic L, Mills JL, et al, for the Diabetes in Early Pregnancy Study. Changes in cholesterol, triglycerides, body weight and blood pressure. Am J Obstet Gynecol 1992;166:513–8.

[57] Hod M, van Dijk DJ, Karp M, et al. Diabetic nephropathy and pregnancy: the effect of ACE inhibitors prior to pregnancy on fetomaternal outcome. Nephrol Dial Transplant 1995;10: 2328–33.

[58] Victor A. Normal blood sugar variation during pregnancy. Acta Obstet Gynecol Scand 1974;53:37–40.

[59] Parretti E, Carignani L, Cioni R, et al. Sonographic evaluation of fetal growth and body composition in women with different degrees of normal glucose metabolism. Diabetes Care 2003;26:2741.

[60] Yogev Y, Ben-Haroush A, Chen R, et al. Diurnal glycemic profile in obese and normal weight nondiabetic pregnant women. Am J Obstet Gynecol 2004;191:949.

[61] Ben-Haroush A, Yogev Y, Chen R, et al. The postprandial glucose profile in the diabetic pregnancy. Am J Obstet Gynecol 2004;191:576.

[62] Peterson CM, Jovanovic LB, Brownlee M, et al. Closing the loop: practical and theoretical. Diabetes Care 1980;3:318.

[63] Combs CA, Gunderson E, Kitzmiller JL, et al. Relationship of fetal macrosomia to maternal postprandial glucose control during pregnancy. Diabetes Care 1992;15:1251.

[64] Jovanovic L. Insulin therapy in pregnancy. In: Leahy JL, Defalu WT, editors. Insulin therapy. New York: Marcel Dekker, Inc; 2002. p. 139.

[65] Ellison JM, Stegmann JM, Colner SL, et al. Rapid changes in postprandial blood glucose produce concentration differences at finger, forearm, and thigh sampling sites. Diabetes Care 2002;25:961.

[66] Jovanovic L. The role of continuous glucose monitoring in gestational diabetes mellitus. Diabetes Technol Ther 2000;2(Suppl 1):S67.

[67] Kerssen A, de Valk HW, Visser GH. Day-to-day glucose variability during pregnancy in women with Type 1 diabetes mellitus: glucose profiles measured with the Continuous Glucose Monitoring System. BJOG 2004;111:919.

[68] Boden G, Master RW, Gordon SS, et al. Monitoring metabolic control in diabetic outpatients with glycosylated hemoglobin. Ann Intern Med 1980;92:357.

[69] Ditzel J, Kjaergaard JJ. Haemoglobin AIc concentrations after initial insulin treatment for newly discovered diabetes. BMJ 1978;1:741.

[70] Karlsson J, Kjellmer I. The outcome of diabetic pregnancies in relation to the mother's blood sugar level. Am J Obstet Gynecol 1972;112:213.

[71] Rohlfing CL, Wiedmeyer HM, Little RR, et al. Defining the relationship between plasma glucose and HbA(1c): analysis of glucose profiles and HbA(1c) in the Diabetes Control and Complications Trial. Diabetes Care 2002;25:275.

[72] de Veciana M, Major CA, Morgan MA, et al. Postprandial versus preprandial blood glucose monitoring in women with gestational diabetes mellitus requiring insulin therapy. N Engl J Med 1995;333:1237.

[73] Singer DE, Coley CM, Samet JH, et al. Tests of glycemia in diabetes mellitus. Their use in establishing a diagnosis and in treatment. Ann Intern Med 1989;110:125.

[74] Coetzee EJ, Jackson WP, Berman PA. Ketonuria in pregnancy–with special reference to calorie-restricted food intake in obese diabetics. Diabetes 1980;29:177.

[75] Sheehan EA, Beck F, Clarke CA, et al. Effects of beta-hydroxybutyrate on rat embryos grown in culture. Experientia 1985;41:273.

[76] Chez RA, Curcio FD III. Ketonuria in normal pregnancy. Obstet Gynecol 1987;69:272.

[77] Wyatt JW, Frias JL, Hoyme HE, et al, for the IONS study group. Congenital anomaly rate in offspring of pre-gestational diabetic women treated with insulin lispro during pregnancy. Diabet Med 2004;22(6):803–7.

[78] Coustan DR, Reece EA, Sherwin RS, et al. A randomized clinical trial of insulin pump vs. intensive conventional therapy in diabetic pregnancies. JAMA 1986;255:631.

[79] Rudolf MC, Coustan DR, Sherwin RS, et al. Efficacy of the insulin pump in the home treatment of pregnant patients. Diabetes 1981;30:891.

[80] Bornstein K, Jovanovic L. Type 1 diabetic woman and safe insulin protocols. In: Ruderman N, editor. ADA handbook on exercise in diabetes. Alexandria (VA): American Diabetes Association. Inc; 2002. pp. 511–32.

[81] Kitzmiller JL, Cloherty JP, Younger MD, et al. Diabetic pregnancy and perinatal morbidity. Am J Obstet Gynecol 1978;131(5):560–80.

[82] Landon MB, Gabbe SG, Brunner JP, et al. Doppler umbilical artery velocimetry in pregnancy complicated by insulin-dependent diabetes mellitus. Obstet Gynecol 1989;73:961.

[83] Benedetti TJ, Gabbe SG. Shoulder dystocia: a complication of fetal macrosomia and prolonged second stage of labor with mid-pelvic delivery. Obstet Gynecol 1978;52:526.

[84] Golditch IM, Kirkman K. The large fetus: management and outcome. Obstet Gynecol 1978; 52:26.

[85] Shepard MJ, Richards VA. An evaluation of two equations for predicting fetal weight by ultrasound. Am J Obstet Gynecol 1982;142:47.

[86] Milunsky A. Prenatal diagnosis of neural tube defects: VIII. the importance of serum alpha-fetoprotein screening in diabetic pregnant women. Am J Obstet Gynecol 1982;142:1030.

[87] Reece EA, Hobbins JC. Ultrasonography and diabetes mellitus in pregnancy. In: Sanders RG, editor. The principles and practice of ultrasonography in obstetrics and gynecology. 3rd edition. Norwalk (CT): Appleton-Century-Crofts; 1985. p. 297.

[88] Bracero L, Schulman H, Fleischer A. Umbilical artery velocimetry in diabetes and pregnancy. Obstet Gynecol 1986;68:654.

[89] Jovanovic L, Peterson CM. Insulin and glucose requirements during the first stage of labor in insulin-dependent diabetic women. Am J Med 1983;75:607.

[90] Jovanovic L. Glucose and insulin requirements during labor and delivery: the case for normoglycemia in pregnancies complicated by diabetes. Endocr Pract 2004;10:40–5.

[91] Jovanovic L, Peterson CM. Maternal milk and plasma glucose and insulin levels: studies in normal and diabetic subjects. J Am Coll Nutr 1989;8:125–31.

ELSEVIER
SAUNDERS

Endocrinol Metab Clin N Am
35 (2006) 99–116

ENDOCRINOLOGY
AND METABOLISM
CLINICS
OF NORTH AMERICA

Pituitary Disorders During Pregnancy

Mark E. Molitch, MD*

*Division of Endocrinology, Metabolism, and Molecular Medicine, Department of Medicine,
Northwestern University Feinberg School of Medicine, Chicago, IL, USA*

Anterior pituitary gland and pregnancy

Pituitary adenomas are common in women, constituting 5.7% of intracranial (malignant and nonmalignant) neoplasms, with an age-adjusted incidence rate of 0.82 cases/100,000 person-years [1]. These adenomas may cause problems in women because of oversecretion of hormones by the tumor and hypopituitarism. Hormonal dysfunction caused by pituitary adenomas may affect fertility and pregnancy outcome if pregnancy does ensue. In addition, the pregnancy itself alters hormone secretion and pituitary function, complicating the evaluation of patients with pituitary neoplasms. The need for preventing harm to the developing fetus influences therapeutic decisions for the mother.

During pregnancy, the normal pituitary gland enlarges considerably as a result of the estrogen-stimulated hyperplasia and hypertrophy of the prolactin-producing lactotrophs [2,3]. Concomitantly, prolactin levels increase gradually throughout gestation [4]. The elevated prolactin levels found at term prepare the breast for lactation. The finding of amenorrhea associated with hyperprolactinemia could be due to pregnancy and not due to pathologic hyperprolactinemia.

MRI scans of the pituitary during pregnancy show a size increase secondary to the lactotroph hyperplasia, with the peak size occurring in the first 3 days postpartum when gland heights of 12 mm may be seen [5–7]. After delivery, there is a rapid involution of the gland so that normal pituitary size is found by 6 months postpartum [6,7]. This stimulatory effect of pregnancy on the pituitary has important implications for a patient with a prolactinoma who desires pregnancy.

* Division of Endocrinology, Metabolism, and Molecular Medicine, Department of Medicine, Northwestern University Feinberg School of Medicine, 303 East Chicago Avenue, Tarry 15-731, Chicago, IL 60611.

E-mail address: molitch@northwestern.edu

Beginning in the second half of pregnancy, pituitary growth hormone (GH) secretion decreases, and the circulating level of a GH variant made by the syncytiotrophoblastic epithelium of the placenta increases to 10 to 20 ng/mL [8,9]. The decreased production of normal pituitary GH likely is caused by negative feedback effects of insulin-like growth factor type 1, which is stimulated by the placentally produced GH variant [8,9]. In patients with acromegaly who have autonomous GH secretion and become pregnant, both forms of GH persist in the blood throughout pregnancy [10].

During gestation, cortisol levels progressively increase, resulting in a 2 to 3 fold increase by term [11]. Most of the elevation of cortisol levels is due to the estrogen-induced increase in cortisol-binding globulin levels [12]. The bioactive "free" fraction also is elevated 3-fold, and the cortisol production rate is increased so that there is a 2 to 3 fold elevation in urinary free cortisol level [11,12]. Adrenocorticotropic hormone (ACTH) levels have been variously reported as being normal, suppressed, or elevated early in gestation [11,13]. Later in the pregnancy, however, there is a progressive increase, followed by a final surge of ACTH and cortisol levels during labor [11]. ACTH does not cross the placenta, but it is manufactured by the placenta [13]. The amounts of ACTH in serum that are of placental compared with pituitary origin at various stages of gestation are unknown. Corticotropin-releasing hormone (CRH) also is produced by the placenta and is released into maternal plasma [14]. The CRH is bioactive and may release ACTH from the placenta, in a paracrine fashion, and from the maternal pituitary [14]. The role of placental CRH in regulating ACTH and cortisol secretion during pregnancy in humans is unclear.

Thyroid-stimulating hormone (TSH) levels decrease in the first trimester, in response to the increased thyroid hormone levels that are stimulated by human chorionic gonadotropin, but return to the normal range by the third trimester [15]. In response to placental sex steroid production, hypothalamic gonadotropin releasing hormone (GnRH) and pituitary gonadotropin (follicle-stimulating hormone and luteinizing hormone) levels decline in the first trimester of pregnancy, with a blunted gonadotropin response to GnRH [16].

Prolactinoma

Hyperprolactinemia is responsible for about one third of all cases of female infertility [17]. Hyperprolactinemia impairs the hypothalamic-pituitary-ovarian axis at several levels, the primary site of inhibition being at the hypothalamus, where it inhibits the pulsatile secretion of GnRH [18]. The differential diagnosis of hyperprolactinemia is extensive [18].

For patients with prolactinomas, the choice of therapy may have important consequences for decisions regarding pregnancy. Transsphenoidal surgery is curative in 50% to 60% of cases and rarely causes hypopituitarism when it is performed on women with microadenomas. For patients with macroadenomas, surgery cures a much smaller number with a considerably greater risk of causing hypopituitarism and may affect fertility [18].

Dopamine agonists, including bromocriptine, pergolide (approved for the treatment of Parkinson's disease but not hyperprolactinemia in the United States), quinagolide (not approved in the United States), and cabergoline, have become the primary mode of therapy for almost all patients with prolactinomas. Bromocriptine, pergolide, and quinagolide can restore ovulatory menses in 70% to 80% of women, and cabergoline can restore ovulatory menses in greater than 90% [18–20]. When this restoration has been accomplished, and if pregnancy is desired, mechanical contraception is used until the first two or three cycles have occurred so that an intermenstrual interval can be established. In this way, a woman knows when she has missed a menstrual period, a pregnancy test can be performed quickly, and the precise gestational age of the fetus can be known. In this way, these drugs will have been given for only about 3 to 4 weeks of the gestation. Because of its long half-life in the body, however, cabergoline cessation at that point still results in a further fetal exposure for an additional 1 or more weeks.

In addition to their efficacy in lowering prolactin levels, the dopamine agonists often reduce tumor size of prolactin-secreting macroadenomas. Bromocriptine reduces the size by 50% or more in 50% to 75% of patients [18,20,21]. Pergolide reduces the size in 80% to 90% of patients, and cabergoline achieves such reductions in greater than 90% of patients in some series [18,20–23].

Effects of pregnancy on prolactinoma growth

In women with prolactinomas, the stimulatory effect of the hormonal milieu of pregnancy may result in significant tumor enlargement during gestation (Fig. 1). A review summarized 16 series reported during the years 1979–1985 totaling 246 women with microadenomas and 91 women with macroadenomas who became pregnant [24]. Subsequently, three series totaling an additional 130 women with microadenomas and 60 women with macroadenomas have been reported [25–27]. When these data are combined [24–27], only 6 of the 376 women (1.3%) with microadenomas had symptoms of tumor enlargement (headaches or visual disturbances or both) (Table 1). In no case was surgical intervention necessary. These series included 86 patients with macroadenomas who had not had prior surgery or irradiation. Of these, 20 (23.2%) had symptomatic tumor enlargement. During pregnancy, surgery was required in 4 patients, and bromocriptine was required in 15. Seventy-one women with macroadenomas had been treated with irradiation or surgery before pregnancy; only 2 of the 71 (2.8%) had symptomatic tumor enlargement. If tumor enlargement occurs, reinstitution of bromocriptine and cabergoline usually is successful in reducing the size of the tumor, but transsphenoidal surgery may be necessary [24,28].

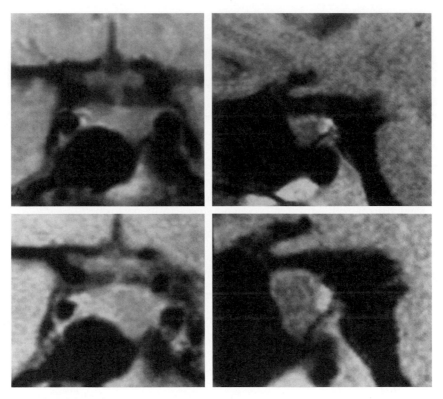

Fig. 1. Coronal and sagittal MRI scans of an intrasellar prolactin-secreting macroadenoma in a woman before conception (*top*) and at 7 months of gestation (*bottom*). Note the marked tumor enlargement at the latter point, at which time the patient was complaining of headaches. (*From* Molitch ME. Medical treatment of prolactinomas. Endocrinol Metab Clin North Am 1999;28:143–70.)

Effects of hyperprolactinemia and its treatment on pregnancy

Bromocriptine taken for only the first few weeks of gestation has not been associated with any increase in spontaneous abortions, ectopic pregnancies, trophoblastic disease, multiple pregnancies, or congenital malformations (Table 2) [29,30]. Long-term follow-up studies of 64 children between ages 6 months and 9 years whose mothers took bromocriptine in this fashion have shown no ill effects [31]. Experience with the use of bromocriptine

Table 1
Effect of pregnancy on prolactinomas

Tumor type	Prior therapy	No. of patients	Symptomatic enlargementa
Microadenomas	None	376	6 (1.3%)
Macroadenomas	None	86	20 (23.2%)
Macroadenomas	Yes	71	2 (2.8%)

Table 2
Effect of bromocriptine on pregnancies

Criteria	Bromocriptine		Normal population (%)
	No.	%	
Pregnancies	*6239*	*100.0*	*100.0*
Spontaneous abortion	620	9.9	10.0–15.0
Termination	75	1.2	—
Ectopic	31	0.5	0.5–1.0
Hydatidiform moles	11	0.2	0.05–0.7
Deliveries (known duration)	*4139*	*100.0*	*100.0*
At term (> 38 wk)	3620	87.5	85.0
Preterm (< 38 wk)	519	12.5	15.0
Deliveries (known outcome)	*5120*	*100.0*	*100.0*
Single births	5031	9.3	8.7
Multiple births	89	1.7	1.7
Infants (known details)	*5213*	*100.0*	*100.0*
Normal	5030	96.5	95.0
Who have malformations	93	1.8	3.0–4.0
Who have perinatal disorders	90	1.7	>2.0

Data from Krupp P, Monka C, Richter K The safety aspects of infertility treatments. In. Program of the Second World Congress of Gynecology and Obstetrics. Rio de Janeiro, Brazil, August 1988. p. 9.

throughout gestation is limited to only slightly more than 100 women, but no abnormalities were noted in the infants except one with an undescended testicle and one with a talipes deformity [32]. Because bromocriptine crosses the placenta [33], however, it should not be used any longer than necessary during pregnancy.

Pergolide has been shown to cross the placenta in mice, but no teratogenicity was seen in doses of 60 mg/kg/d [34]. Detailed data are available on the safety during early gestation for only one patient treated with pergolide for Parkinson's disease [35]. In this pregnancy, no teratogenicity or developmental abnormalities were found in the child, but the authors stated in this report that, "in premarketing studies of pergolide for endocrine disorders, two major and three minor congenital abnormalities were described among 38 pregnancies, but a causal relationship has not been established" [35]. Other information from the manufacturer (Eli Lilly & Co) stated that they had only limited data on pregnancies in which the fetus was exposed to pergolide, finding that 7.2% of pregnancy outcomes resulted in spontaneous abortions, 7.2% in minor malformations, 14.3% in intentional abortions, and 28.6% in healthy infants; for 43.4%, no information was available [36]. This limited information is sufficient to recommend against using pergolide when a woman wishes to get pregnant.

Some early publications reported no detrimental effects on pregnancy or fetal development in women who became pregnant during treatment with quinagolide [37]. A more recent review of 176 pregnancies, in which quinagolide was maintained for a median duration of 37 days, reported 24 spontaneous abortions, 1 ectopic pregnancy, and 1 stillbirth at 31 weeks' gestation [38]. Nine fetal malformations were reported in this group: spina bifida, trisomy 13, Down syndrome, talipes, cleft lip, arrhinencephaly, and Zellweger syndrome [38]. Quinagolide also should not be used if pregnancy is desired.

Cabergoline has been shown to cross the placenta in animal studies [16], but such data are lacking in humans. Data on exposure of the fetus or embryo during the first several weeks of pregnancy have been reported in more than 350 cases, and such use has not shown an increased percentage of spontaneous abortion, premature delivery, multiple gestation, or congenital abnormalities [39–43]. No alterations in newborn weights were observed [39–43]. Available data from 107 infants followed for 1 to 72 months showed normal physical and mental development [39].

With respect to using a dopamine agonist to facilitate ovulation and fertility, bromocriptine has the largest safety database and has a proven safety record for pregnancy. Although the database for cabergoline use in pregnancy is much smaller, it does not seem to exert any deleterious effects on pregnant women, and the incidence of malformation in their offspring is not greater than in the general population. For a woman who is intolerant to bromocriptine and who is doing well with cabergoline, continuation of cabergoline for facilitating pregnancy seems reasonable. The safety databases for pergolide and quinagolide are limited, but they seem to raise considerable concerns, so these drugs should not be used when fertility is desired. The effects of transsphenoidal surgery during gestation are not known specifically, but would not be expected to be significantly different from the effects of other types of surgery (unless hypopituitarism should ensue) [44].

Management of prolactinoma in pregnancy

The risks of surgery versus medical therapy for prolactinoma should be explained in detail to each patient. For patients with microadenomas or intrasellar macroadenomas, bromocriptine or cabergoline therapy generally is preferred to surgery because it is safe for the fetus when discontinued early in gestation, and it poses only a small risk of tumor enlargement for the mother. Such patients should be seen each trimester and assessed for symptoms such as headaches or visual problems; visual field testing needs to be done only when clinically indicated. When the tumor is large or extends to the optic chiasm or into the cavernous sinus, the following approaches should be considered: (1) preoperative surgical debulking, (2) intensive monitoring without bromocriptine therapy, or (3) continuous bromocriptine therapy. The safety of the last approach has not been established, but based on the few cases cited earlier, it probably is not harmful. Patients with macroadenomas should be seen monthly for such assessments, and visual fields should be tested each trimester. Prolactin levels, which normally increase in pregnancy, may not increase in women with prolactinomas [45]. Prolactin levels may not always increase with pregnancy-induced tumor enlargement [45]; periodic measurements of prolactin levels are of little benefit.

When there is evidence of tumor enlargement during pregnancy, bromocriptine therapy should be reinstituted immediately and the dosage increased as rapidly as tolerated. Such therapy must be monitored closely. If there is no response to bromocriptine, switching to cabergoline, transsphenoidal surgery, or delivery (if the pregnancy is far enough advanced) should be considered [24].

Although suckling stimulates prolactin secretion in normal women for the first few weeks to months postpartum, there are no data to suggest that breastfeeding can cause tumor growth. There seems to be no reason to discourage nursing in women with prolactinomas.

Acromegaly

Reports of pregnancy in patients with acromegaly are uncommon (< 100 cases) [46–54], perhaps because 30% to 40% of such patients have hyperprolactinemia [55]. Correction of hyperprolactinemia with bromocriptine may be necessary to permit ovulation and conception in these patients [47,53].

Diagnosis of acromegaly during pregnancy

Conventional radioimmunoassays for GH cannot distinguish between normal pituitary GH and the placental GH variant [8]. Special radioimmunoassays using antibodies that recognize specific epitopes on the two hormones [8] must be used. When such specific assays are not available, it may be necessary to wait until after delivery to assess pituitary GH secretion accurately because the placental variant decreases to undetectable levels within 24 hours [8]. There are two differences between the secretion of the placental GH variant and the secretion of pituitary GH during acromegaly, however, that may allow a distinction to be made during pregnancy. First, pituitary GH secretion in acromegaly is highly pulsatile, with 13 to 19 pulses per 24 hours [56], whereas secretion of the pregnancy GH variant is nonpulsatile [9]. Second, in acromegaly, about 70% of patients have a GH response to thyrotropin-releasing hormone [57], whereas the placental GH variant does not respond to this hormone [10].

Effects of pregnancy on tumor size and acromegaly

Only two patients with tumors secreting GH have been reported to have enlargement of their tumors with a resultant visual field defect in one during pregnancy [25,58]. Patients with acromegaly should be monitored for symptomatic tumor enlargement in a fashion similar to that for patients with prolactin-secreting macroadenomas. There is some evidence that pregnancy may cause an exacerbation of acromegaly in a few cases [47], but this does not seem to be a sufficient enough risk to advise against pregnancy.

Effects of acromegaly on pregnancy

Certain complications of acromegaly are potentially harmful to the mother and the fetus. Carbohydrate intolerance is present in 50% of patients with acromegaly, and overt diabetes is seen in 10% to 20% [55]. Insulin resistance secondary to the increased levels of GH may increase the risk of gestational diabetes. There is increased salt retention, and hypertension occurs in 25% to 35% of patients. In addition, cardiac disease is present in about one third of patients. There may be a specific cardiomyopathy associated with acromegaly, and coronary artery disease may be increased [55]. The risks for gestational diabetes, hypertension, and heart disease likely are increased in women with acromegaly during pregnancy.

Management of acromegaly and pregnancy

The considerations regarding the use of bromocriptine and cabergoline in women with prolactinomas also apply to women with acromegaly. For most patients, these drugs should not be continued during pregnancy. Data on the use of octreotide during pregnancy are limited. Only 14 pregnant patients treated with octreotide, octreotide long-acting-release, and lanreotide have been reported; no malformations were found in their children [54]. Octreotide crosses the placenta [59] and can affect developing fetal tissues. It does not bind with high affinity to the placenta and has no effect on the placental GH variant [60]. Because octreotide crosses the placenta, and because data documenting safety are limited, it is recommended that octreotide and other somatostatin analogues be discontinued if pregnancy is considered, and that contraception be used when these drugs are administered. Considering the prolonged nature of the course of most patients with acromegaly, interruption of medical therapy for 9 to 12 months should not have a particularly adverse effect on the long-term outcome. These drugs can control tumor growth, and for enlarging tumors, their reintroduction during pregnancy may be warranted versus operating.

Cushing's syndrome

Slightly more than 100 cases of Cushing's syndrome in pregnancy have been reported [61–76]. The distribution of causes of Cushing's syndrome in pregnancy differs markedly from that in the nonpregnant population. Less than 50% of pregnant patients described had pituitary adenomas, a similar number had adrenal adenomas, and more than 10% had adrenal carcinomas [61–73]. Only three reports have described pregnancies associated with the ectopic ACTH syndrome [63,67]. In many cases, the hypercortisolism first became apparent during pregnancy, with improvement after parturition, leading to the speculation that unregulated placental CRH was instrumental in causing this pregnancy-induced exacerbation [62,63,67,73]. Rarely, recurrent Cushing's syndrome may be associated with pregnancy only to remit completely after delivery; the cause for this has not been found [74,75].

Diagnosis of Cushing's syndrome during pregnancy

Diagnosing Cushing's syndrome during pregnancy may be difficult. Both conditions may be associated with weight gain in a central distribution, fatigue, edema, emotional upset, glucose intolerance, and hypertension. The striae associated with the weight gain and increased abdominal girth are usually white in normal pregnancy and red or purple in Cushing's syndrome. Hirsutism and acne may point to excessive androgen production.

The laboratory evaluation of Cushing's syndrome during pregnancy is not straightforward. Elevated total and free serum cortisol and ACTH levels and urinary free cortisol excretion are compatible with that of normal pregnancy. The overnight dexamethasone test usually shows inadequate suppression during normal pregnancy [64]. At least in the latter part of the third trimester, the elevated cortisol levels are not suppressed during the low-dose dexamethasone test, but are suppressed during the high-dose test, similar to what is observed in patients with Cushing's syndrome [62]. ACTH levels are normal to elevated in pregnant patients with all forms of Cushing's syndrome [61–66]. These normal rather than suppressed levels of ACTH in patients with adrenal adenomas may result from the production of ACTH by the placenta or from the nonsuppressible stimulation of pituitary ACTH by placental CRH.

A persistent circadian variation in the elevated levels of total and free serum cortisol during normal pregnancy may be most helpful in distinguishing Cushing's syndrome from the hypercortisolism of pregnancy because this finding is characteristically absent in all forms of Cushing's syndrome [12]. Salivary cortisol measurements may be useful in this regard, but normal limits for midnight levels of salivary cortisol during pregnancy have not yet been standardized [73]. In many cases, MRI of the pituitary (without contrast enhancement) or ultrasound of the adrenal may be required, although MRI of the pituitary in patients with Cushing's syndrome is often nondiagnostic. Little experience has been reported with newer techniques, such as CRH stimulation testing or petrosal venous sinus sampling during pregnancy. Ross and colleagues [65] found the typical exaggerated ACTH response to CRH in a woman with Cushing's syndrome, but Mellor and colleagues [72] found only a doubling of cortisol levels in response to CRH; neither patient had ill effects from such testing. In two patients studied by Lindsay and colleagues [76], ACTH levels increased more than threefold, but cortisol level increases were less than twofold. CRH testing during petrosal sinus sampling was performed without ill effects in one woman by Pinette and colleagues [68] and in four women by Lindsay and colleagues

[76], but catheterization was performed via the direct jugular vein approach rather than the femoral vein approach to minimize fetal irradiation; in these cases, clearly increased central-to-peripheral ACTH gradients were found.

Effects of Cushing's syndrome on pregnancy

Cushing's syndrome is associated with a fetal mortality of 25% from spontaneous abortion, stillbirth, and early neonatal death because of extreme prematurity [61–73,76]. Premature labor occurs in more than 50% of cases, regardless of cause [61–73,76]. The passage of cortisol across the placenta occasionally results in suppression of the fetal adrenals [69]. This passage seems to be uncommon, but the neonate should be tested for this potential problem and given exogenous corticosteroids until the results of the evaluation are known.

Maternal complications also may occur. Hypertension develops in most patients. Diabetes and myopathy are frequent. Postoperative wound infection and dehiscence are common after cesarean section. The pregnancy seems to induce an amelioration of Cushing's syndrome in some patients, but an exacerbation in others [61–67,73].

Management of Cushing's syndrome during pregnancy

In data from the literature summarized from two reviews [61,64], fetal loss rates of 9% and 24% and premature labor rates of 20% and 47% were found in 11 and 17 women who were treated during pregnancy compared with fetal loss rates of 30% and 38% and premature labor rates of 48% and 72% in 26 and 43 women in whom treatment was delayed. Treatment during pregnancy has been advocated [61,64,76].

Medical therapy for Cushing's syndrome during pregnancy is not very effective [63,64,73]. A few case reports have documented the efficacy of metyrapone [76]. Ketoconazole has been given to two patients with complications of intrauterine growth retardation, but no malformations or other perinatal disorders [70,71]. Use of other drugs, such as aminoglutethimide, mitotane, bromocriptine, and cyproheptadine, has been limited [73]; because of potential toxicity to the fetus, aminoglutethimide and mitotane should be avoided. Transsphenoidal resection of a pituitary ACTH-secreting adenoma has been performed successfully in several patients during the second trimester [62,65,68,69,72,73,76]. Although any surgery poses risks for the mother and fetus [44], with Cushing's syndrome, the risks of not operating seem to be considerably higher than the risks of proceeding with surgery.

Thyroid-stimulating hormone–secreting tumors

Only three cases of pregnancy occurring in women with TSH-secreting tumors have been reported [77–79]. In one of these cases, octreotide, which had been stopped, had to be reinstituted to control tumor size [77], and in a second, octreotide was continued during pregnancy for tumor size control. The most pressing issue with such tumors is the need to control hyperthyroidism during pregnancy, and that can be done with standard antithyroid drugs [78]. With growing macroadenomas, octreotide may be necessary for tumor size control [77,79].

Clinically nonfunctioning adenomas

Pregnancy would not be expected to influence tumor size in patients with clinically nonfunctioning adenomas, and only two cases have been reported in which tumor enlargement during pregnancy resulted in a visual field defect [25,80]. The lactotroph hyperplasia that occurs during pregnancy can be quite significant, however [2,3]. MRI obtained during pregnancy and the immediate postpartum period has shown that this hyperplasia may cause the normal pituitary to increase to 12 mm in height [5–7]. It would be expected that if this lactotroph hyperplasia were to occur in a patient with a preexisting clinically nonfunctioning adenoma, this hyperplasia could push up the clinically nonfunctioning adenoma to cause chiasmal compression or headaches. In the second case reported, the patient responded rapidly to bromocriptine treatment, probably owing to shrinkage of the lactotroph hyperplasia with decompression of the chiasm and probably with little or no direct effect on the tumor itself [80]. Most clinically nonfunctioning adenomas are gonadotroph adenomas [81]. Two patients have been reported who had gonadotroph adenomas secreting intact follicle-stimulating hormone with a resultant ovarian hyperstimulation syndrome [82,83]; both became pregnant, one after having the follicle-stimulating hormone hypersecretion controlled by bromocriptine [82] and the second after surgical removal of the tumor [83].

Hypopituitarism

Hypopituitarism may occur because of tumor compression of the hypothalamus or pituitary stalk or from prior neurosurgery. Hormone deficits can be partial or complete, and loss of gonadotropin secretion is common. Induction of ovulation may be difficult, and a variety of techniques have been used, including administration of human chorionic gonadotropin and follicle-stimulating hormone (in the past as human menopausal gonadotropin) [84–87], pulsatile GnRH [88–90], and in vitro fertilization [91].

In women, the only hormone replacements to be considered during pregnancy are thyroid and adrenal hormones. Because of the increased thyroxine turnover that occurs during pregnancy, thyroxine levels decrease, and TSH levels increase with a fixed thyroxine dose over the course of gestation [15,92]. The average increase in thyroxine needed in these patients is about 0.05 mg/d. Because patients with hypothalamic-pituitary dysfunction may not elevate their TSH levels normally in the face of increased need for thyroxine, it may be appropriate to increase the thyroxine supplementation by 0.025 mg after the first trimester and by an additional 0.025 mg after the second trimester. There are no data to support this approach, however.

Because the cortisol production rate normally is increased in pregnancy [11,12], the dose of long-term glucocorticoid replacement theoretically ought to be increased during pregnancy. This dose increase does not seem to be necessary in practice, however, and patients usually can be kept on their standard replacement doses of glucocorticoids. Additional glucocorticoids are needed for the stress of labor and delivery, such as 75 mg of hydrocortisone intravenously every 8 hours with rapid tapering postpartum. If there is significant stress during the pregnancy, such as infection, that would require prolonged high doses of glucocorticosteroids, the steroid of choice is prednisolone, which does not cross the placenta [93]. Even high doses of prednisone are generally quite safe [94], however, and suppression of neonatal adrenal function in offspring of women taking prednisone during pregnancy is rare [95]. Glucocorticoids also may pass to the neonate in breast milk, but the amounts (0.14% of maternal blood levels) are not sufficient to alter neonatal adrenal function, even with large maternal doses of prednisone [96].

Lymphocytic hypophysitis

Lymphocytic hypophysitis usually presents in the peripartum period as a mass lesion indistinguishable from a pituitary adenoma. It is characterized by massive infiltration of the pituitary by lymphocytes and plasma cells with destruction of the normal parenchyma. The disorder is thought to have an autoimmune basis. Most cases occur in association with pregnancy, and women present during pregnancy or postpartum with symptoms of varying degrees of hypopituitarism or symptoms related to the mass lesion, such as headaches or visual field defects. Mild hyperprolactinemia and diabetes insipidus also may be found. On CT or MRI, a sellar mass is found, which may extend in an extrasellar fashion and may cause visual field defects. The condition usually is confused with that of a pituitary tumor and cannot be distinguished from a tumor except by biopsy. By virtue of the hypopituitarism it produces, lymphocytic hypophysitis also can be confused clinically with Sheehan's syndrome except that there is no history of obstetric hemorrhage [97,98].

The diagnosis of lymphocytic hypophysitis should be considered in women with symptoms of hypopituitarism or mass lesions of the sella during pregnancy or postpartum, especially in the absence of a history of obstetric hemorrhage. An evaluation of pituitary function and CT or MRI are warranted. If prolactin levels are only modestly elevated (< 150 ng/mL) in the presence of a large mass, the diagnosis is unlikely to be an enlarging prolactinoma and more likely to be hypophysitis or a nonsecreting tumor.

Hormone replacement therapy should be instituted promptly when hypopituitarism is determined to be present. For unclear reasons, there seems to be a particular predilection for impaired ACTH secretion, and this axis must be evaluated carefully and treated to avoid adrenal insufficiency [99]. Unless there are visual field defects, uncontrollable headaches, or radiologic evidence of progressive enlargement of the sellar mass, rapid surgical intervention is not warranted because some women may undergo a spontaneous regression of the mass and return of pituitary function [99–101]. Surgery generally does not result in improvement in endocrine function, however [102,103]. Although high doses of glucocorticoids have been advocated to reduce the inflammation [103], there have been no controlled studies documenting the benefit of this approach, and the author does not recommend this.

Sheehan's syndrome

Sheehan's syndrome consists of pituitary necrosis secondary to ischemia occurring within hours of delivery [104,105]. It is usually secondary to hypotension and shock from an obstetric hemorrhage. Pituitary enlargement during pregnancy apparently predisposes to the risk for ischemia with occlusive spasm of the arteries to the anterior pituitary and stalk [104,105]. The degree of ischemia and necrosis dictates the subsequent patient course. Modern obstetric techniques have resulted in Sheehan's syndrome being found rarely in current practice [106].

Acute necrosis is suspected in the setting of an obstetric hemorrhage in which hypotension and tachycardia persist after adequate replacement of blood products. In addition, the woman fails to lactate and may have hypoglycemia [104,105,107]. Investigation should include levels of ACTH, cortisol, prolactin, and free thyroxine. The ACTH stimulation test would be normal because the adrenal cortex would not be atrophied. Thyroxine levels may prove normal initially because the hormone has a half-life of 7 days. Prolactin levels are usually low, although they are generally 5- to 10-fold elevated in the puerperium. Treatment with saline and stress doses of corticosteroids should be instituted immediately after drawing the blood tests. Additional pituitary testing with subsequent therapy should be delayed until recovery. Diabetes insipidus also may occur secondary to vascular occlusion with atrophy and scarring of the neurohypophysis [108].

When milder forms of infarction occur, the diagnosis of Sheehan's syndrome may be delayed for months or years [107,108]. These women generally have a history of amenorrhea, decreased libido, failure to lactate, breast atrophy, loss of pubic and axillary hair, fatigue, and symptoms of secondary adrenal insufficiency with nausea, vomiting, diarrhea, and abdominal pain [107,108]. Some women experience only partial hypopituitarism and may have normal menses and fertility [109]. Although women may have episodes of transient polydipsia and polyuria, many have impaired urinary concentrating ability and deficient vasopressin secretion [110]. CT or MRI generally reveal partial or completely empty sellae [111].

References

[1] Central Brain Tumor Registry of the United States (CTBRUS). Statistical report: primary brain tumors in the US 1997–2001.Available at: http://www.cbtrus.org/. Accessed April 8, 2005.

[2] Goluboff LG, Ezrin C. Effect of pregnancy on the somatotroph and the prolactin cell of the human adenohypophysis. J Clin Endocrinol Metab 1969;29:1533–8.

[3] Scheithauer BW, Sano T, Kovacs KT, et al. The pituitary gland in pregnancy: a clinicopathologic and immunohistochemical study of 69 cases. Mayo Clin Proc 1990;65:461–74.

[4] Rigg LA, Lein A, Yen SSC. Pattern of increase in circulating prolactin levels during human gestation. Am J Obstet Gynecol 1977;129:454–6.

[5] Gonzalez JG, Elizondo G, Saldivar D, et al. Pituitary gland growth during normal pregnancy: an in vivo study using magnetic resonance imaging. Am J Med 1988;85:217–20.

[6] Elster AD, Sanders TG, Vines FS, Chen MYM. Size and shape of the pituitary gland during pregnancy and post partum: measurement with MR imaging. Radiology 1991;181: 531–5.

[7] Dinç H, Esen F, Demirci A, et al. Pituitary dimensions and volume measurements in pregnancy and post partum: MR assessment. Acta Radiol 1998;39:64–9.

[8] Frankenne F, Closset J, Gomez F, et al. The physiology of growth hormones (GHs) in pregnant women and partial characterization of the placental GH variant. J Clin Endocrinol Metab 1988;66:1171–80.

[9] Eriksson L, Frankenne F, Eden S, et al. Growth hormone 24-h serum profiles during pregnancy lack of pulsatility for the secretion of the placental variant. Br J Obstet Gynaecol 1989;106:949–53.

[10] Beckers A, Stevenaert A, Foidart J-M, et al. Placental and pituitary growth hormone secretion during pregnancy in acromegalic women. J Clin Endocrinol Metab 1990;71:725–31.

[11] Carr BR, Parker CR Jr, Madden JD, et al. Maternal plasma adrenocorticotropin and cortisol relationships throughout human pregnancy. Am J Obstet Gynecol 1981;139:416–22.

[12] Nolten WE, Lindheimer MD, Rueckert PA, et al. Diurnal patterns and regulation of cortisol secretion in pregnancy. J Clin Endocrinol Metab 1980;51:466–72.

[13] Rees LH, Burke CW, Chard T, et al. Possible placental origin of ACTH in normal human pregnancy. Nature 1975;254:620–2.

[14] Sasaki A, Shinkawa O, Yoshinaga K. Placental corticotropin-releasing hormone may be a stimulator of maternal pituitary adrenocorticotropic hormone secretion in humans. J Clin Invest 1989;84:1997–2001.

[15] Glinoer D. The regulation of thyroid function in pregnancy: pathways of endocrine adaptation from physiology to pathology. Endocr Rev 1997;18:404–33.

[16] Jeppsson S, Rannevik G, Liedholm P, Thorell JI. Basal and LHRH stimulated secretion of FSH during pregnancy. Am J Obstet Gynecol 1977;127:32–6.

[17] Kredentser JV, Hoskins CF, Scott JZ. Hyperprolactinemia: a significant factor in female infertility. Am J Obstet Gynecol 1981;139:264–7.

[18] Molitch ME. Disorders of prolactin secretion. Endocrinol Metab Clin North Am 2001;30: 585–610.

[19] Webster J, Piscitelli G, Polli A, et al. A comparison of cabergoline and bromocriptine in the treatment of hyperprolactinemic amenorrhea. N Engl J Med 1994;331:904–9.

[20] Molitch ME. Dopamine resistance of prolactinomas. Pituitary 2003;6:19–27.

[21] Bevan JS, Webster J, Burke CW, Scanlon MF. Dopamine agonist and pituitary tumor shrinkage. Endocr Rev 1992;13:220–40.

[22] Biller BMK, Molitch ME, Vance ML, et al. Treatment of prolactin-secreting macroadenomas with the once-weekly dopamine agonist cabergoline. J Clin Endocrinol Metab 1996;81: 2338–43.

[23] Colao A, DiSarno A, Landi ML, et al. Macroprolactinoma shrinkage during cabergoline treatment is greater in naïve patients than in patients pretreated with other dopamine agonists: a prospective study of 110 patients. J Clin Endocrinol Metab 2000;85:2247–52.

[24] Molitch ME. Pregnancy and the hyperprolactinemic woman. N Engl J Med 1985;312: 1364–70.

[25] Kupersmith MJ, Rosenberg C, Kleinberg D. Visual loss in pregnant women with pituitary adenomas. Ann Intern Med 1994;121:473–7.

[26] Rossi AM, Vilska S, Heinonen PK. Outcome of pregnancies in women with treated or untreated hyperprolactinemia. Eur J Obstet Gynaecol Reprod Biol 1995;63:143–6.

[27] Musolino NRC, Bronstein MD. Prolactinomas and pregnancy. In: Bronstein MD, editor. Pituitary tumors and pregnancy. Norwell (MA): Kluwer Academic Publishers; 2001. p. 91–108.

[28] Liu C, Tyrrell JB. Successful treatment of a large macroprolactinoma with cabergoline during pregnancy. Pituitary 2001;4:179–85.

[29] Krupp P, Monka C, Richter K. The safety aspects of infertility treatments. In: Program of the Second World Congress of Gynecology and Obstetrics, Rio de Janeiro, Brazil, 1988. p. 9.

[30] Krupp P, Monka C. Bromocriptine in pregnancy: safety aspects. Klin Wochenschr 1987;65: 823–7.

[31] Raymond JP, Goldstein E, Konopka P, et al. Follow-up of children born of bromocriptine-treated mothers. Horm Res 1985;22:239–46.

[32] Konopka P, Raymond JP, Merceron RE, Seneze J. Continuous administration of bromocriptine in the prevention of neurological complications in pregnant women with prolactinomas. Am J Obstet Gynecol 1983;146:935–8.

[33] Bigazzi M, Ronga R, Lancranjan I, et al. A pregnancy in an acromegalic woman during bromocriptine treatment: effects on growth hormone and prolactin in the maternal, fetal, and amniotic compartments. J Clin Endocrinol Metab 1979;48:9–12.

[34] Buelke-Sam J, Byrd RA, Johnson JA, et al. Developmental toxicity of the dopamine agonist pergolide mesylate in CD-1 mice: I. gestational exposure. Neurotoxicol Teratol 1991;13: 283–95.

[35] De Mari M, Zenzola A, Lamberti P. Antiparkinsonian treatment in pregnancy. Mov Disord 2002;17:428–9.

[36] Acharya V. Review of pregnancy reports in patients on pergolide treatment. Data on file. Indianapolis (IN): Eli Lilly & Co; 2004.

[37] Morange I, Barlier A, Pellegrini I, et al. Prolactinomas resistant to bromocriptine: long-term efficacy of quinagolide and outcome of pregnancy. Eur J Endocrinol 1996;135: 413–20.

[38] Webster J. A comparative review of the tolerability profiles of dopamine agonists in the treatment of hyperprolactinaemia and inhibition of lactation. Drug Saf 1996;14:228–38.

[39] Robert E, Musatti L, Piscitelli G, Ferrari CI. Pregnancy outcome after treatment with the ergot derivative, cabergoline. Reprod Toxicol 1996;10:333–7.

[40] Garceau R. Pregnancies reported to Pharmacia Upjohn in patients receiving cabergoline. Data on file. Kalamazoo (MI): Pharmacia & Upjohn; 1997.

[41] Verhelst J, Abs R, Maiter D, et al. Cabergoline in the treatment of hyperprolactinemia: a study in 455 patients. J Clin Endocrinol Metab 1999;84:2518–22.

[42] Ricci E, Parazzini F, Motta T, et al. Pregnancy outcome after cabergoline treatment in early weeks of gestation. Reprod Toxicol 2002;16:791–3.

[43] Musolino NRC, Bronstein MD. Prolactinomas and pregnancy. In: Bronstein MD, editor. Pituitary tumors and pregnancy. Norwell (MA): Kluwer Academic Publishers; 2001. p. 91–108.

[44] Brodsky JB, Cohen EN, Brown BW Jr, et al. Surgery during pregnancy and fetal outcome. Am J Obstet Gynecol 1980;138:1165–7.

[45] Divers WA, Yen SSC. Prolactin-producing microadenomas in pregnancy. Obstet Gynecol 1983;62:425–9.

[46] Colao A, Merola B, Ferone D, Lombardi G. Acromegaly. J Clin Endocrinol Metab 1997; 82:2777–81.

[47] Herman-Bonert V, Seliverstow M, Melmed S. Pregnancy in acromegaly: successful therapeutic outcome. J Clin Endocrinol Metab 1998;83:727–31.

[48] Mozas J, Ocón E, López de la Torre M, et al. Successful pregnancy in a woman with acromegaly treated with somatostatin analog (octreotide) prior to surgical resection. Int J Gynecol Obstet 1999;65:71–3.

[49] DeMenis E, Billeci D, Marton E. Uneventful pregnancy in an acromegalic patient treated with slow-release lanreotide: a case report. J Clin Endocrinol Metab 1999;84:1489.

[50] Hierl T, Ziegler R, Kasperk C. Pregnancy in persistent acromegaly. Clin Endocrinol (Oxf) 2000;53:262–3.

[51] Neal JM. Successful pregnancy in a woman with acromegaly treated with octreotide. Endocr Pract 2000;6:148–50.

[52] Fassnacht M, Capeller B, Arlt W, et al. Octreotide LAR treatment throughout pregnancy in an acromegalic woman. Clin Endocrinol (Oxf) 2001;55:411–5.

[53] Bronstein MD, Salgado LR, Musolino NR. Medical management of pituitary adenomas: the special case of management of the pregnant woman. Pituitary 2002;5:99–107.

[54] Serri O, Lanoie G. Successful pregnancy in a woman with acromegaly treated with octreotide long-acting release. Endocrinologist 2003;13:17–9.

[55] Molitch ME. Clinical manifestations of acromegaly. Endocrinol Metab Clin North Am 1992;21:597–614.

[56] Barkan AL, Stred SE, Reno K, et al. Increased growth hormone pulse frequency in acromegaly. J Clin Endocrinol Metab 1989;69:1225–33.

[57] Chang-DeMoranville BM, Jackson IMD. Diagnosis and endocrine testing in acromegaly. Endocrinol Metab Clin North Am 1992;21:649–68.

[58] Okada Y, Morimoto I, Ejima K, et al. A case of active acromegalic woman with a marked increase in serum insulin-like growth factor-1 levels after delivery. Endocr J 1997;44:117–20.

[59] Caron P, Gerbeau C, Pradayrol L. Maternal-fetal transfer of octreotide. N Engl J Med 1995;333:601–2.

[60] Caron P, Buscail L, Beckers A, et al. Expression of somatostatin receptor SST4 in human placenta and absence of octreotide effect on human placental growth hormone concentration during pregnancy. J Clin Endocrinol Metab 1997;82:3771–6.

[61] Bevan JS, Gough MH, Gillmer MD, Burke CW. Cushing's syndrome in pregnancy: the timing of definitive treatment. Clin Endocrinol (Oxf) 1987;27:225–33.

[62] Casson IF, Davis JC, Jeffreys RV, et al. Successful management of Cushing's disease during pregnancy by transsphenoidal adenectomy. Clin Endocrinol (Oxf) 1987;27:423–8.

[63] Aron DC, Schnall AM, Sheeler LR. Cushing's syndrome and pregnancy. Am J Obstet Gynecol 1990;162:244–52.

[64] Buescher MA, McClamrock HD, Adashi EY. Cushing's syndrome in pregnancy. Obstet Gynecol 1992;79:130–7.

[65] Ross RJ, Chew SL, Perry L, et al. Diagnosis and selective cure of Cushing's disease during pregnancy by transsphenoidal surgery. Eur J Endocrinol 1995;132:722–6.

[66] Chico A, Manzanares JM, Halperin I, et al. Cushing's disease and pregnancy. Eur J Obstet Gynaecol Reprod Biol 1996;64:143–6.

[67] Guilhaume B, Sanson ML, Billaud L, et al. Cushing's syndrome and pregnancy: aetiologies and prognosis in twenty-two patients. Eur J Med 1992;1:83–9.

[68] Pinette MG, Pan YQ, Oppenheim D, et al. Bilateral inferior petrosal sinus corticotropin sampling with corticotropin-releasing hormone stimulation in a pregnant patient with Cushing's syndrome. Am J Obstet Gynecol 1994;171:563–4.

[69] Kreines K, DeVaux WD. Neonatal adrenal insufficiency associated with maternal Cushing's syndrome. Pediatrics 1971;47:516–9.

[70] Amado JA, Pesquera C, Gonzalez EM, et al. Successful treatment with ketoconazole of Cushing's syndrome in pregnancy. Postgrad Med J 1990;66:221–3.

[71] Berwaerts J, Verhelst J, Mahler C. Abs R. Cushing's syndrome in pregnancy treated by ketoconazole: case report and review of the literature. Gynecol Endocrinol 1999;13: 175–82.

[72] Mellor A, Harvey RD, Pobereskin LH, Sneyd JR. Cushing's disease treated by trans-sphenoidal selective adenomectomy in mid-pregnancy. Br J Anaesth 1998;80:850–2.

[73] Madhun ZT, Aron DC. Cushing's disease in pregnancy. In: Bronstein MD, editor. Pituitary tumors and pregnancy. Norwell (MA): Kluwer Academic Publishers; 2001. p. 149–72.

[74] Wallace C, Toth EL, Lewanczuk RZ, Siminoski K. Pregnancy-induced Cushing's syndrome in multiple pregnancies. J Clin Endocrinol Metab 1996;81:15–21.

[75] Hána V, Dokoupilová M, Marek J, Plavka R. Recurrent ACTH-independent Cushing's syndrome in multiple pregnancies and its treatment with metyrapone. Clin Endocrinol (Oxf) 2001;54:277–81.

[76] Lindsay JR, Jonklaas J, Oldfield EH, Nieman LK. Cushing's syndrome during pregnancy: personal experience and review of the literature. J Clin Endocrinol Metab 2005;90: 3077–83.

[77] Caron P, Gerbeau C, Pradayrol L, et al. Successful pregnancy in an infertile woman with a thyrotropin-secreting macroadenoma treated with the somatostatin analog (octreotide). J Clin Endocrinol Metab 1996;81:1164–8.

[78] Blackhurst G, Strachan MW, Collie D, et al. The treatment of a thyrotropin-secreting pituitary macroadenoma with octreotide in twin pregnancy. Clin Endocrinol (Oxf) 2002;56: 401–4.

[79] Chaiamnuay S, Moster M, Katz MR, Kim YN. Successful management of a pregnant woman with a TSH secreting pituitary adenoma with surgical and medical therapy. Pituitary 2003;6:109–13.

[80] Masding MG, Lees PD, Gawne-Cain ML, Sandeman DD. Visual field compression by a non-secreting pituitary tumour during pregnancy. J R Soc Med 2003;96:27–8.

[81] Molitch ME. Clinically non-functioning adenomas. In: Bronstein MD, editor. Pituitary tumors and pregnancy. Norwell (MA): Kluwer Academic Publishers; 2001. p. 123–9.

[82] Murata Y, Ando H, Nagasaka T, et al. Successful pregnancy after bromocriptine therapy in an anovulatory woman complicated with ovarian hyperstimulation caused by follicle-stimulating hormone-producing plurihormonal pituitary microadenoma. J Clin Endocrinol Metab 2003;88:1988–93.

[83] Sugita T, Seki K, Nagai Y, et al. Successful pregnancy and delivery after removal of gonadotrope adenoma secreting follicle-stimulating hormone in a 29-year-old amenorrheic woman. Gynecol Obstet Invest 2005;59:138–43.

[84] Golan A, Abramov L, Yedwab G, David MP. Pregnancy in panhypopituitarism. Gynecol Obstet Invest 1990;29:232–4.

[85] Verdu LI, Martin-Caballero C, Garcia-Lopez G, Cueto MJ. Ovulation induction and normal pregnancy after panhypopituitarism due to lymphocytic hypophysitis. Obstet Gynecol 1998;91:850–2.

[86] Volz J, Heinrich U, Volz-Köster S. Conception and spontaneous delivery after total hypophysectomy. Fertil Steril 2002;77:624–5.

[87] Kitajima Y, Endo T, Yamazaki K, et al. Successful twin pregnancy in panhypopituitarism caused by suprasellar germinoma. Obstet Gynecol 2003;102:1205–7.

[88] Gompel A, Mauvais-Jarvis P. Induction of ovulation with pulsatile GnRH in hypothalamic amenorrhea. Hum Reprod 1988;3:473–7.

[89] Martin KA, Hall JE, Adams JM, Crowley WF Jr. Comparison of exogenous gonadotropins and pulsatile gonadotropin-releasing hormone for induction of ovulation in hypogonadotropic amenorrhea. J Clin Endocrinol Metab 1993;77:125–9.

[90] Hall JE, Martin KA, Whitney HA, et al. Potential for fertility with replacement of hypothalamic gonadotropin-releasing hormone in long term female survivors of cranial tumors. J Clin Endocrinol Metab 1994;79:1166–72.

[91] Suganuma N, Furuhashi M, Ando T, et al. Successful pregnancy and delivery after in vitro fertilization and embryo transfer in a patient with primary hypopituitarism. Fertil Steril 2000;73:1057–8.

[92] Mandel SJ, Larsen PR, Seely EW, Brent GA. Increased need for thyroxine during pregnancy in women with primary hypothyroidism. N Engl J Med 1990;323:91–6.

[93] Beitins IZ, Bayard F, Ances IG, et al. The transplacental passage of prednisone and prednisolone in pregnancy near term. J Pediatr 1972;81:936–45.

[94] Turner ES, Greenberger PA, Patterson R. Management of the pregnant asthmatic patient. Ann Intern Med 1980;93:905–18.

[95] Kenny FM, Preeyasombat C, Spaulding JS, Migeon CJ. Cortisol production rate: IV. infants born of steroid-treated mothers and of diabetic mothers: infants with trisomy syndrome and with anencephaly. Pediatrics 1966;37:960–6.

[96] McKenzie SA, Selley JA, Agnew JE. Secretion of prednisolone into breast milk. Arch Dis Child 1975;50:894–6.

[97] Thodou E, Asa SL, Kontogeorgos G, et al. Lymphocytic hypophysitis: clinicopathological findings. J Clin Endocrinol Metab 1995;80:2302–11.

[98] Pressman EK, Zeidman SM, Reddy UM, et al. Differentiating lymphocytic adenohypophysitis from pituitary adenoma in the peripartum patient. J Reprod Med 1995;40:251–9.

[99] Gillam M, Molitch ME. Lymphocytic hypophysitis. In: Bronstein MD, editor. Pituitary tumors and pregnancy. Norwell (MA): Kluwer Academic Publishers; 2001. p. 131–48.

[100] Leiba S, Schindel B, Weinstein R, et al. Spontaneous postpartum regression of pituitary mass with return of function. JAMA 1986;255:230–2.

[101] McGrail KM, Beyerl BD, Black PM, et al. Lymphocytic adenohypophysitis of pregnancy with complete recovery. Neurosurgery 1987;20:791–3.

[102] Leung GK, Lopes MB, Thorner MO, et al. Primary hypophysitis: a single-center experience in 16 cases. J Neurosurg 2004;101:262–71.

[103] Caturegli P, Newschaffer C, Olivi A, et al. Autoimmune hypophysitis. Endocr Rev 2005; 26(5):599–614.

[104] Sheehan HL, Davis JC. Pituitary necrosis. Br Med Bull 1968;24:59–70.

[105] Keleştimur F. Sheehan's syndrome. Pituitary 2003;6:181–8.

[106] Feinberg E, Molitch M, Peaceman A. Frequency of Sheehan's syndrome. Fertil Steril 2005;84:975–9.

[107] Ozbey N, Inanc S, Aral F, et al. Clinical and laboratory evaluation of 40 patients with Sheehan's syndrome. Isr J Med Sci 1994;30:826–9.

[108] Sheehan HL. The neurohypophysis in post-partum hypopituitarism. J Pathol Bacteriol 1963;85:145–69.

[109] Grimes HG, Brooks MH. Pregnancy in Sheehan's syndrome: report of a case and review. Obstet Gynecol Surv 1980;35:481–8.

[110] Iwasaki Y, Oiso Y, Yamauchi K, et al. Neurohypophyseal function in post-partum hypopituitarism: impaired plasma vasopressin response to osmotic stimuli. J Clin Endocrinol Metab 1989;68:560–5.

[111] Bakiri F, Bendib S-E, Maoui R, et al. The sella turcica in Sheehan's syndrome: computerized tomographic study in 54 patients. J Endocrinol Invest 1991;14:193–6.

**ELSEVIER
SAUNDERS**

Endocrinol Metab Clin N Am
35 (2006) 117–136

ENDOCRINOLOGY
AND METABOLISM
CLINICS
OF NORTH AMERICA

Thyroid Disorders During Pregnancy

Shane O. LeBeau, MD[a], Susan J. Mandel, MD, MPH[b],*

[a]*Division of Endocrinology and Metabolism, Department of Medicine, University of
Pittsburgh Medical Center, Pittsburgh, PA, USA*
[b]*Division of Endocrinology, Diabetes, and Metabolism, University of Pennsylvania School of
Medicine, Philadelphia, PA, USA*

Thyroid disorders are common among women of childbearing years. Thyroid dysfunction often is overlooked in pregnant women, however, because of nonspecific symptoms and the hypermetabolic state of normal pregnancy. Compounding the diagnosis further is the alteration in thyroid physiology that normally occurs during gestation. A clinician first must consider thyroid dysfunction a possibility, then differentiate normal physiologic changes from true disease. When thyroid dysfunction is recognized, proper management is essential for a healthy pregnancy. Abnormalities in maternal thyroid function can adversely affect the fetus directly by way of the transplacental passage of abnormal maternal hormone concentrations, thyroid-stimulating hormone (TSH) receptor antibodies, or prescribed antithyroid medications and indirectly by way of the altered maternal gravid physiology.

Normal gravid thyroid physiology

Several alterations in thyroid physiology occur during normal pregnancy. These changes take place at different times of gestation, are reversible postpartum, and collectively stimulate the maternal thyroid gland. Hypothyroid women who receive levothyroxine replacement require a 25% to 47% average dosage increase during pregnancy to maintain normal serum TSH concentrations [1–3]. Thyroidal stimulation is supported further by the findings of increased serum thyroid stimulating hormone (TSH) and thyroglobulin concentrations, relative hypothyroxinemia, and occasional goiter formation in pregnant women from areas of borderline iodine sufficiency [4].

---

* Corresponding author. Division of Endocrinology, Diabetes, and Metabolism, Department of Medicine, University of Pennsylvania School of Medicine, 415 Curie Boulevard, 611 CRB, Philadelphia, PA 19104.

E-mail address: smandel@mail.med.upenn.edu (S.J. Mandel).

0889-8529/06/$ - see front matter © 2005 Elsevier Inc. All rights reserved.
doi:10.1016/j.ecl.2005.09.009   *endo.theclinics.com*

The most recognized alteration in maternal thyroid physiology is the increase in thyroxine-binding globulin (TBG). This increase begins early in the first trimester, plateaus during midgestation, and persists until shortly after delivery [5]. Elevated TBG results from a decrease in its hepatic clearance, owing to estrogen-induced sialylation [6]. The increased concentration of TBG expands the extrathyroidal pool, triggering a concomitant increase in maternal thyroid hormone synthesis and elevation of total thyroxine (T_4) and triiodothyronine (T_3) levels [5]. In addition to TBG, maternal glomerular filtration rate is increased during early gestation and maintained throughout pregnancy; this results in an increased renal clearance of iodide, which indirectly stimulates the maternal thyroid machinery [7]. Lastly, transplacental passage of T_4 and iodide and placental metabolism of iodothyronines stimulate the maternal thyroid by depleting the maternal circulation of thyroid hormone and its precursors [8].

In addition to indirect stimuli, there is strong evidence that human chorionic gonadotropin (hCG) has intrinsic thyrotropic activity. A significant degree of homology exists between the hormone-specific β-subunits and the extracellular receptor binding domains of hCG and TSH [9,10]. hCG secretion begins shortly after conception, peaks around gestational week 10, and gradually declines thereafter to a nadir by about week 20 [5]. It is believed that the high serum concentrations of hCG during early pregnancy directly activate the TSH receptor. This belief is substantiated by the finding that serum hCG concentrations during early pregnancy are negatively correlated with serum TSH concentrations and positively correlated with free T_4 concentrations [5,11]. Serum TSH concentrations vary throughout pregnancy, with the first-trimester values being lower than the values before conception and during the second and third trimesters [12]. Using an assay with a detection limit of 0.05 mU/L, researchers found that during the first trimester, 9% of pregnant women without thyrotoxic symptoms had subnormal serum TSH concentrations (> 0.05 mU/L, but < 0.4 mU/L), whereas an additional 9% had suppressed concentrations (< 0.05 mU/L) [13]. Ultimately, the nadir of maternal serum TSH levels mirrors the peak in hCG concentrations [5]. A more recent study has reported the upper 95% confidence interval (CI) for serum TSH levels in the first trimester to be 2.5 mU/L [14].

Although consistent patterns of total T_4 and TSH during pregnancy are well documented, the same is not true for free T_4 concentrations, particularly during the first trimester. Free T_4 concentrations during this time have been reported to be higher, lower, and the same as concentrations before conception [5]. These discrepant findings are likely due to a combination of shortcomings in methodology and dietary iodine intake among study participants [12]. Based on the available data, it is likely that free T_4 and T_3 concentrations increase slightly during the first trimester in response to elevated hCG. Subsequently, free T_4 values decline as pregnancy progresses and nadir during the third trimester with measured values in commercial assays that may be lower than the assays' published reference ranges [12]. Curr-ently, none of the manufacturers of the automated free T_4 assays has pro-vided trimester-specific reference ranges. Until this information is available, the serum total T_4 concentration may be a better reflection of T_4 production during pregnancy. To account for the increased thyroid hormone production during gestation, the normal reference range for total T_4 should be adjusted by a factor of 1.5 for pregnant patients [12,15].

Hypothyroidism

Screening studies have shown that an elevated serum TSH concentration is found in 2.5% of pregnancies [16,17]. In an iodine-sufficient environment, hypothyroidism during pregnancy is caused primarily by Hashimoto's thy-roiditis and prior radioactive iodine treatment or surgical ablation of Graves' disease [18]. Nevertheless, the clinician should keep in mind the less common causes (eg, overtreatment of hyperthyroidism with thiona-mides, transient hypothyroidism owing to postpartum thyroiditis, medi-cations that alter the absorption or metabolism of levothyroxine, and pituitary/hypothalamic disease) because the diagnosis and management of these patients may be different.

Diagnosis

The diagnosis of hypothyroidism during pregnancy is crucial because of its potential adverse effects on the mother and the child. Only 20% to 30% of patients with overt hypothyroidism develop symptoms consistent with disease, however, whereas most patients with subclinical disease are entirely asymptomatic [19,20]. When symptoms do exist, the diagnosis often is over-looked, and a woman's complaints may be attributed to pregnancy itself. The diagnosis of primary hypothyroidism is made by documenting an ele-vated serum TSH concentration; however, most commercial laboratories have not established trimester-specific reference ranges. Patients with central hypothyroidism resulting from pituitary or hypothalamic disease do not manifest an elevated serum TSH level during pregnancy.

Pregnancy outcome

Despite the association between overt hypothyroidism and infertility, hy-pothyroid women may become pregnant [21]. The likelihood that either ma-ternal or fetal complications will arise depends on the severity of disease and adequacy of treatment. Gestational hypertension occurs more often in overtly hypothyroid women (36%) than in women with subclinical disease (25%) or the general population (8%) [22]. A separate study reported a markedly increased use of cesarean section because of fetal distress among women who were severely hypothyroid (56%) at their initial antenatal visit compared with women who were mildly hypothyroid or euthyroid (3%) [23]. In addition, some investigators have found that women with overt hypothyroidism are more likely to develop placental abruption, anemia, and postpartum hemorrhage than women with subclinical disease, although these findings have been disputed [19]. A prospective study of women with untreated subclinical hypothyroidism found that compared with euthyroid women, they were three times more likely (95% CI 1.8–8.2) to develop placental abruption and 1.8 times more likely (95% CI 1.1–2.3) to experience preterm labor (< 37 completed weeks) [24]. Finally, very preterm delivery (< 32 completed weeks) was reported to occur more frequently (odds ratio [OR] 3.13; 95% CI 1.02–9.63) in women with a serum TSH level greater than 3 mU/L at 16 weeks [25]. This analysis included adjustments for gestational hypertension.

The children of hypothyroid women also can be adversely affected. Research has shown that the incidence of low-birth-weight neonates is markedly increased in cases of overt hypothyroidism (22%) compared with subclinical disease (9%) and the general population (7%) [22]. Although some experts attribute these findings to premature delivery, others believe there is an association between maternal thyroid status and somatic development, as supported by a report of severe growth retardation reversal in the fetus of a hypothyroid woman (TSH 72 mU/L) after adequate levothyroxine replacement. In this particular case, the fetal biparietal diameter and femur length were below the third decile and normalized over the course of 10 weeks after an increase in levothyroxine and normalization of maternal serum TSH [26].

Research also shows the significant role of maternal thyroid hormone in fetal neurologic development. Although the fetal thyroid does not begin to function until approximately 12 weeks' gestation, T_3 is present in the fetal brain by 7 weeks [27–29]. It is thought that this T_3 originates from intracellular deiodination of transplacentally transferred maternal T_4 [29]. An association between maternal hypothyroidism and impaired cognitive function among offspring was first described in the 1960s [30]. Investigators compared the results of several neuropsychological testing parameters between children born to mothers who were hypothyroid (TSH > 98th percentile) and euthyroid (TSH < 98th percentile) at 17 weeks' gestation [14]. After correcting for socioeconomic factors, the 62 children born to hypothyroid mothers scored an average of 4 points lower ($P = .06$) on the Wechsler Intelligence Scale for Children (full-scale IQ test) compared with controls. The decrease in IQ was more significant (7 points; $P = .005$), when only the children of untreated hypothyroid mothers (48 children) were compared with the control group. Because the IQ scores of the children born to levothyroxine-treated hypothyroid mothers (14 children) did not differ from controls, the authors hypothesized that perhaps first-trimester maternal thyroid hormone levels were adequate earlier in gestation when the fetal need may have been greatest [14]. Pop et al [31] performed a similar study in which they compared development between children born to women with hypothyroxinemia (free $T_4 \leq$ 10th percentile) and normal serum TSH concentrations ($<$ 2.2 mU/L) at gestational week 12 with children of controls (free T_4 50th–90th percentiles and normal TSH). They found a significant delay in mental and motor development for 1-year-olds and 2-year-olds born to the women with hypothyroxinemia. Infants of mothers with hypothyroxinemia at 12 weeks that normalized during pregnancy did not differ significantly from controls. In addition, infants in the control group whose mothers became hypothyroxinemic after 12 weeks of gestation did not show impaired development [31]. The potential influences of iodine nutrition and other maternal comorbidities were not addressed in this study. Although the relative contribution of maternal versus fetal thyroid hormone to neurologic development is not fully understood, these findings suggest that maternal hormone is important during the first trimester, before the fetal thyroid gland begins to function, and later in gestation.

Treatment

The treatment of hypothyroidism during pregnancy depends on the timing of diagnosis, the severity of disease, and possibly the cause of thyroid dysfunction (Box 1). The starting levothyroxine dose for women with overt hypothyroidism should be 2 μg/kg/d) [12]. This dosage is higher than that required for full replacement in nonpregnant patients and accounts for the increased thyroidal demand of normal pregnancy. If the initial serum TSH level is only slightly elevated (ie, TSH $<$ 10 mU/L), an initial dose of 0.1 mg/d of levothyroxine may be sufficient [32].

The likelihood that hypothyroid women who receive levothyroxine replacement will need a dosage increase may depend on the cause of their thyroid dysfunction. In one study, 76% of hypothyroid women versus 47% of women with Hashimoto's thyroiditis required an increase in levothyroxine dosage during pregnancy [2]. In addition, because women with Hashimoto's thyroiditis may have residual thyroid function that can respond partially to the stimulatory effects of pregnancy, they require a smaller mean dosage increase (25%) than hypothyroid women (45%) [2].

As previously discussed, the stimulatory effects in pregnancy begin early in the first trimester and persist until delivery. Maternal requirements must be monitored closely throughout gestation. A serum TSH level should be checked as soon as pregnancy is confirmed. In a prospective study, the median time for dosage increase was 8 weeks' gestation [1]. In addition, 25% of women with a normal TSH concentration during the first trimester and 37% with a normal TSH in the second trimester eventually require an increase in levothyroxine dosage [2]. Women with a serum TSH level less than 2.5 mU/L at initial screening should have their thyroid function re-evaluated every 3 to 4 weeks during the first half of pregnancy and every 6 weeks during the latter half.

Box 1. Guidelines for clinical management of maternal hypothyroidism during pregnancy

1. Check serum TSH level as soon as pregnancy is confirmed.
2. For newly diagnosed hypothyroid women, initial levothyroxine dosage is based on severity of hypothyroidism. For overt hypothyroidism, administer 2 μg/kg/d. If TSH is < 10 mU/L, initial dose of 0.1 mg/d may be sufficient.
3. For previously diagnosed hypothyroid women, monitor serum TSH every 3–4 weeks during first half of pregnancy and every 6 weeks thereafter.
4. Adjust levothyroxine dosage to maintain serum TSH ≤ 2.5 mU/L.
5. Monitor serum TSH and total T_4 levels 3–4 weeks after every dosage adjustment. When levothyroxine dosage achieves equilibrium, resume monitoring TSH alone.
6. Levothyroxine ingestion should be separated from prenatal vitamins containing iron, iron and calcium supplements, and soy products by at least 4 hours to ensure adequate absorption.
7. After delivery, reduce levothyroxine to prepregnancy dosage, and check serum TSH in 6 weeks.

Levothyroxine dosage should be adjusted to maintain a maternal serum TSH concentration 2.5 mU/L or less [12]. Kaplan [2] proposed a set of guidelines for adjusting levothyroxine replacement according to the elevation in serum TSH:

1. Serum TSH concentration < 10 mU/L, increase 0.05 mg/d.
2. Serum TSH concentration = 10–20 mU/L, increase 0.075 mg/d.
3. Serum TSH concentration > 20 mU/L, increase 0.1 mg/d.

Thyroid function should be re-evaluated by serum TSH and total T_4 measurements 3 to 4 weeks after every change in dosage. The normal range for total T_4 concentrations during pregnancy is 1.5 times the nonpregnant range [12]. When a levothyroxine dosage equilibrium has been achieved, a clinician may resume monitoring maternal thyroid function with serum TSH concentrations alone. As with all patients on levothyroxine therapy, pregnant women should be instructed to separate dosage ingestion from prenatal vitamins containing iron, iron and calcium supplements, and soy products by approximately 4 hours to ensure adequate absorption. In addition, for adequate iodine nutrition, it is important to check that the prenatal vitamin contains the recommended daily requirement for pregnancy (220 μg/day) [33]. Women should resume their prepregnancy levothyroxine dosage immediately after delivery and have their serum TSH level re-evaluated in 6 weeks.

Euthyroidism with autoimmune thyroid disease

The prevalence of thyroid autoimmunity among euthyroid women of childbearing age is quite high. According to data from the third National Health and Nutrition Examination Survey, 12.6% and 13.6% of women 39 years old or younger, without known thyroid disease, tested positive for thyroperoxidase (12.6%) and thyroglobulin (13.6%) antibodies [34]. These women may be at an increased risk for several pregnancy-related complications, including spontaneous miscarriage, subclinical hypothyroidism, and postpartum thyroiditis [35]. (Postpartum thyroiditis is not discussed in this article.)

A meta-analysis of 10 prospective studies of euthyroid women revealed that women with antithyroid antibodies were more than twice as likely to experience a miscarriage (odds ratio 2.30; 95% CI 1.80–2.95) [36]. The presence of these antithyroid antibodies is not associated with that of other organ-specific antibodies [37]. Although the nature of the association between thyroid autoimmunity and increased incidence of miscarriage is unknown, several possible hypotheses exist. Some investigators believe that the presence of antibodies signifies a generalized heightened autoimmune state that adversely affects the fetoplacental unit [36]. Others speculate that the link is related to subtle hypothyroidism among affected women [35].

Euthyroid women with thyroid autoimmunity may experience an increase in serum TSH levels during pregnancy compared with controls [35]. Although most of these women likely maintain normal serum TSH concentrations, one study reported that 16% of these women developed subclinical hypothyroidism during pregnancy based on an elevated TSH [38]. This study was conducted in a region of borderline iodine sufficiency and requires validation. Nevertheless, it suggests that the presence of antithyroid antibodies may signify a lack of thyroidal reserve in response to the stimulatory effects of pregnancy. The authors recommend initiating levothyroxine therapy in women with antithyroid antibodies before pregnancy if the serum TSH level is greater than 2.5 mU/L. Serum TSH should be monitored throughout pregnancy in all antithyroid antibody–positive women, with initiation or adjustment of levothyroxine to maintain the TSH concentration at 2.5 mU/L or less.

Hyperthyroidism

The prevalence of hyperthyroidism during pregnancy ranges from 0.1% to 0.4%, with Graves' disease accounting for 85% of cases [32,39]. Single toxic adenoma, multinodular toxic goiter, and subacute thyroiditis constitute most of the remaining cases during pregnancy, whereas exogenous thyroid hormone and hydatidiform molar disease are extremely rare [40].

Gestational thyrotoxicosis and hyperemesis gravidarum

As discussed previously, research strongly suggests that the high serum concentrations of hCG during early pregnancy activate the TSH receptor [5,11,41,42]. The stimulatory effect of hCG results in a wide spectrum of clinical scenarios ranging from a slight decrease in maternal TSH concentration (18% of women without thyrotoxic symptoms) [13] to transient thyrotoxicosis, known as gestational thyrotoxicosis (elevated serum free T_4 and suppressed serum TSH levels).

Hyperemesis gravidarum is a syndrome affecting some pregnant women and is defined by severe nausea and vomiting leading to a 5% loss of body weight, dehydration, and ketosis. Of women with hyperemesis gravidarum, 60% have a subnormal serum TSH level (< 0.4 mU/L), and nearly 50% have an elevated serum free T_4 concentration [43]. In addition, the severity of symptoms experienced by a woman with hyperemesis gravidarum is positively correlated with maternal free T_4 levels [43]. Despite the apparent correlation, hyperemesis gravidarum does not seem to be directly related to thyroid function. Only 12% of such women have an elevated free T_3 index [43]. Some investigators believe that another compound stimulated by the increased concentrations of hCG (eg, estradiol) may be the causative agent [43]. Whether symptomatic or not, gestational thyrotoxicosis usually resolves spontaneously by 20 weeks' gestation when hCG declines. Treatment with antithyroid medications is generally not necessary. If gestational thyrotoxicosis continues beyond 20 weeks, a repeat evaluation for other causes of hyperthyroidism should be considered.

Graves' disease

Graves' disease is the most common cause of hyperthyroidism during pregnancy [32,39]. Similar to other autoimmune diseases, the activity level of Graves' disease may fluctuate during gestation, with exacerbation during the first trimester and gradual improvement during the latter half. Patients with Graves' disease also may experience an exacerbation shortly after delivery [44]. With this possibility in mind, there are several different clinical scenarios by which a woman may present with Graves' disease during pregnancy. First, a woman with stable Graves' disease receiving thionamide therapy may experience an exacerbation during early pregnancy. Second, a woman in remission may experience a relapse of disease. Lastly, a woman without prior history may be diagnosed with Graves' disease de novo during pregnancy.

Diagnosis

The diagnosis of Graves' disease may be difficult to make clinically because of the presence of hypermetabolic symptoms in normal pregnancy, such as palpitations, irritability, and heat intolerance. The thyroid examination is often different from that of normal pregnancy, hyperemesis gravidarum, and gestational thyrotoxicosis. Women with Graves' disease usually have a goiter (with or without bruit), but the accompanying autoimmune syndromes of ophthalmopathy and possibly dermopathy are still quite rare.

Laboratory studies also are helpful, revealing a suppressed serum TSH level and usually elevated free and total T_4 serum concentrations. As described previously, however, 60% of women with hyperemesis gravidarum have a subnormal serum TSH, and nearly 50% have an elevated serum free T_4 concentration [45]. In situations in which doubt exists, measurement of serum total T_3 concentration and T_3 resin uptake may be helpful because only 12% of women with hyperemesis gravidarum have an elevated free T_3 index [45]. Finally, TSH receptor antibodies are usually present with Graves' disease and may aid in confirming the diagnosis.

Pregnancy outcome

The risk of complications for the mother and the child is related to the duration and control of maternal hyperthyroidism. The highest incidence occurs in cases with the poorest control, and the lowest incidence occurs in cases with adequate treatment [40,46–48]. The frequency of preterm labor is highest among untreated mothers (88%) compared with partially treated mothers (25%) and adequately treated mothers (8%) [46]. In addition, untreated women are twice as likely to develop preeclampsia during pregnancy than women receiving antithyroid medication [40]. As for the fetus, stillbirth is much more common among untreated women (50%) than either partially treated women (16%) or adequately treated women (0%) [46]. Finally, studies have indicated that children born to mothers with uncontrolled hyperthyroidism are more likely to be small for gestational age and to have congenital malformations unrelated to thionamide therapy [47,48].

Treatment

The most important thing to remember when treating Graves' disease during pregnancy is that two patients are involved, the mother and fetus. The goal of therapy is to control maternal disease, while minimizing to potential for fetal hypothyroidism and hyperthyroidism (Box 2).

Thionamides

Thionamide antithyroid drugs, propylthiouracil (PTU) and methimazole (MMI), are the mainstay of treatment of Graves' disease during pregnancy. These medications decrease thyroid hormone production by inhibiting

---

Box 2. Guidelines for clinical management of maternal hyperthyroidism during pregnancy

1. Use the lowest dosage of thionamide (preferably PTU) to maintain maternal total T_4 concentrations in the upper one third of normal to slightly elevated range for pregnancy. Normal range of total T_4 during pregnancy is estimated to be 1.5 times the nonpregnant state [46].
2. Monitor maternal total T_4 serum concentration every 2–4 weeks, and titrate thionamide as necessary. Monitoring serum TSH may become useful later.
3. Measure TSH receptor antibodies (thyroid-stimulating immunoglobulins or TSH receptor binding inhibitory immunoglobulins) at 26–28 weeks to assess risk of fetal/neonatal hyperthyroidism. TSH receptor antibody measurement is crucial in hypothyroid levothyroxine-treated women with a prior history of Graves' disease, who do not appear thyrotoxic.
4. Perform fetal ultrasound at weeks 26–28 to assess potential fetal response to thionamide treatment and effect of TSH receptor antibodies on fetal thyroid function.
5. Consider thyroidectomy if persistently high doses of thionamide (PTU > 600 mg/d or MMI > 40 mg/d) are required, or if the patient cannot tolerate thionamide therapy.
6. β-Adrenergic blocking agents and low doses of iodine may be used perioperatively to control hyperthyroid state.
7. Check fetal cord blood at delivery for TSH and T_4.

---

iodine organification and iodotyrosine coupling by thyroidal peroxidase. A study found the median time to normalization of maternal thyroid function to be 7 weeks with PTU and 8 weeks with MMI [49].

Although equally effective, concern exists regarding a possible difference in the transplacental passage of the thionamides. PTU is known to be more highly bound to albumin than MMI [32]. This fact has led some authors to theorize that MMI crosses the placenta in higher concentrations and may place the fetus at greater risk of hypothyroidism. Convincing evidence of this phenomenon has not been established. One study of six women, without thyroid disease, receiving a single injection of either sulphur-35 [35S]-PTU or [35S]-MMI before therapeutic abortion in the first half of pregnancy, revealed that PTU may cross the placenta to a lesser degree than MMI [50]. A perfusion study conducted on placental tissue from women without thyroid disease, undergoing cesarean section at term, revealed similar placental transfer kinetics for PTU and MMI [51].

To minimize the occurrence of fetal hypothyroidism, the clinician must assume that both thionamides cross the placenta. Data concerning a correlation between maternal antithyroid drug dosage and fetal thyroid function are conflicted, however. Three studies [47,52,53] reported a direct relationship between maternal dosage and fetal function, whereas four studies [54–57] showed a lack of correlation. The most recent study reported that 21% of the neonates born to mothers taking less than 100 mg of PTU daily and 14% of neonates born to mothers taking less than 10 mg of MMI daily still had an elevated serum TSH level at birth [57].

The lack of correlation between maternal thionamide dosage and fetal thyroid function is multifactorial. Absorption of antithyroid medications and serum concentrations are different for each mother. Additionally, each woman with Graves' disease has a different titer of TSH receptor antibodies. Research has shown a strong correlation between maternal TSH receptor antibodies and fetal and neonatal exposure [28,53,58]. These antibodies may be either stimulatory or inhibitory; however, most women with Graves' disease possess immunoglobulins that stimulate the fetal thyroid. Stimulation becomes clinically relevant near the end of the second trimester and continues until delivery [27].

In light of the role that TSH receptor antibodies play and the lack of correlation between thionamide dose and fetal thyroid function, it is not surprising that a better means of following therapy exists. Momotani et al [56] reported that treatment decisions could be made safely according to maternal thyroid status in women not previously treated with ablative therapy. According to their work, when maternal serum free T_4 concentrations were either slightly elevated or within the upper third of normal, 95% of neonates had cord free T_4 values within the normal range. Conversely, when maternal serum free T_4 concentrations were either within the bottom two thirds of normal or below the lower limit of normal, 36% and 100% of neonates had free T_4 concentrations below normal [56].

Avoiding fetal hypothyroidism from thionamide treatment of maternal Graves' disease is crucial. Excessive treatment may result in fetal TSH stimulation, goiter formation, and possibly respiratory compromise after delivery owing to tracheal compression. Fetal hypothyroidism resulting from overtreatment of maternal Graves' disease potentially could affect neurocognitive development (see earlier) In addition to following maternal thyroid hormone concentrations, fetal response to therapy should be evaluated by ultrasound during gestational weeks 26 to 28. If a fetal goiter is identified, the clinician must determine whether it is due to fetal hypothyroidism or hyperthyroidism (see later). This decision usually can be made clinically. If the mother is biochemically hyperthyroid and the fetus is tachycardic, fetal hyperthyroidism is more likely [59]. If the mother's serum total T_4 or free T_4 values are in the mid-normal to lower range, however, it is more likely that the fetus is hypothyroid [56]. If the fetal goiter is related to hypothyroidism, rapid improvement may occur after a decrease, or discontinuation, of thionamide treatment [60]. If improvement is not apparent, consideration should be given to more aggressive diagnostic testing, such as periumbilical blood sampling, with treatment tailored to the specific findings (eg, intra-amniotic levothyroxine therapy for persistent hypothyroidism) [61,62].

Aside from the hypothyroidism, the other potential side effects of thionamide therapy must be considered. The maternal side effects are the same for any individual taking these medications, the most common being a rash. As for the fetus/neonate, several cross-sectional studies have found no effect on cognitive or somatic development among infants exposed to PTU or MMI [63–66]. Several rare birth defects have been observed in neonates born to mothers taking MMI during pregnancy (eg, aplasia cutis, choanal atresia, esophageal atresia, and minor dysmorphic features) [67,68]. None of these findings has been reported with PTU. The authors prefer PTU as first-line therapy. If a woman is unable to tolerate PTU, the authors prescribe MMI, especially after first-trimester organogenesis.

Treatment guidelines

The initial dosage of antithyroid medication depends on the severity of disease. PTU should be used preferentially given the multiple case reports of congenital defects and dysmorphic features occurring in infants exposed to MMI [67,68]. If one is allergic or intolerant of PTU, however, MMI should be substituted (especially after first-trimester organogenesis) before recommending thyroidectomy. Antithyroid medication should be titrated to maintain maternal T_4 concentrations within the upper third, or slightly above, of the normal range for pregnancy. Because pregnancy reference ranges have not been reported for most free T_4 assays, the authors recommend using the serum total T_4 concentration for thionamide dose titration. In addition, the authors adopt a pregnancy reference range for total T_4 to be 1.5 times the nonpregnant reference range owing to thyroidal stimulation during pregnancy (see section on normal gravid thyroid physiology) [15]. Clinicians should re-evaluate maternal thyroid function every 2 to 4 weeks and adjust thionamide therapy accordingly. Serum TSH levels are not helpful in the management of Graves' disease during early pregnancy because of the lag time that exists between the normalization of thyroid hormones and TSH, but may be useful later in gestation when the disease is controlled. The authors do not exceed 600 mg/d of PTU or 40 mg/d of MMI for extended periods. One should continue to titrate PTU to the lowest possible dose that maintains control. Graves' disease may ameliorate as pregnancy progresses. As a result, thionamide therapy may be discontinued in 30% of women during the final weeks of pregnancy [69]. Cord blood testing for TSH and T_4 is recommended in all infants born to mothers with active Graves' disease. In addition, to assess the risk for fetal or neonatal hyperthyroidism, measurement of TSH receptor antibodies at 26 to 28 weeks' gestation is recommended (see later).

β-Adrenergic blockers

β-Adrenergic blockers are used often in the treatment of hyperthyroidism because of the presence of adrenergic signs and symptoms (eg, tachycardia, palpitations, and diaphoresis). A retrospective analysis reported, however, an increased frequency of first-trimester miscarriages in mothers treated for 6 to 12 weeks with a thionamide and propranolol (24%) compared with a thionamide alone (5.5%) [70]. This difference existed despite similar thyroid hormone concentrations. Although this was a small study, the authors recommend avoiding β-adrenergic blocking agents if possible in the first trimester.

Iodides

Because of past reports of neonatal hypothyroidism after exposure to iodine, its use during pregnancy has been severely limited. Most published work consists of case reports, however, in which euthyroid mothers were exposed to iodine-rich food, medicine, contrast media, or disinfectant agents or hyperthyroid mothers were simultaneously treated with iodine and thionamides [71]. A study investigating the use of low-dose iodine (6–40 mg/d of potassium iodide) for the treatment of Graves' disease during pregnancy revealed improved maternal thyroid function and normal neonatal outcome [71]. Specifically, none of the neonates exposed to potassium iodide exhibited a goiter, and only 6% had an elevated TSH by way of the cord blood. Although this evidence does not make iodine a first-line therapy for pregnant women with Graves' disease, it does suggest that low-dose potassium iodide may be considered in special circumstances, such as in preparation for thyroidectomy or in thionamide-intolerant patients refusing surgery.

Surgery

Subtotal thyroidectomy for the treatment of Graves' disease during pregnancy is reserved for specific situations: when persistently high dosages of thionamides (PTU > 600 mg/d, MMI > 40 mg/d) are required to control maternal disease, if a patient is allergic or intolerant of both thionamides, if a patient is noncompliant with medical therapy, or if compressive symptoms occur in the mother because of goiter size [32]. Historically, it has been recommended that surgery occur during the second trimester, before gestational week 24, in an attempt to minimize the risk of miscarriage [59]. Women who are persistently hyperthyroid before surgery should be prepared with a β-adrenergic blocking agent and a 10- to 14-day course of potassium iodide with the intent of treating the hyperthyroid state and minimizing the potential for perioperative disease exacerbation.

Radioactive iodine therapy

Radioactive iodine therapy is contraindicated for the treatment of Graves' disease during pregnancy. Fetal tissue is more radiosensitive than adult tissue and may be susceptible to congenital defects during early development [72]. Additionally, the fetal thyroid gland begins to concentrate iodine after gestational week 10, predisposing the fetus/neonate to congenital hypothyroidism [73,74].

Fetal or neonatal hyperthyroidism

Fetal or neonatal hyperthyroidism occurs in 1% of pregnancies complicated by active or previously ablated Graves' disease [75]. In both instances, hyperthyroidism results from the transplacental passage of maternal TSH receptor antibodies that stimulate the fetal (or neonatal) thyroid gland. The passage of immunoglobulins and the potential for fetal hyperthyroidism become clinically significant at the end of the second trimester [76]. Commercial assays for thyroid-stimulating immunoglobulins may not be as helpful as levels of TSH receptor binding inhibitory immunoglobulins. Thyroid-stimulating immunoglobulin levels greater than 35% and TSH receptor binding inhibitory immunoglobulin levels greater than 40% have been associated with fetal thyrotoxicosis [53,58,77]. If either antibody titer is suspiciously high, a careful fetal ultrasound examination should be performed. In the presence of fetal tachycardia and goiter, fetal thyrotoxicosis should be suspected [59]. The necessity of cordocentesis to confirm the diagnosis in the clinical setting of fetal tachycardia and a mother with either active or previously treated Graves' disease is controversial [58,78].

There are two possible clinical scenarios in which fetal Graves' disease is observed. First, a woman may have active Graves' disease. In this case, the maternal thyroid function serves as a "biosensor" that reflects the fetal thyroid. Maternal and fetal thyroid synthetic function are subject to stimulation by the thyroid-stimulating antibodies and inhibition by the maternal thionamide medication. If the maternal hyperthyroidism is controlled appropriately, fetal thyrotoxicosis should not occur. The second scenario concerns a woman who is hypothyroid on levothyroxine replacement therapy after either radioactive iodine or thyroidectomy for Graves' disease. Although she is still producing thyroid-stimulating antibodies, her thyroid function tests do not reflect their stimulatory influence. The transplacental passage of these antibodies still may affect the fetus, however, resulting in fetal thyrotoxicosis. In this situation, the maternal thyroid does not serve as a "biosensor" for the fetal thyroid. The fetal thyroid is exposed only to the stimulating antibodies without the concomitant inhibitory effect of the maternal thionamide therapy.

Treatment of fetal hyperthyroidism begins by increasing the dosage of maternal thionamide if the mother has active Graves' disease or initiating PTU therapy in the case of previously ablated mothers. PTU should be initiated at 150 mg/d and crosses the placenta to inhibit the synthesis of fetal thyroid hormone. The fetus should be re-evaluated for clinical improvement (heart rate, goiter resolution) by ultrasound in 2 weeks [28]. It is crucial to remember that although fetal tachycardia is seen with fetal hyperthyroidism, fetal bradycardia may not be present with fetal hypothyroidism resulting from overtreatment from maternal PTU. As soon as the fetal heart rate normalizes, the PTU dose should be reduced systemically with frequent monitoring of fetal heart rate to maintain it in the normal range. Many patients with Graves' disease have a continued decrease in thyroid-stimulating antibody production after 32 weeks, and often PTU can be stopped before delivery [44]. For previously ablated hyperthyroid mothers, levothyroxine therapy may need to be increased if hypothyroxinemia develops while treating fetal hyperthyroidism with PTU.

Although maternal TSH receptor antibody titers usually decline toward delivery, neonatal thyrotoxicosis still may be observed if the stimulating antibodies are present in high titers near term [53,58]. Neonatal manifestations of hyperthyroidism may not be apparent until after a few days of life if a mother was maintained on thionamide treatment until delivery [79]. Affected neonates require antithyroid medication until the maternal antibodies are cleared from their system at approximately 3 months of age, after which time, signs of hyperthyroidism resolve, and thyroid function testing normalizes [79].

Thyroid nodules and thyroid cancer

The prevalence of clinically apparent thyroid nodules is higher in women than in men [80,81]. In addition, the incidence of nodular disease increases with age to a greater extent in women [82–84]. A retrospective study suggested that the increased prevalence of thyroid nodules among women may be related to pregnancy. The prevalence of nodular disease, as detected by ultrasonography, was three times as high in women who had experienced at least one pregnancy compared with women who had never been pregnant [85]. A more recent prospective study found that the incidence of incipient thyroid nodules increased from 15% during the first trimester to 24% 3 months postpartum, whereas existing nodules experienced a significant amount of growth during the same time period [86]. Despite the increase in thyroid nodule formation and growth, there is no evidence to suggest that thyroid cancer arises de novo more frequently during pregnancy than in the nonpregnant state.

The evaluation of a thyroid nodule discovered during pregnancy is similar to that of the nonpregnant patient. A laboratory evaluation of thyroid function should be obtained, keeping in mind normal gravid thyroid physiology. At the same time, sonographic evaluation should be performed to characterize the nodule further, and a subsequent fine-needle aspiration should be performed (with or without ultrasound guidance) if indicated [87]. The spectrum of cytologic results is the same as in the nonpregnant state [88]. Nodules with benign cytology should be observed and followed by an endocrinologist after delivery. Nodules with cytologic findings consistent with follicular neoplasm may require further evaluation after delivery with radioactive iodine imaging, which is contraindicated during pregnancy, and possibly surgery. If the fine-needle aspiration cytology is consistent with thyroid cancer, surgery is recommended. Currently, there is no consensus on the appropriate timing of surgery. Some experts recommend operating during the second trimester, before 24 weeks' gestation, to minimize the risk of miscarriage [21]. Thyroid cancer discovered during pregnancy is not more aggressive, however, than that diagnosed in a similar aged group of nonpregnant women, leading other experts to advocate postponing definitive surgery until after delivery in most patients [89,90]. A retrospective study of pregnant women with differentiated thyroid cancer found there to be no difference in either recurrence or survival rates between women operated on during or after their pregnancy [90].

The authors have adopted a clinical practice influenced by both schools of thought. If a malignant nodule is discovered early in pregnancy, it should be monitored with repeat ultrasound at midtrimester. If the nodule has grown significantly, surgery should be considered with the assistance of an experienced anesthesiologist. Postoperative radioactive iodine therapy, if indicated, must be delayed until after the delivery. Conversely, if the nodule size is stable, or the malignancy is not discovered until the second half of pregnancy, surgery can occur after the patient has delivered. In all women with cytology indicative of papillary thyroid cancer, regardless of surgical timing, levothyroxine suppression therapy should be initiated to maintain the serum TSH in the subnormal, but detectable, range (ie, 0.1–0.3 mU/L). In addition, women with previously diagnosed or treated differentiated thyroid cancer require an increased levothyroxine dosage during pregnancy. The recommended schedule for serum TSH testing is the same as that outlined for hypothyroid women (see Box 1). The authors adopt a therapeutic target for serum TSH of 0.1 to 0.8 mU/L for patients with papillary or follicular thyroid cancer, depending on their risk of recurrence, and less than 2.5 mU/L for patients with medullary thyroid cancer.

Summary

Thyroid disorders are common among pregnant women. Diagnosis of thyroid dysfunction is complicated, however, by nonspecific symptoms, the hypermetabolic state of pregnancy, and normal gravid thyroid physiology, which results in alterations of maternal serum TSH and thyroxine concentrations. If untreated, hypothyroidism and hyperthyroidism may adversely affect the mother and fetus. In cases of primary hypothyroidism, maternal serum TSH concentrations should be monitored throughout pregnancy, and the levothyroxine dosage should be adjusted to maintain maternal serum TSH levels at 2.5 mU/L or less. Conversely, in cases of true hyperthyroidism (e.g., Graves' disease), maternal thyroid function should be evaluated every 2 to 4 weeks, and thionamide therapy (preferably PTU) should be given, titrated to achieve maternal serum total T_4 concentration within the upper one third of normal to slightly elevated range for pregnancy. Fetal ultrasonography and measurement of maternal serum TSH receptor antibody concentrations should be employed to prevent fetal/neonatal complications. Finally, the evaluation of nodular thyroid disease and cancer is similar in pregnant and nonpregnant patients. Use of radioactive iodine is contraindicated during pregnancy, however, and should be postponed until after delivery.

References

[1] Alexander EK, Marqusee E, Lawrence J, et al. Timing and magnitude of increases in levothyroxine requirements during pregnancy in women with hypothyroidism. N Engl J Med 2004;351:241.

[2] Kaplan M. Monitoring thyroxine treatment during pregnancy. Thyroid 1992;2:147.

[3] Mandel SJ, Larsen PR, Seely EW, et al. Increased need for thyroxine during pregnancy in women with primary hypothyroidism. N Engl J Med 1990;323:91.

[4] Glinoer D, Delange F, Laboureur I, et al. Maternal and neonatal thyroid function at birth in an area of marginally low iodine intake. J Clin Endocrinol Metab 1992;75:800.

[5] Glinoer D, DeNayer P, Bourdoux P, et al. Regulation of maternal thyroid during pregnancy. J Clin Endocrinol Metab 1990;71:276.

[6] Ain KB, Mori Y, Refetoff S. Reduced clearance rate of thyroxine-binding globulin (TGB) with increased sialylation: a mechanism for estrogen-induced elevation of serum TBG concentration. J Clin Endocrinol Metab 1987;65:689.

[7] Dworkin H, Jacquez J, Beierwaltes W. Relationship of iodine ingestion to iodine excretion in pregnancy. J Clin Endocrinol Metab 1966;26:1329.

[8] Burrow GN, Fisher DA, Larsen PR. Maternal and fetal thyroid function. N Engl J Med 1994;331:1072.

[9] Hershman JM. Physiological and pathological aspects of the effect of human chorionic gonadotropin on the thyroid. Best Pract Res Clin Endocrinol Metab 2004;18:249.

[10] Smits G, Govaerts C, Nubourgh I, et al. Lysine 183 and glutamic acid 157 of the TSH receptor: two interacting residues with a key role in determining specificity toward TSH and human CG. Mol Endocrinol 2002;16:722.

[11] Kimura M, Amino N, Tamaki H, et al. Physiologic thyroid activation in normal early pregnancy is induced by circulating hCG. Obstet Gynecol 1990;75:775.

[12] Mandel SJ, Spencer CA, Hollowell JG. Are detection and treatment of thyroid insufficiency in pregnancy feasible? Thyroid 2005;15:44.

[13] Glinoer D, DeNayer P, Robyn C, et al. Serum levels of intact human chorionic gonadotropin (HCG) and its free α and β subunits, in relation to maternal thyroid stimulation during normal pregnancy. J Endocrinol Invest 1993;16:881.

[14] Haddow JE, Palomaki GE, Allan WC, et al. Maternal thyroid deficiency during pregnancy and subsequent neuropsychological development of the child. N Engl J Med 1999;341:549.

[15] Demers L, Spencer CA. Laboratory medicine practice guidelines: laboratory support for the diagnosis and monitoring of thyroid disease. Thyroid 2003;13:6.

[16] Glinoer D. The regulation of thyroid function in pregnancy: pathways of endocrine adaptation from physiology to pathology. Endocr Rev 1997;18:404.

[17] Klein RZ, Haddow JE, Faix JD, et al. Prevalence of thyroid deficiency in pregnant women. Clin Endocrinol (Oxf) 1991;35:41.

[18] Neale D, Burrow G. Thyroid disease and pregnancy. Obstet Gynecol Clin North Am 2004; 31:893.

[19] Davis LE, Leveno KJ, Cunningham FG. Hypothyroidism complicating pregnancy. Obstet Gynecol 1988;72:108.

[20] Montoro M, Collea JV, Frasier SD, et al. Successful outcome of pregnancy in women with hypothyroidism. Ann Intern Med 1981;94:31.

[21] Mestman JH, Goodman TM, Montoro MM. Thyroid disorders of pregnancy. Endocrinol Metab Clin North Am 1995;24:41.

[22] Leung AS, Millar LK, Koonings PP, et al. Perinatal outcome in hypothyroid pregnancies. Obstet Gynecol 1993;81:349.

[23] Wasserstrum N, Anania CA. Perinantal consequences of maternal hypothyroidism in early pregnancy and inadequate replacement. Clin Endocrinol (Oxf) 1995;42:353.

[24] Casey B, Dashe JS, Wells CE, et al. Subclinical hypothyroidism and pregnancy outcomes. Obstet Gynecol 2005;105:239.

[25] Stagnaro-Green A, Chen X, Bogden JD, et al. The thyroid and pregnancy: a novel risk factor for very preterm delivery. Thyroid 2005;15:351.

[26] Rotondi M, Caccavale C, DiSerio C, et al. Successful outcome of pregnancy in a thyroidectomized parathyroidectomized young woman affected by severe hypothyroidism. Thyroid 1999;9:1037.

[27] Fisher D. Endocrinology of fetal development. In: Wilson JD, Foster DW, editors. Textbook of endocrinology. Philadelphia: Saunders; 1999. p. 2073–102.

[28] Fisher DA. Fetal thyroid function: diagnosis and managment of fetal thyroid disorders. Clin Obstet Gynecol 1997;40:16.

[29] Morreale de Escobar G, Obregon MJ, Escobar del Rey F. Maternal thyroid hormones early in pregnancy and fetal brain development. Best Pract Res Clin Endocrinol Metab 2004;18:225.

[30] Man EB, Jones WS. Thyroid function in human pregnancy: V. incidence of maternal serum low butanol-extractable iodines and of normal gestational TBG and TPBA capacities: retardation of 8-month-old infants. Am J Obstet Gynecol 1969;104(6):898–908.

[31] Pop VJ, Brouwers EP, Vader HL, et al. Maternal hypothyroxinaemia during early pregnancy and subsequent child development: a 3-year follow-up study. Clin Endocrinol (Oxf) 2003;59:282.

[32] Mandel SJ. Thyroid disease and pregnancy. In: Copper DS, editor. Medical management of thyroid disease. New York: Marcel Dekker; 2001. p. 387–418.

[33] Smallridge RC, Ladenson PW. Hypothyroidism in pregnancy: consequences to neonatal health. J Clin Endocrinol Metab 2001;86:2349.

[34] Hollowell JG, Staehling NW, Flanders WD, et al. Serum TSH, T4, and thyroid antibodies in the United States population (1988 to 1994): National Health and Nutrition Examination Survey (NHANES III). J Clin Endocrinol Metab 2002;82:489.

[35] Stagnaro-Green A, Glinoer D. Thyroid autoimmunity and the risk of miscarriage. Best Pract Res Clin Endocrinol Metab 2004;18:167.

[36] Prummel MF, Wiersinga WM. Thyroid autoimmunity and miscarriage. Eur J Endocrinol 2004;150:751.

[37] Stagnaro-Green A, Roman SH, Cobin RH, et al. Detection of at-risk pregnancy by means of highly sensitive assays for thyroid autoantibodies. JAMA 1990;264:1422.

[38] Glinoer D, Riahi M, Grün J, et al. Risk of subclinical hypothyroidism in pregnant women with asymptomatic autoimmune thyroid disorders. J Clin Endocrinol Metab 1994;79:197.

[39] Glinoer D. Thyroid hyperfunction during pregnancy. Thyroid 1998;8:859.

[40] Millar LK, Wing DA, Leung AS, et al. Low birth weight and preeclampsia in pregnancies complicated by hyperthyroidism. Obstet Gynecol 1994;84:946.

[41] Yoshikawa N, Nishikawa M, Horimoto M, et al. Thyroid-stimulating activity in sera of normal pregnant women. J Clin Endocrinol Metab 1989;69:891.

[42] Yoshimura M, Hershman JM. Thyrotropic action of human chorionic gonadotropin. Thyroid 1995;5:425.

[43] Goodwin TM, Montoro M, Mestman JH, et al. The role of chorionic gonadotropin in transient hyperthyroidism of hyperemesis gravidarum. J Clin Endocrinol Metab 1992;75:1333.

[44] Amino N, Tanizawa O, Mori H, et al. Aggravation of thyrotoxicosis in early pregnancy and after delivery in Graves' disease. J Clin Endocrinol Metab 1982;55:108.

[45] Goodwin GM, Montoro M, Mestman JH. Transient hyperthyroidism and hyperemesis gravidarum: clinical aspects. Am J Obstet Gynecol 1992;167:648.

[46] Davis LE, Lucas MJ, Hankins GDV, et al. Thyrotoxicosis complicating pregnancy. Am J Obstet Gynecol 1989;160:63.

[47] Mitsuda N, Tamaki H, Amino N, et al. Risk factors for developmental disorders in infants born to women with Graves' disease. Obstet Gynecol 1992;80:359.

[48] Momotani N, Ito K, Hamada N, et al. Maternal hyperthyroidism and congenital malformation in the offspring. Clin Endocrinol (Oxf) 1984;20:695.

[49] Wing DA, Millar LK, Koonings PP, et al. A comparison of propylthiouracil versus methimazole in the treatment of hyperthyroidism in pregnancy. Am J Obstet Gynecol 1994;170:90.

[50] Marchant B, Brownlie BEW, McKay Hart D, et al. The placental transfer of propylthiouracil, methimazole and carbimazole. J Clin Endocrinol Metab 1977;45:1187.

[51] Mortimer R, Cannell G, Addison R, et al. Methimazole and propylthiouracil equally cross the perfused human term placental lobule. J Clin Endocrinol Metab 1997;82:3099.

[52] Lamberg BA, Ikonen E, Teramo K, et al. Treatment of maternal hyperthyroidism with antithyroid agents and changes in thyrotrophin and thyroxine in the newborn. Acta Endocrinol (Copenh) 1981;97:186.

[53] Mortimer RH, Tyack SA, Galligan JP, et al. Graves' disease in pregnancy: TSH receptor binding inhibiting immunoglobulins and maternal and neonatal thyroid function. Clin Endocrinol (Oxf) 1990;32:141.

[54] Cheron RG, Kaplan MM, Larsen PR, et al. Neonatal thyroid function after propylthiouracil therapy for maternal Graves' disease. N Engl J Med 1981;304:525.

[55] Gardner DF, Cruikshank DP, Hays PM, et al. Pharmacology of propylthiouracil (PTU) in pregnant hyperthyroid women: correlation of maternal PTU concentrations with cord serum thyroid function test. J Clin Endocrinol Metab 1986;62(21):217–20.

[56] Momotani N, Noh J, Oyanagi H, et al. Antithyroid drug therapy for Graves' disease during pregnancy. N Engl J Med 1986;315:24.

[57] Momotani N, Noh JY, Ishikawa N, et al. Effects of propylthiouracil and methimazole on fetal thyroid status in mothers with graves' hyperthyroidism. J Clin Endocrinol Metab 1997;82:3633.

[58] Peleg D, Cada S, Peleg A, et al. The relationship between maternal serum thyroid-stimulating immunoglobulin and fetal and neonatal thyrotoxicosis. Obstet Gynecol 2002;99:1040.

[59] Mestman JH. Hyperthyroidism in pregnancy. Best Pract Res Clin Endocrinol Metab 2004; 18:267.

[60] Ochoa-Maya M, Frates NC, Lee-Parritz A, et al. Resolution of fetal goiter after discontinuation of propylthiouracil in a pregnant woman with Graves' hyperthyroidism. Thyroid 1999;9:1111.

[61] Davidson KM, Richards DS, Schatz DA, et al. Successful in utero treatment of fetal goiter and hypothyroidism. N Engl J Med 1991;324:543.

[62] Van Loon AJ, Derksen J, Bos AF, et al. In utero diagnosis and treatment of fetal goitrous hypothyroidism, caused by maternal use of propylthiouracil. Prenat Diagn 1995;15:599.

[63] Burrow GN, Klatskin EH, Genel M. Intellectual development in children whose mothers received propylthiouracil during pregnancy. Yale J Biol Med 1978;51:151.

[64] Eisenstein Z, Weiss M, Katz Y, et al. Intellectual capacity of subjects exposed to methimazole or propylthiouracil in utero. Eur J Pediatr 1992;1:558.

[65] McCarroll AM, Hutchinson M, McAuley R, et al. Long-term assessment of children exposed in utero to carbimazole. Arch Dis Child 1976;51:532.

[66] Messer PM, Hauffa BP, Olbricht T, et al. Antithyroid drug treatment of Graves' disease in pregnancy: long-term effects on somatic growth, intellectual development and thyroid function of the offspring. Acta Endocrinol (Copenh) 1990;123:311.

[67] Clementi M, Gianantonio ED, Pelo E, et al. Methimazole embryopathy: delineation of the phenotype. Am J Med Genet 1999;83:43.

[68] Mandel SJ, Brent GA, Larsen PR. Review of antithyroid drug use during pregnancy and report of a case of aplasia cutis. Thyroid 1994;4:129.

[69] Mestman JH. Hyperthyroidism in pregnancy. Clin Obstet Gynecol 1997;40:45.

[70] Sherif IH, Oyan WT, Bosairi S, et al. Treatment of hyperthyroidism in pregnancy. Acta Obstet Gynecol Scand 1991;70:461.

[71] Momotani N, Hisaoka T, Noh J, et al. Effects of iodine on thyroid status of fetus versus mother in treatment of Graves' disease complicated by pregnancy. J Clin Endocrinol Metab 1992;75:738.

[72] Masiukiewicz US, Burrow GN. Hyperthyroidism in pregnancy: diagnosis and treatment. Thyroid 1999;9:647.

[73] Evans P, Webster J, Evans W, et al. Radioiodine treatments in unsuspected pregnancy. Clin Endocrin 1998;48:281.

[74] Stoffer SS, Hamburger JI. Inadvertent ^{131}I therapy for hyperthyroidism in the first trimester of pregnancy. J Nucl Med 1976;17:146.

[75] Burrow GN. Thyroid function and hyperfunction during gestation. Endocr Rev 1993;14:194.

[76] Polak M, Le Gac I, Vuillard E, et al. Fetal and neonatal thyroid function in relation to maternal Graves' disease. Best Pract Res Clin Endocrinol Metab 2004;18:289.

[77] Matsuura N, Fujiedu K, Iida Y, et al. TSH-receptor antibodies in mothers with Graves' disease and outcome in their offspring. Lancet 1988;331:14.

[78] Kilpatrick S. Umbilical blood sampling in women with thyroid disease in pregnancy: is it necessary? Obstet Gynecol 2003;189:1.

[79] Skuza KA, Sills IN, Stene M, et al. Prediction of neonatal hyperthyroidism in infants born to mothers with Graves' disease. J Pediatr 1996;128:264.

[80] Stoffer R, Welsh J, Hellwig C, et al. Nodular goiter: incidence morphology before and after iodine prophylaxis, and clinical diagnosis. Arch Intern Med 1960;106:10.

[81] Vander JB, Gaston EA, Dawber TR. The significance of nontoxic thyroid nodules. Ann Intern Med 1968;69:537.

[82] Hintze G, Windeler J, Baumert J, et al. Thyroid volume and goiter prevalence in the elderly as determined by ultrasound and their relationships to laboratory indices. Acta Endocrinol (Copenh) 1991;124:12.

[83] Knudsen N, Perrild H, Christiansen E, et al. Thyroid structure and size and two year follow-up of solitary cold thyroid nodules in an unselected population with borderline iodine deficiency. Eur J Endocrinol 2000;142:224.

[84] Mazzaferri EL. Management of a solitary thyroid nodule. N Engl J Med 1993;328:553.

[85] Struve CW, Haupt S, Ohlen S. Influence of frequency of previous pregnancies on the prevalence of thyroid nodules in women without clinical evidence of thyroid disease. Thyroid 1993;3:7.

[86] Kung A, Chau M, Lao T, et al. The effect of pregnancy on thyroid nodule formation. J Clin Endocrinol Metab 2002;87:1010.

[87] Mandel SJ. A 64-year-old woman with a thyroid nodule. JAMA 2004;292:2632.

[88] Tan GH, Gharib H, Goellner JR, et al. Management of thyroid nodules in pregnancy. Arch Intern Med 1996;156:2317.

[89] Herzon FS, Morris DM, Segal MN, et al. Coexistent thyroid cancer and pregnancy. Arch Otolaryngol Head Neck Surg 1994;120:1191.

[90] Moosa M, Mazzaferri EL. Outcome of differentiated thyroid cancer diagnosed in pregnant women. J Clin Endocrinol Metab 1997;82:2862.

ELSEVIER
SAUNDERS

Endocrinol Metab Clin N Am
35 (2006) 137–155

ENDOCRINOLOGY
AND METABOLISM
CLINICS
OF NORTH AMERICA

Fertility in Polycystic Ovary Syndrome

Shrita M. Patel, MD[a], John E. Nestler, MD[b],*

[a]Division of Endocrinology, Diabetes, and Metabolism, Center for Clinical Epidemiology
and Biostatistics, University of Pennsylvania School of Medicine, Philadelphia, PA, USA
[b]Division of Endocrinology and Metabolism, Department of Internal Medicine,
Medical College of Virginia, Virginia Commonwealth University, Richmond, VA, USA

Polycystic ovary syndrome (PCOS) is the most common cause of anovulatory infertility in the United States, affecting 5% to 10% of women of reproductive age [1,2]. It is typically characterized by hyperandrogenism and chronic anovulation. Hyperandrogenism may present as hirsutism, acne, or male-pattern alopecia. Anovulation manifests as irregular menstrual cycles, usually amenorrhea or oligomenorrhea, and infertility [3]. In the past, abnormally regulated luteinizing hormone (LH) levels alone were believed to account for these symptoms. However, recent evidence suggests that hyperinsulinemic insulin resistance plays a pathogenic role in PCOS by increasing circulating ovarian androgen concentrations, perhaps via P450c17α stimulation [4,5], thus impeding ovulation [6–8]. Obese as well as lean women with PCOS manifest insulin resistance independent of fat mass [6,9]. Presumably as a result of their insulin resistance, women with PCOS have also been found to be at increased risk for the development of type 2 diabetes mellitus [10], dyslipidemia [11], and possibly cardiovascular disease.

The presence of hyperinsulinemic insulin resistance in PCOS creates an interesting paradox because peripheral tissues, such as skeletal muscle, are resistant to insulin in terms of glucose metabolism, whereas the ovary remains sensitive to insulin with regard to stimulation of testosterone biosynthesis, suggesting tissue-specific differences in insulin sensitivity. The exact underlying mechanism of insulin resistance in PCOS remains poorly characterized. Although recent studies have implicated a post-insulin receptor

* Corresponding author. Division of Endocrinology and Metabolism, Department of Internal Medicine, Medical College of Virginia, Virginia Commonwealth University, PO Box 980111, Richmond, VA 23298–0111.
   E-mail address: nestler@hsc.vcu.edu (J.E. Nestler).

0889-8529/06/$ - see front matter © 2005 Elsevier Inc. All rights reserved.
doi:10.1016/j.ecl.2005.09.005

defect as the likely mechanism [12–15], further work must be done to elucidate a specific target. Of note, attention is concurrently being focused on the
possibility of PCOS as a genetic disorder, expressing itself only after interaction with other environmental factors [16–18].

Infertility treatment in polycystic ovary syndrome

Seventy-five percent of women with PCOS suffer from infertility, which is
primarily related to anovulation and a high rate of early miscarriage [19].
Several modalities are available to restore ovulation in affected women.
Therapeutic options target direct and indirect stimulation of the ovaries
by follicle-stimulating hormone (FSH) and, more recently, amelioration of
insulin resistance.

In obese women with PCOS, weight loss as a means of improving insulin
sensitivity is often a primary goal because loss of 5% to 10% of body weight
over 6 months is sufficient to re-establish ovarian function in more than
50% of patients [19]. Unfortunately, weight loss is difficult for many patients, and it is even more difficult to maintain. Furthermore, lean patients
with PCOS do not benefit from such measures. Therefore, drug therapy is
often warranted in most patients with PCOS.

Clomiphene citrate, an indirect stimulator of FSH secretion, has long been
used to treat anovulatory infertility in women with PCOS. Ovulation is restored in approximately 80% of patients who are given clomiphene, approximately half of whom become pregnant, usually within the first three cycles of
treatment [19]. The apparent discrepancy between ovulation and pregnancy
rates may be explained by clomiphene's antiestrogenic effects at the level of
the endometrium and cervical mucus, perhaps preventing spermatic penetra-
tion and embryonic implantation. Alternatively, recent evidence suggests
that insulin resistance may adversely affect expression of endometrial cell-
surface proteins involved in implantation and maintenance of pregnancy
[20], irrespective of clomiphene treatment. Nevertheless, clomiphene is
a safe oral medication with few adverse effects other than an increased multiple pregnancy rate [21]. For those who do not respond to clomiphene,
adjuvant therapy with dexamethasone has proven beneficial by way of suppressing adrenal androgen secretion and reducing LH levels [22]; however,
side effects of long-term glucocorticoid use often make it unappealing.

Another option for infertility treatment is direct gonadotropin therapy
with FSH. The current approach uses a low-dose step-up protocol that,
when compared with conventional dosing, yields an improved pregnancy
rate while significantly decreasing the incidence of multiple pregnancies
and the ovarian hyperstimulation syndrome (OHSS) [19]. Although clinically
effective, this approach requires a high degree of skill, extensive hormone
and ultrasound monitoring, low tolerance of multiple follicles, and high
cost [21]. Multiple cycles of therapy may be required.

Aside from weight loss, other therapies for anovulatory infertility that target insulin resistance have become widely popular in recent years because of the growing recognition that insulin resistance likely hampers fertility and decreases the efficacy of other pharmacologic therapies in PCOS. Of the insulin-sensitizing drugs, metformin, an oral biguanide used to treat type 2 diabetes mellitus, is the most comprehensively evaluated drug, with proven effectiveness in lean as well as obese women with PCOS [4,5,23]. An improvement in insulin sensitivity and reduction in circulating insulin by metformin may enhance ovulation in PCOS by decreasing intraovarian concentrations of androgens, normalizing gonadotropin secretory dynamics, or a combination of these and other processes.

The efficacy of metformin monotherapy in promoting ovulation and fertility in PCOS was recently confirmed in a meta-analysis by Lord and colleagues [24]. The meta-analysis consisted of 13 randomized controlled clinical trials that included 428 women with PCOS. Ovulation was achieved in 46% of women with PCOS who received metformin compared with 24% who received placebo (odds ratio [OR] = 3.88, 95% confidence interval [CI]: 2.25 6.69) [24]. Subsequently, a pilot study comparing metformin and life-style modification showed no difference in ovulation rates between the two groups; however, the study had a 39% dropout rate, potentially biasing the results [25]. A further study showed that the addition of metformin to a hypocaloric diet in obese women with PCOS resulted in improvement in menstrual irregularity when compared with the placebo and hypocaloric diet arm [26]. Similarly, in clomiphene-resistant patients, the combination of clomiphene and metformin has been shown to improve ovulation [27] and pregnancy rates [24,28] when compared with clomiphene alone.

Newer insulin sensitizers known as the thiazolidinediones (TZDs) have also received attention with regard to their potential role in the treatment of PCOS. Troglitazone, the first drug of this class, has been shown to improve ovulation rates, hyperandrogenemia, and insulin resistance compared with placebo [29]. Its mechanism of action, although partially systemic, is also thought to involve direct ovarian action because thecal cells possess the peroxisome proliferator–activated receptor-γ (PPARγ) nuclear receptors that these drugs target. In thecal cell cultures, troglitazone impedes stimulation of androgen biosynthesis by the combination of LH and insulin [30]. However, troglitazone was withdrawn from the worldwide market because of hepatocellular toxicity.

Rosiglitazone is another TZD that is commercially available, and it has also been shown to normalize menses and improve insulin resistance in women with PCOS [31]. Additionally, when rosiglitazone was administered to nonobese women who had PCOS with normal insulin sensitivity, ovulation frequency and androgen levels improved compared with placebo even though insulin parameters did not change [32]. This supports the theory that TZDs as a class may have direct inhibitory effects on ovarian androgen biosynthesis. Pioglitazone, the most recently developed TZD, also improved ovulation frequency, hyperandrogenism, and insulin resistance [33]. When added to metformin in metformin nonresponders, pioglitazone continued to improve these parameters [34].

More invasive options exist in case these treatments fail. Laparoscopic ovarian drilling (LOD) involves puncturing the ovary, ideally in three to six places, with electrocoagulation or a laser [35], simulating ovarian wedge resection. LOD most benefits lean women who have PCOS with high LH concentrations [19]. After surgery, LH concentrations fall significantly. An advantage of laparoscopy is that tubal patency can be checked simultaneously in a single procedure. Disadvantages include surgical complications and anesthetic risks. Additionally, concerns have been raised that LOD may result in adhesions leading to tubal obstruction [21]. Similar pregnancy rates were found with LOD after 6 to 12 months of follow-up compared with three to six cycles of gonadotropin therapy, with a lower incidence of multiple pregnancies and OHSS with LOD [36]. Notably, when LOD was compared with metformin therapy in clomiphene-resistant women, ovulation rates were similar between the two groups. Pregnancy, miscarriage, and live birth rates were significantly improved in the latter group, however, suggesting an overall superior benefit in reproductive outcomes with metformin therapy [37], perhaps because of the favorable effects of metformin on the endometrium or oocyte.

In vitro fertilization (IVF) offers a last resort in women with PCOS resistant to these strategies. Although there are some questions regarding oocyte and embryo quality in women with PCOS as a cause of lower fertilization rates, some believe that this is compensated for by the increased number of available oocytes in these women [38]. Also, future therapies such as in vitro maturation of oocytes and the use of aromatase inhibitors, such as letrozole, are currently being developed [19].

Given these strategies, it is clear that lifestyle modification, clomiphene citrate, and metformin are safe, effective, and low-cost options for improving fertility in women with PCOS. At present, the optimal initial pharmacologic approach to the treatment of infertility in PCOS is unknown. This question should soon be answered by the Pregnancy in Polycystic Ovary Syndrome (PPCOS) study, which is a National Institutes of Health (NIH)–sponsored multicenter, randomized, double-blind clinical trial whose purpose is to establish which of the following drug regimens results in the highest live birth rate in women with PCOS: metformin XR, clomiphene, or the combination of these two drugs.

Insulin resistance and normal pregnancy

Insulin resistance, mediated by human placental lactogen (HPL), progesterone, cortisol, and estradiol in pregnancy, and compensatory hyperinsulinemia increase throughout normal gestation and are maximal in the third trimester [39]. Corresponding markers of insulin resistance increase as well, including plasma concentrations of triglycerides, small dense low-density lipoprotein (LDL) particles, free fatty acids, plasminogen activator inhibitor-1 (PAI-1), tissue plasminogen activator antigen (TPA Ag), vascular cell adhesion molecules (VCAMs), leptin, and tumor necrosis factor–α (TNF-α) [39]. Thus, normal pregnancy itself is a state of heightened insulin resistance. Further, in women with PCOS, pregnancy may augment the preexisting insulin resistance and hyperinsulinemia, resulting in fatal and nonfatal complications.

Complications of pregnancy in polycystic ovary syndrome

Early pregnancy loss

Early pregnancy loss (EPL), defined as miscarriage of a clinically recognized pregnancy during the first trimester, occurs in 10% to 15% of normal women. Women with PCOS, however, suffer a threefold higher risk [40]. Multiple studies support this link, many of which initially implicated elevated plasma LH levels as the main culprit [41–44]. In one study, long-term pituitary suppression with a gonadotropin-releasing hormone analogue (GnRHa) decreased the miscarriage rate in patients with PCOS compared with gonadotropin treatment alone [45]. A subsequent study by Clifford and coworkers [46] reported that suppression of endogenous LH release before conception in women with elevated LH levels and a history of recurrent miscarriage did not improve the live birth rate, however.

Thereafter, investigators turned to alternative hypotheses to explain the increased risk of EPL in PCOS. One hypothesis involved hyperandrogenemia as a potential risk factor. A retrospective study of women with a history of recurrent miscarriage found that they had elevated androgen levels compared with normal fertile controls [47]. Further, there were no differences in plasma LH levels between the two groups. One possible explanation for the association between androgen excess and EPL is that high androgen levels antagonize estrogen and thereby adversely affect endometrial development and embryonic implantation [47]. This work was supported by a prospective study that found similar results [48].

Another hypothesis suggested high plasminogen activator inhibitor activity (PAI-Fx) as a risk factor for EPL in women with PCOS. A study of 41 women with PCOS revealed that PAI-Fx positively correlated with the number of miscarriages [49]. Further, PAI-Fx was shown to be an independent reversible risk factor for miscarriage in women with PCOS, presumably because it induces a hypofibrinolytic state causing placental insufficiency [49].

Arguably, the most compelling hypothesis has come from research on the effect of obesity on miscarriage rates. An early retrospective cohort study found that moderate obesity in women with PCOS, treated with low-dose gonadotropin, was associated with an increased risk of miscarriage [50]. Subsequently, Fedorcsak and colleagues [51] studied a cohort of 383 lean and obese women who conceived after IVF or intracytoplasmic sperm injection (ICSI) to determine their miscarriage rates. Obese women were again found to have an increased risk of EPL (22% versus 12%; $P = .03$) and a decreased live birth rate compared with lean women. Obesity, characterized by hyperinsulinemic insulin resistance, was shown to be an independent risk factor for EPL [51].

Investigators have examined the effects of insulin-sensitizing drugs on the rate of miscarriage in PCOS. Glueck and colleagues [52] performed a prospective cohort pilot study of women with PCOS, comparing those treated with metformin before conception who continued the drug throughout pregnancy with historical controls who did not receive metformin. Results showed that the rate of first trimester pregnancy loss was 39% in the historical controls but only 11% in the metformin group. Ten women in the metformin group had had previous pregnancies while not receiving metformin. In this subcohort, the miscarriage rate decreased from 73% to 10% with the addition of metformin ($P < .002$). Overall, no evidence of teratogenicity was noted in the metformin group. Before metformin therapy, fasting serum insulin levels correlated positively with PAI activity ($r = 0.60$, $P = .004$). Over a median treatment period of 6 months (before conception), a reduction in fasting serum insulin was also positively correlated with a reduction in PAI activity ($r = 0.65$, $P = .04$), suggesting that hyperinsulinemia and PAI activity may be closely related; perhaps both can help to explain the etiology of EPL in PCOS.

Glueck and coworkers [53] went on to complete a follow-up prospective study confirming that EPL decreased from 62% to 26% ($P < .0001$) when women with PCOS continued metformin throughout pregnancy. Again, no teratogenic adverse events occurred. In this study, PAI activity was again lower on metformin compared with premetformin entry levels. However, logistic regression revealed that entry fasting serum insulin was the only significant variable associated with total (previous and current) first trimester miscarriage (OR = 1.32 for each 5-µIU/mL increment in insulin, 95% CI: 1.09–1.60, $P = .005$).

A larger retrospective study of women with PCOS performed by an independent group also showed a decrease in EPL in those who continued metformin throughout pregnancy compared with controls (8.8% versus 42%; $P < .001$) [40]. This trend remained significant in the subgroup analysis of women with a prior history of miscarriage. No adverse fetal outcomes were noted in the metformin group, except for 1 of 62 live births that suffered from achondroplasia, a hereditary condition thought to be unrelated to metformin. Additionally, those women who remained on metformin had significantly decreased serum androgen concentrations and improved insulin sensitivity during pregnancy compared with controls; both are plausible explanations for the decrease in miscarriage rate.

Given the consistency among these studies, insulin resistance seems to play an important role in EPL in women with PCOS. It is plausible that insulin resistance with hyperinsulinemia is the inciting event, which in turn causes hyperandrogenemia and high PAI activity. The resulting abnormal endometrial development and placental blood flow would then create a hostile environment for fetal growth. Also, insulin resistance is associated with decreased uterine vascularity [20]. Recent evidence further suggests that hyperinsulinemia decreases levels of glycodelin and insulin growth factor–binding protein-1 (IGFBP-1) [20], two major endometrial proteins. This has been corroborated in women with PCOS during the first trimester, implicating endometrial epithelial and stromal dysfunction during peri-implantation and early pregnancy as possible mechanisms for EPL in PCOS [20]. When comparing women with PCOS who experienced EPL with those who did not have such a history, serum glycodelin was significantly lower during gestational weeks 3 through 8 ($P < .02$) and serum IGFBP-1 was significantly lower during gestational weeks 9 through 11 ($P = .003$) in the former [20].

Aside from being associated with hyperandrogenemia, increased PAI activity, decreased uterine vascularity, and lower serum glycodelin and IGFBP-1 levels, hyperinsulinemic insulin resistance is most likely also associated with a host of as yet unidentified chemical and hormonal changes that, together, contribute to EPL in women with PCOS.

In summary, metformin may offer an inexpensive and effective treatment for EPL in women with PCOS, even in those with a history of EPL. Metformin is a pregnancy class B drug, and thus is not contraindicated in pregnancy. However, none of the studies to date indicate the duration of time that metformin would need to be administered during pregnancy to prevent EPL, or if simply conceiving while taking metformin might confer full benefit. The latter idea is supported by the finding of a 50% reduction in miscarriages in women with PCOS who underwent mock laparoscopy and were then treated with metformin for 6 months, with the metformin being discontinued when a diagnosis of pregnancy was made, compared with women who underwent LOD and were then treated with a placebo [37].

Of all the insulin sensitizers, metformin may be the safest option, given that the TZDs are pregnancy class C drugs. The safety of metformin in pregnancy has come under question, however. Hellmuth and colleagues [54] performed a cohort study of pregnant diabetic women treated with metformin compared with women treated with sulfonylurea or insulin. They found an increased incidence of preeclampsia and perinatal mortality in the metformin group. The authors acknowledge that the reference group selected was not an ideal one, however, because the women in the metformin group had a significantly higher body mass index (BMI) and worse diabetes control, both of which predispose to preeclampsia, than the women treated with sulfonylurea or insulin. In contrast, Glueck and colleagues [55] performed a recent prospective study to assess the growth and motor-social development in 126 live births to 109 women with PCOS, who conceived on and continued metformin throughout pregnancy. The authors found that metformin was not teratogenic and did not adversely affect birth length and weight, growth, or motor-social development in the first 18 months of life. Several studies have further substantiated this claim [40,56]. Given the conflicting data, however, randomized controlled trials need to be performed to assess metformin's safety profile in pregnancy more definitively.

Gestational diabetes

Gestational diabetes mellitus (GDM), defined as diabetes or impaired glucose tolerance (IGT) with onset in pregnancy, complicates 3% to 5% of all pregnancies in the United States [57]. GDM develops because pregnancy induces or aggravates insulin resistance, thus placing stress on pancreatic β-cells which cannot respond appropriately [58]. Alarmingly, the yearly cumulative incidence of GDM increased between 1991 and 2000, independent of changes in age and ethnicity [59].

Up to 80% of obese and 30% of lean women with PCOS demonstrate insulin resistance before conception, and as many as 30% are affected by IGT later in life [9]. Because of relative infertility, women with PCOS frequently conceive at an older age, which is another risk factor for GDM [58]. Because women with PCOS have multiple risk factors for GDM and its subsequent complications, the existence of a possible association between these clinical entities has been investigated.

A prospective cohort study by Lanzone and coworkers [60] followed 12 women with PCOS who became pregnant after FSH therapy. None of the women had IGT or diabetes at baseline. At 23 to 29 weeks of gestation, a 100-g oral glucose tolerance test (OGTT) was performed on all patients. According to O'Sullivan's criteria, 3 patients developed IGT and 2 developed GDM; all these women had a history of pregestational hyperinsulinemia. Further, the severity of hyperglycemia seemed to be related to the degree of pregestational insulin secretion [60]. The study supported the hypothesis that women with PCOS and pregestational hyperinsulinemia are at increased risk of IGT and GDM and also suggested that there may exist a "dose-response" relation between the level of pregestational hyperinsulinemia and subsequent degree of glycemic dysfunction.

Holte and colleagues [61] went on to characterize potential differences between women who had a 3- to 5-year history of GDM and those with uncomplicated pregnancies, who were matched for age and delivery date. Polycystic ovaries, diagnosed by ultrasound, were found in 41% of the GDM group versus 3% of the control group ($P < .0001$). Hirsutism and irregular menstrual cycles were also more common in the GDM group.

A subgroup analysis of the GDM subjects allowed investigators to determine if significant differences existed between women with polycystic ovaries compared with those with normal ovaries. BMI was similar between the two groups; however, truncal obesity was higher in the polycystic ovary group. No differences in gestational age at delivery, birth weight of the offspring, or mode of delivery between the groups were found. Also, glycemic responses during OGTTs or intravenous glucose tolerance tests during pregnancy were similar. Women with polycystic ovaries showed greater insulin responses during these tests compared with women with normal ovaries, however. Based on the insulin and glucose measurements, the polycystic ovary group demonstrated insulin resistance as the primary problem during the index pregnancy, whereas the normal ovary group demonstrated β-cell dysfunction. Additionally, women with polycystic ovaries had higher plasma androstenedione, testosterone, and free androgen index (FAI) levels independent of BMI and age. Thus, among women with prior GDM, those with polycystic ovaries formed a distinct subgroup that may be more prone to developing various features of the metabolic syndrome compared with women with normal ovaries [61].

A similar study was performed, this time matching the GDM group and controls for age and BMI, which confirmed that polycystic ovaries diagnosed by ultrasound were more common in women with a history of GDM [62]. Of note, by using polycystic ovaries as a surrogate for PCOS, both studies may have overestimated the true prevalence of PCOS in GDM because polycystic ovaries can be found in normal ovulatory women.

Thereafter, investigators' interest in the relation between PCOS and GDM increased. Radon and coworkers [63] performed a retrospective cohort study of GDM in women with PCOS, comparing them with age- and weight-matched controls. The authors showed that GDM developed in 41% of women with PCOS versus 3% of controls (OR = 22.2, 95% CI: 3.8–170), but no comparison had been performed with regard to the ability of obesity or PCOS to predict GDM independently. Mikola and colleagues [64] performed a retrospective cohort study of GDM and preeclampsia in women with PCOS compared with an unselected control population and found that GDM developed in 20% of women with PCOS versus 8.9% of controls ($P < .0001$). After logistic regression analysis, however, BMI greater than 25 kg/m^2 was found to be the strongest predictor of GDM, whereas PCOS remained a lesser but still independent predictor. This information suggests that the intrinsic insulin resistance of PCOS, which is independent of body weight, may explain the increased risk of GDM in patients with PCOS [64]. This idea was supported by Urman and coworkers [65] who found that even when lean patients with PCOS were compared with lean controls, the incidence of GDM remained significantly higher in patients with PCOS.

To clarify further the effect of insulin resistance on the development of GDM, Bjercke and colleagues [66] prospectively followed women with PCOS, grouped by insulin resistance status, and normal controls. GDM was again more frequent in women with PCOS compared with controls (7.7% versus 0.6%; $P < .01$). Surprisingly, however, the development of GDM in women with PCOS was independent of pregestational insulin resistance status. Given the small sample size (23 insulin-resistant and 29 non-insulin-resistant women with PCOS), the authors may have missed a difference if one truly existed. Conversely, if no difference in GDM existed between those with and without pregestational insulin resistance, one might consider other determinants of PCOS as possible explanations.

The hypothesis that PCOS is associated with GDM has not been supported by all studies. For example, a retrospective cohort study by Haakova and coworkers [67] compared pregnant women with PCOS with age- and weight-matched pregnant controls and found no statistical difference in the development of GDM. Nevertheless, consistency among many studies combined with their large magnitudes of effect is supportive evidence in favor of insulin resistance causing women with PCOS to be at increased risk for developing GDM. This effect has been noted independent of age and BMI. Several reports prospectively document insulin resistance preceding GDM, implying a cause-effect relation. Further, the association is biologically feasible because insulin resistance is the main offender implicated in type 2 diabetes mellitus.

Consequences of GDM are significant and include the long-term risk of developing diabetes later in life as well as significant immediate perinatal risks, including macrosomia, hypoglycemia, stillbirth, jaundice, and respiratory distress syndrome. Rates of birth trauma and cesarean section are also increased. Another potential complication is the development of pregnancy-induced hypertensive disorders (PIHDs), such as preeclampsia and gestational hypertension. A recent case-control study examined this relation and found that women with GDM have a 1.5-fold increased risk of developing PIHDs [68]. Ethnicity was found to modify the association, with the greatest risk existing among black women [68].

Given the significant attendant complications, some investigators have examined potential drug therapy to prevent the onset of GDM in women with PCOS. One study compared women with PCOS who conceived while taking metformin and continued taking it throughout pregnancy with women with PCOS who conceived without metformin therapy [58]. GDM developed in 3% of the metformin pregnancies compared with 31% of the nonmetformin pregnancies (OR = 0.093, 95% CI: 0.011–0.795; P = .03). After adjustment for age at delivery, metformin was associated with a 10-fold reduction in GDM in women with PCOS. Further, metformin was shown to decrease BMI, insulin levels, insulin resistance, and insulin secretion; these effects were maintained throughout pregnancy. Metformin did not result in any major fetal malformations or fetal hypoglycemia, again supporting its safety in pregnancy. Nevertheless, the utility of metformin administration to women with PCOS during pregnancy to prevent development of GDM has not been rigorously tested in a randomized clinical trial.

Pregnancy-induced hypertensive disorders

PIHDs complicate 3% to 5% of pregnancies in previously normotensive women [39] and usually develop during the third trimester. Although hypertension in these women typically resolves by 6 weeks postpartum, they are at increased risk of developing essential hypertension later in life. Gestational hypertension is diagnosed as elevated blood pressure without systemic symptoms. Preeclampsia, conversely, is defined by elevated blood pressure in conjunction with proteinuria (urine protein > 300 mg in 24 hours). Other manifestations associated with preeclampsia include disseminated intravascular coagulation, hemolysis, elevated liver function tests, and seizures [39]. Until now, delivery has been the only definitive treatment, increasing risk to the newborn. With new insights into the etiology of this spectrum of illnesses, potentially safer alternatives may become available.

The etiology of PIHDs is likely multifactorial, involving immune, genetic, and placental abnormalities [39]. It has been well described that women with PIHDs demonstrate an exaggerated hyperinsulinemia relative to normal pregnancy [69–72], suggesting that metabolic abnormalities may also be significant. For example, Hamasaki and colleagues [71] reported in a prospective cohort study that the relative risk of developing gestational hypertension in women with hyperinsulinemia compared with normal controls was 1.19 (95% CI: 1.03–1.38) after adjusting for age, parity, and BMI. Additionally, preeclampsia has been shown to be associated with insulin resistance and its ensuing metabolic changes, including glucose intolerance, elevated plasma triglycerides, low high-density lipoprotein (HDL), and increased small dense LDL as well as increased leptin, TNF-α, and PAI-1 [39]. Reduced serum sex hormone–binding globulin (SHBG) levels in the first trimester and elevated total and free testosterone adjusted for BMI are also associated with preeclampsia [39]. It would be reasonable to hypothesize that hyperinsulinemic insulin-resistant women with PCOS may be at increased risk for PIHDs.

One of the earliest studies to describe a relation between women with PCOS and preeclampsia was published in 1982 by Diamant and coworkers [73]. These investigators found the incidence of "preeclamptic toxemia" to be 11 fold higher in pregnant patients with PCOS, all of whom conceived after ovulation induction, compared with a control group. Further, this disorder occurred more frequently in patients with PCOS compared with anovulatory patients in whom PCOS was excluded. The investigators concluded that pregnancies after ovulation induction are associated with a higher incidence of hypertensive disorders compared with controls. Of note, this group had no data on BMI, a potential risk factor for the development of preeclampsia.

Subsequently, a prospective study by Gjonnaess [74] revealed that preeclampsia occurred in 13% of women with PCOS who conceived after LOD, which was higher than in the general population. When the women with PCOS were then stratified by weight, however, an increased risk of preeclampsia was found only in the heavier women, and it was concluded that an increased risk of preeclampsia in women with PCOS was associated with moderate or severe obesity. However, even women who were mildly overweight demonstrated a 13% incidence of preeclampsia suggesting that PCOS itself may play some role in the association.

A retrospective case-control study of preeclampsia in women with PCOS compared with age- and parity-matched controls was performed by de Vries and colleagues [75]. Although the overall incidence of PIHDs was similar between the two groups, the incidence of preeclampsia in women with PCOS was 14% compared with 2.5% in controls ($P = .02$). These findings could not be explained by obesity because BMI was similar between the groups. Further, among patients with PCOS, BMI was similar in those with preeclampsia and those without PIHDs. To account for BMI more accurately, a retrospective cohort study of preeclampsia in women with PCOS compared with age- and weight-matched controls was conducted [63]. In this study, preeclampsia also occurred more frequently in women with PCOS than in controls, with a highly significant OR of 15.0 (95% CI: 1.9–121.5). Although there was a higher degree of parity among the controls, the former study by de Vries and colleagues [75] had controlled for parity and maintained a significant association. These findings were supported by Urman and coworkers [65] who found that even when lean patients with PCOS were compared with lean controls, the incidence of PIHDs remained significantly higher in the patients with PCOS. Thus, some factor other than obesity was contributing to the increased risk of preeclampsia in women with PCOS.

Some experts would argue that different ovulation induction methods, or perhaps ovulation induction itself, may be responsible for the increased risk of preeclampsia seen in women with PCOS. To address this, de Vries and colleagues [75] stratified women with PCOS by treatment regimens for ovulation induction and found no relation between the method used and the development of preeclampsia. Additionally, the incidence of preeclampsia was similar between the patients with PCOS who underwent ovulation induction compared with those who conceived spontaneously. Further, in the previously cited study by Gjonnaess [74], all women with PCOS conceived without ovulation induction. Another study by Kashyap and colleagues [76] examined patients with PCOS and infertile controls, all of whom were given gonadotropin therapy with human menopausal gonadotropin (hMG) for ovulation induction. Women in both groups had similar age, BMI, parity, and other gestational hypertension risk factors. Pregnant patients with PCOS had a 31.8% incidence of gestational hypertension compared with a 3.7% incidence in the infertile controls (OR = 12.1, 95% CI: 1.3–566.8; $P = .016$). Collectively, the evidence suggests that neither type of ovulation induction method nor ovulation induction itself contributes to the development of PIHDs in women with PCOS. These findings again support PCOS as a potential independent risk factor for PIHDs.

In 2002, Bjercke and colleagues [66] prospectively assessed the impact of insulin resistance on the development of PIHDs in women with PCOS. Controls consisted of women with singleton pregnancies who had conceived after assisted reproduction. Overall, the frequency of gestational hypertension was significantly increased in pregnancies in women with PCOS compared with controls (11.5% versus 0.3%; $P < .05$), and preeclampsia was found more frequently among insulin-resistant patients with PCOS than in non-insulin-resistant patients with PCOS (22% versus 7%; $P < .05$) and controls. BMI was similar among the insulin-resistant and non–insulin-resistant women with PCOS. This was the first prospective study in women with PCOS to support the association between hyperinsulinemia and PIHDs proposed earlier by other investigators.

Nonetheless, some of the available data do not support the proposed hypothesis. A study by Mikola and coworkers [64] found no significant difference in the incidence of preeclampsia between women with PCOS and a normal control population. After multiple logistic regression, nulliparity was the only significant risk factor for preeclampsia; BMI greater than 25 kg/m², multiple pregnancy, and PCOS had no predictive value. When de Vries and colleagues [75] matched cases and controls for parity, however, women with PCOS maintained a significant association with preeclampsia. A more recent study by Haakova and coworkers [67] also retrospectively analyzed the relationship between women with PIHDs and women with PCOS. Although a trend toward increased PIHDs occurred in the women with PCOS, no statistically significant difference was found when compared with age- and weight-matched controls.

Clearly, the limited data on the association between PCOS and PIHDs are conflicting. The effects of age, BMI, ovulation induction, and parity have been studied, however, and the magnitude of association among positive studies remains quite large.

Taken one step further, the impact of insulin resistance in women with PCOS who develop preeclampsia has also been examined, suggesting a possible mechanistic link. Several reports document hyperinsulinemia or hyperglycemia developing before preeclampsia, providing support for insulin resistance in disease pathogenesis [69,77,78]. Additionally, insulin resistance or its associated features have been shown to occur many years after a preeclamptic first pregnancy [79–82]. Persistence of insulin resistance postpartum further suggests a role for its causality in the development of preeclampsia [82]. Laivuori and colleagues [83] found an association between preeclamptic pregnancy and the existence of hyperandrogenemia 17 years after delivery, suggesting that these women could have had hyperinsulinemic PCOS during their reproductive years (although all reportedly had normal menstruation) and may be at risk for its metabolic consequences after menopause.

Several theoretic mechanisms exist whereby hyperinsulinemia could predispose to PIHDs in women with PCOS. For example, hyperinsulinemia may increase renal sodium reabsorption [84] and stimulate the sympathetic nervous system [85]. Insulin resistance or associated hyperglycemia may impair endothelial function [86]. Endothelial dysfunction may decrease prostacyclin production [87]. Studies in animal models have shown that androgens increase vasoconstriction in response to pressors [88] and also decrease the synthesis of prostacyclin [89], potentially playing a further role in the development of PIHDs. Interestingly, the plasma total renin level was found to be higher in normotensive women with PCOS compared with healthy controls, independent of insulin resistance [90]. Although many possible theories exist, more studies need to be done to confirm a mechanistic link between hyperinsulinemia and preeclampsia.

Preeclampsia may have acute and chronic consequences. Acute problems primarily revolve around delivery complications and increased perinatal morbidity. Chronic effects, however, are more difficult to study because women who develop these problems often have a remote diagnosis of PIHD that is difficult to ascertain [39]. One study was able to show that the risk of hypertension is increased almost threefold after 2 to 24 years of follow-up in women with a history of preeclampsia or eclampsia compared with controls [91]. Other long-term consequences that have been reported include hypertriglyceridemia, hyperuricemia, hyperandrogenemia, and abnormal brachial artery flow-mediated (endothelium-dependent) dilatation [39], consistent with the effects of insulin resistance.

Given this increase in cardiovascular risk factors, some investigators have attempted to determine if mortality attributable to cardiovascular causes is increased among women with a prior history of preeclampsia. One study found that mortality attributable to cardiovascular causes was increased among Norwegian women who had preeclampsia and preterm delivery (ie, severe preeclampsia) compared with preeclamptic women with term delivery or women with preterm delivery alone [92]. Another study found that women with a discharge diagnosis of preeclampsia were twice as likely to be admitted to the hospital for or to die from ischemic heart disease compared with women with uncomplicated pregnancies [93]. These findings suggest that preeclampsia may serve as a marker for future cardiovascular disease. Whether this association is independent of obesity and other predictors of cardiovascular risk still remains to be seen.

Given the available evidence, it is possible to imagine that interventions targeted at improving insulin sensitivity may decrease the likelihood of preeclampsia and later life complications, including risk of cardiovascular events. For instance, weight reduction before pregnancy and avoidance of excessive weight gain during pregnancy may contribute to improved insulin sensitivity and decreased risk for developing preeclampsia. When lifestyle modification cannot be maintained, however, incentive to use insulin-sensitizing drug therapy, such as metformin, may exist. Studies that examine the effect of metformin on the incidence of preeclampsia and its complications in women with PCOS are currently needed.

Future directions

In summary, infertility in PCOS has multiple facets (eg, anovulation, decreased implantation), and several treatment options exist including those that target insulin resistance. Once pregnancy is achieved, however, women are faced with several potential complications, including EPL, GDM, and PIHDs. All these disorders are potentially linked by their association with hyperinsulinemia and insulin resistance. Hence, it is notable that preliminary studies suggest that metformin, which is an insulin-sensitizing agent that is a pregnancy class B drug, may decrease the risk of EPL and GDM in women with PCOS. Furthermore, given the long-term metabolic consequences of PCOS, including type 2 diabetes, hyperlipidemia, and cardiovascular disease, some experts speculate as to whether administering metformin during pregnancy may not only prevent pregnancy complications but also retard or prevent some of these long-term health risks. In fact, the occurrence of EPL, GDM, and PIHDs may be identified as predictors of cardiovascular risk in women with PCOS.

Although it is reassuring that metformin administration during pregnancy appears to be safe, rigorous randomized controlled trials must be conducted to confirm metformin's efficacy and safety under these conditions before its use during pregnancy can be recommended.

References

[1] Knochenhauer ES, Key TJ, Kahsar-Miller M, et al. Prevalence of the polycystic ovary syndrome in unselected black and white women of the southeastern United States: a prospective study. J Clin Endocrinol Metab 1998;83(9):3078–82.

[2] Asuncion M, Calvo RM, San Millan JL, et al. A prospective study of the prevalence of the polycystic ovary syndrome in unselected Caucasian women from Spain. J Clin Endocrinol Metab 2000;85(7):2434–8.

[3] Franks S. Polycystic ovary syndrome. N Engl J Med 1995;333(13):853–61.

[4] Nestler JE, Jakubowicz DJ. Decreases in ovarian cytochrome P450c17alpha activity and serum free testosterone after reduction of insulin secretion in polycystic ovary syndrome. N Engl J Med 1996;335(9):617–23.

[5] Nestler JE, Jakubowicz DJ. Lean women with polycystic ovary syndrome respond to insulin reduction with decreases in ovarian P450c17alpha activity and serum androgens. J Clin Endocrinol Metab 1997;82(12):4075–9.

[6] Chang RJ, Nakamura RM, Judd HL, et al. Insulin resistance in nonobese patients with polycystic ovarian disease. J Clin Endocrinol Metab 1983;57(2):356–9.

[7] Franks S, Gilling-Smith C, Watson H, et al. Insulin action in the normal and polycystic ovary. Endocrinol Metab Clin North Am 1999;28(2):361–78.

[8] Dunaif A. Insulin resistance and the polycystic ovary syndrome: mechanism and implications for pathogenesis. Endocr Rev 1997;18(6):774–800.

[9] Dunaif A, Segal KR, Futterweit W, et al. Profound peripheral insulin resistance, independent of obesity, in polycystic ovary syndrome. Diabetes 1989;38(9):1165–74.

[10] Legro RS, Kunselman AR, Dodson WC, et al. Prevalence and predictors of risk for type 2 diabetes mellitus and impaired glucose tolerance in polycystic ovary syndrome: a prospective, controlled study in 254 affected women. J Clin Endocrinol Metab 1999;84(1):165–9.

[11] Talbott E, Clerici A, Berga SL, et al. Adverse lipid and coronary heart disease risk profiles in young women with polycystic ovary syndrome: results of a case-control study. J Clin Epidemiol 1998;51(5):415–22.

[12] Rosenbaum D, Haber RS, Dunaif A. Insulin resistance in polycystic ovary syndrome: decreased expression of GLUT-4 glucose transporters in adipocytes. Am J Physiol 1993;264: E197–202.

[13] Dunaif A, Wu X, Lee A, et al. Defects in insulin receptor signaling in vivo in the polycystic ovary syndrome (PCOS). Am J Physiol Endocrinol Metab 2001;281(2): E392–9.

[14] Book CB, Dunaif A. Selective insulin resistance in the polycystic ovary syndrome. J Clin Endocrinol Metab 1999;84(9):3110–6.

[15] Nestler JE, Jakubowicz DJ, Reamer P, et al. Ovulatory and metabolic effects of D-chiro-inositol in the polycystic ovary syndrome. N Engl J Med 1999;340(17):1314–20.

[16] Legro RS, Driscoll D, Strauss JF, et al. Evidence for a genetic basis for hyperandrogenemia in polycystic ovary syndrome. Proc Natl Acad Sci USA 1998;95(25):14956–60.

[17] Franks S, McCarthy M. Genetics of ovarian disorders: polycystic ovary syndrome. Rev Endocr Metab Disord 2004;5(1):69–76.

[18] Franks S, Gharani N, Waterworth D, et al. Genetics of polycystic ovary syndrome. Mol Cell Endocrinol 1998;145(1–2):123–8.

[19] Homburg R. The management of infertility associated with polycystic ovary syndrome. Reprod Biol Endocrinol 2003;(1):109.

[20] Jakubowicz DJ, Essah PA, Seppala M, et al. Reduced serum glycodelin and insulin-like growth factor-binding protein-1 in women with polycystic ovary syndrome during first trimester of pregnancy. J Clin Endocrinol Metab 2004;89(2):833–9.

[21] Norman RJ. Metformin—comparison with other therapies in ovulation induction in polycystic ovary syndrome [editorial]. J Clin Endocrinol Metab 2004;89(10):4797–800.

[22] Parsanezhad ME, Alborzi S, Motazedian S, et al. Use of dexamethasone and clomiphene citrate in the treatment of clomiphene citrate-resistant patients with polycystic ovary syndrome and normal dehydroepiandrostenedione sulfate levels: a prospective, double-blind, placebo-controlled trial. Fertil Steril 2002;78(5):1001–4.

[23] Fleming R, Hopkinson ZE, Wallace M, et al. Ovarian function and metabolic factors in women with oligomenorrhea treated with metformin in a randomized double-blind placebo-controlled trial. J Clin Endocrinol Metab 2002;87(2):569–74.

[24] Lord JM, Flight I, Norman RJ. Metformin in polycystic ovary syndrome: systematic review and meta-analysis. BMJ 2003;327(7421):951–5.

[25] Hoeger KM, Kochman L, Wixom N, et al. A randomized, 48-week, placebo-controlled trial of intensive lifestyle modification and/or metformin therapy in overweight women with polycystic ovary syndrome: a pilot study. Fertil Steril 2004;82(2):421–9.

[26] Pasquali R, Gambineri A, Biscotti D, et al. Effect of long-term treatment with metformin added to hypocaloric diet on body composition, fat distribution, and androgen and insulin levels in abdominally obese women with and without the polycystic ovary syndrome. J Clin Endocrinol Metab 2000;85(8):2767–74.

[27] Nestler JE, Jakubowicz DJ, Evans WS, et al. Effects of metformin on spontaneous and clomiphene-induced ovulation in the polycystic ovary syndrome. N Engl J Med 1998;338(26): 1876–80.

[28] Kashyap S, Wells GA, Rosenwaks Z. Insulin-sensitizing agents as primary therapy for patients with polycystic ovary syndrome. Hum Reprod 2004;19(11):2474–83.

[29] Azziz R, Ehrmann D, Legro RS, et al. Troglitazone improves ovulation and hirsutism in the polycystic ovary syndrome: a multicenter, double-blind, placebo-controlled trial. J Clin Endocrinol Metab 2001;86(4):1626–32.

[30] Veldhuis J, Zhang G, Garmey J. Troglitazone, an insulin-sensitizing thiazolidinedione, represses combined stimulation by LH and insulin of de novo androgen biosynthesis by thecal cells in vitro. J Clin Endocrinol Metab 2002;87(3):1129–33.

[31] Belli SH, Graffigna MN, Oneto A, et al. Effect of rosiglitazone on insulin resistance, growth factors, and reproductive disturbances in women with polycystic ovary syndrome. Fertil Steril 2004;81(3):624–9.

[32] Baillargeon JP, Jakubowicz DJ, Iuorno MJ, et al. Effects of metformin and rosiglitazone, alone and in combination, in nonobese women with polycystic ovary syndrome and normal indices of insulin sensitivity. Fertil Steril 2004;82(4):893–902.

[33] Brettenthaler N, De Geyter C, Huber PR, et al. Effect of the insulin sensitizer pioglitazone on insulin resistance, hyperandrogenism, and ovulatory dysfunction in women with polycystic ovary syndrome. J Clin Endocrinol Metab 2004;89(8):3835–40.

[34] Glueck CJ, Moreira A, Goldenberg N, et al. Pioglitazone and metformin in obese women with the polycystic ovary syndrome not optimally responsive to metformin. Hum Reprod 2003;18(8):1618–25.

[35] Saleh AM, Khalil HS. Review of nonsurgical and surgical treatment and the role of insulin-sensitizing agents in the management of infertile women with polycystic ovary syndrome. Acta Obstet Gynecol Scand 2004;83(7):614–21.

[36] Farquhar C, Lilford R, Marjoribanks J, et al. Laparoscopic "drilling" by diathermy or laser for ovulation induction in anovulatory polycystic ovary syndrome. Cochrane Database Syst Rev 2005;(3):CD001122.

[37] Palomba S, Orio F Jr, Nardo LG, et al. Metformin administration versus laparoscopic ovarian diathermy in clomiphene citrate-resistant women with polycystic ovary syndrome: a prospective parallel randomized double-blind placebo controlled trial. J Clin Endocrinol Metab 2004;89(10):4801–9.

[38] Urman B, Tiras B, Yakin K. Assisted reproduction in the treatment of polycystic ovary syndrome. Reprod Biomed Online 2004;8(4):419–30.

[39] Seely EW, Solomon CG. Insulin resistance and its potential role in pregnancy-induced hypertension. J Clin Endocrinol Metab 2003;88(6):2393–8.

[40] Jakubowicz DJ, Iuorno MJ, Jakubowicz S, et al. Effects of metformin on early pregnancy loss in the polycystic ovary syndrome. J Clin Endocrinol Metab 2002,87(2):524–9.

[41] Regan L, Owen EJ, Jacobs HS. Hypersecretion of luteinising hormone, infertility, and miscarriage. Lancet 1990;336(8724):1141–4.

[42] Watson H, Kiddy DS, Hamilton-Fairley D, et al. Hypersecretion of luteinizing hormone and ovarian steroids in women with recurrent early miscarriage. Hum Reprod 1993;8(6): 829–33.

[43] Homburg R, Armar NA, Eshel A, et al. Influence of serum luteinising hormone concentrations on ovulation, conception, and early pregnancy loss in polycystic ovary syndrome. BMJ 1988;297(6655):1024–6.

[44] Balen AH, Tan S, MacDougall J, et al. Miscarriage rates following in-vitro fertilization are increased in women with polycystic ovaries and reduced by pituitary desensitization with buserelin. Hum Reprod 1993;8(6):959–64.

[45] Homburg R, Levy T, Berkovitz D, et al. Gonadotropin-releasing hormone agonist reduces the miscarriage rate for pregnancies achieved in women with polycystic ovarian syndrome. Fertil Steril 1993;59(3):527–31.

[46] Clifford K, Rai R, Watson H, et al. Does suppressing luteinising hormone secretion reduce the miscarriage rate? Results of a randomised controlled trial. BMJ 1996;312(7045): 1508–11.

[47] Okon MA, Laird SM, Tuckerman EM, et al. Serum androgen levels in women who have recurrent miscarriages and their correlation with markers of endometrial function. Fertil Steril 1998;69(4):682–90.

[48] Tulppala M, Stenman UH, Cacciatore B, et al. Polycystic ovaries and levels of gonadotrophins and androgens in recurrent miscarriage: prospective study in 50 women. Br J Obstet Gynaecol 1993;100(4):348–52.

[49] Glueck CJ, Wang P, Fontaine RN, et al. Plasminogen activator inhibitor activity: an independent risk factor for the high miscarriage rate during pregnancy in women with polycystic ovary syndrome. Metabolism 1999,48(12):1589–95.

[50] Hamilton-Fairley D, Kiddy D, Watson H, et al. Association of moderate obesity with a poor pregnancy outcome in women with polycystic ovary syndrome treated with low dose gonadotrophin. Br J Obstet Gynaecol 1992;99(2):128–31.

[51] Fedorcsak P, Storeng R, Dale PO, et al. Obesity is a risk factor for early pregnancy loss after IVF or ICSI. Acta Obstet Gynecol Scand 2000;79(1):43–8.

[52] Glueck CJ, Phillips H, Cameron D, et al. Continuing metformin throughout pregnancy in women with polycystic ovary syndrome appears to safely reduce first-trimester spontaneous abortion: a pilot study. Fertil Steril 2001;75(1):46–52.

[53] Glueck CJ, Wang P, Goldenberg N, et al. Pregnancy outcomes among women with polycystic ovary syndrome treated with metformin. Hum Reprod 2002;17(11):2858–64.

[54] Hellmuth E, Damm P, Molsted-Pedersen L. Oral hypoglycaemic agents in 118 diabetic pregnancies. Diabet Med 2000;17(7):507–11.

[55] Glueck CJ, Goldenberg N, Pranikoff J, et al. Height, weight, and motor-social development during the first 18 months of life in 126 infants born to 109 mothers with polycystic ovary syndrome who conceived on and continued metformin through pregnancy. Hum Reprod 2004;19(6):1323–30.

[56] Coetzee EJ, Jackson WP. The management of non-insulin-dependent diabetes during pregnancy. Diabetes Res Clin Pract 1985;1(5):281–7.

[57] Ferrara A, Hedderson MM, Quesenberry CP, et al. Prevalence of gestational diabetes mellitus detected by the National Diabetes Data Group or the Carpenter and Coustan plasma glucose thresholds. Diabetes Care 2002;25(9):1625–30.

[58] Glueck CJ, Wang P, Kobayashi S, et al. Metformin therapy throughout pregnancy reduces the development of gestational diabetes in women with polycystic ovary syndrome. Fertil Steril 2002;77(3):520–5.

[59] Ferrara A, Kahn HS, Quesenberry CP, et al. An increase in the incidence of gestational diabetes mellitus: Northern California, 1991–2000. Obstet Gynecol 2004;103(3):526–33.

[60] Lanzone A, Caruso A, Di Simone N, et al. Polycystic ovary disease: a risk factor for gestational diabetes? J Reprod Med 1995;40(4):312–6.

[61] Holte J, Gennarelli G, Wide L, et al. High prevalence of polycystic ovaries and associated clinical, endocrine, and metabolic features in women with previous gestational diabetes mellitus. J Clin Endocrinol Metab 1998;83(4):1143–50.

[62] Anttila L, Karjala K, Penttila TA, et al. Polycystic ovaries in women with gestational diabetes. Obstet Gynecol 1998;92(1):13–6.

[63] Radon PA, McMahon MJ, Meyer WR. Impaired glucose tolerance in pregnant women with polycystic ovary syndrome. Obstet Gynecol 1999;94(2):194–7.

[64] Mikola M, Hiilesmaa V, Halttunen M, et al. Obstetric outcome in women with polycystic ovary syndrome. Hum Reprod 2001;16(2):226–9.

[65] Urman B, Sarac E, Dogan L, et al. Pregnancy in infertile PCOD patients. J Reprod Med 1997;42(8):501–5.

[66] Bjercke S, Dale PO, Tanbo T, et al. Impact of insulin resistance on pregnancy complications and outcome in women with polycystic ovary syndrome. Gynecol Obstet Invest 2002;54(2):94–8.

[67] Haakova L, Cibula D, Rezabek K, et al. Pregnancy outcome in women with PCOS and in controls matched by age and weight. Hum Reprod 2003;18(7):1438–41.

[68] Bryson CL, Ioannou GN, Rulyak SJ, et al. Association between gestational diabetes and pregnancy-induced hypertension. Am J Epidemiol 2003;158(12):1148–53.

[69] Joffe GM, Esterlitz JR, Levine RJ, et al. The relationship between abnormal glucose tolerance and hypertensive disorders of pregnancy in healthy nulliparous women. Am J Obstet Gynecol 1998;179(4):1032–7.

[70] Suhonen L, Teramo K. Hypertension and pre-eclampsia in women with gestational glucose intolerance. Acta Obstet Gynecol Scand 1993;72(4):269–72.

[71] Hamasaki T, Yasuhi I, Hirai M, et al. Hyperinsulinemia increases the risk of gestational hypertension. Int J Gynaecol Obstet 1996;55(2):141–5.

[72] Bauman WA, Maimen M, Langer O. An association between hyperinsulinemia and hypertension during the third trimester of pregnancy. Am J Obstet Gynecol 1988;159(2):446–50.

[73] Diamant YZ, Rimon E, Evron S. High incidence of preeclamptic toxemia in patients with polycystic ovarian disease. Eur J Obstet Gynecol Reprod Biol 1982;14(3):199–204.

[74] Gjonnaess H. The course and outcome of pregnancy after ovarian electrocautery in women with polycystic ovarian syndrome: the influence of body-weight. Br J Obstet Gynaecol 1989; 96(6):714–9.

[75] de Vries MJ, Dekker GA, Schoemaker J. Higher risk of preeclampsia in the polycystic ovary syndrome: a case control study. Eur J Obstet Gynecol Reprod Biol 1998;76(1):91–5.

[76] Kashyap S, Claman P. Polycystic ovary disease and the risk of pregnancy-induced hypertension. J Reprod Med 2000;45(12):991–4.

[77] Solomon CG, Carroll JS, Okumura K, et al. Higher cholesterol and insulin levels are associated with increased risk for pregnancy-induced hypertension. Am J Hypertens 1999;12(3): 276–82.

[78] Solomon CG, Graves SW, Greene MF, et al. Glucose intolerance as a predictor of hypertension in pregnancy. Hypertension 1994;23(6 Pt 1):717–21.

[79] Fuh MMT, Yin C-S, Pei D, et al. Resistance to insulin-mediated glucose uptake and hyperinsulinemia in women who had preeclampsia during pregnancy. Am J Hypertens 1995;8(7): 768–71.

[80] Nisell H, Erikssen C, Persson B, et al. Is carbohydrate metabolism altered among women who have undergone a preeclamptic pregnancy? Gynecol Obstet Invest 1999;48(4):241–6.

[81] He S, Silveira A, Hamsten A, et al. Haemostatic, endothelial, and lipoprotein parameters and blood pressure levels in women with a history of preeclampsia. Thromb Haemost 1999;81(4):538–42.

[82] Laivuori H, Tikkanen MJ, Ylikorkala O. Hyperinsulinemia 17 years after preeclamptic first pregnancy. J Clin Endocrinol Metab 1996;81(8):2908–11.

[83] Laivuori H, Kaaja R, Rutanen E-M, et al. Evidence of high circulating testosterone in women with prior preeclampsia. J Clin Endocrinol Metab 1998;83(2):344–7.

[84] Defronzo RA. The effect of insulin on renal sodium metabolism. A review with clinical implications. Diabetologia 1981;21(3):165–71.

[85] Rowe JW, Young JB, Minaker KL, et al. Effect of insulin and glucose infusions on sympathetic nervous system activity in normal man. Diabetes 1981;30(3):219–25.

[86] Calles-Escandon J, Cipolla M. Diabetes and endothelial dysfunction: a clinical perspective. Endocr Rev 2001;22(1):36–52.

[87] Report of the National High Blood Pressure Education Program Working Group on High Blood Pressure in Pregnancy. Am J Obstet Gynecol 2000;183(1 Suppl):S1–22.

[88] Baker PJ, Ramey ER, Ramwell PW. Androgen-mediated sex differences of cardiovascular responses in rats. Am J Physiol 1978;235(2):H242–6.

[89] Wakasugi M, Noguchi T, Kazama YI, et al. The effects of sex hormones on the synthesis of prostacyclin (PGI2) by vascular tissues. Prostaglandins 1989;37(4):401–10.

[90] Hacihanefioglu B, Seyisoglu H, Karsidag K, et al. Influence of insulin resistance on total renin level in normotensive women with polycystic ovary syndrome. Fertil Steril 2000;73(2): 261–5.

[91] Sibai BM, el-Nazer A, Gonzalez-Ruiz A. Severe preeclampsia-eclampsia in young primigravid women: subsequent pregnancy outcome and remote prognosis. Am J Obstet Gynecol 1986;155(5):1011–6.

[92] Irgens HU, Reisaeter L, Irgens LM, et al. Long term mortality of mothers and fathers after pre-eclampsia: population based cohort study. BMJ 2001;323(7323):1213–7.

[93] Smith GC, Pell JP, Walsh D. Pregnancy complications and maternal risk of ischaemic heart disease: a retrospective cohort study of 129,290 births. Lancet 2001;357(9273):2002–6.

ELSEVIER
SAUNDERS

Endocrinol Metab Clin N Am
35 (2006) 157–171

ENDOCRINOLOGY
AND METABOLISM
CLINICS
OF NORTH AMERICA

Hypertension in Pregnancy

Caren G. Solomon, MD, MPH[a], Ellen W. Seely, MD[b],*

[a]*Divisions of General Medicine and Women's Health, Harvard Medical School,
Brigham and Women's Hospital, Boston, MA, USA*
[b]*Endocrinology, Diabetes, and Hypertension Division, Harvard Medical School,
Brigham and Women's Hospital, Boston, MA, USA*

Hypertension complicates 5% to 10% of pregnancies and is a major cause of maternal and neonatal morbidity and mortality. Pregnancy-related hypertension has been classified into four categories by the National High Blood Pressure Education Program Working Group Report on High Blood Presure in Pregnancy (Box 1) [1]. New-onset hypertension in pregnancy includes preeclampsia and gestational hypertension. The diagnosis of either condition requires at least measurement of two elevated blood pressures ($\geq$ 140 mm Hg systolic or $\geq$ 90 mm Hg diastolic) in the second half of pregnancy in a previously normotensive woman. Preeclampsia is distinguished by the presence of proteinuria [2] and often is accompanied by other systemic manifestations. Proteinuria in pregnancy is formally defined as 300 mg or more of protein in a 24-hour specimen. If there is insufficient time to collect a 24-hour urine specimen, measurement of protein and creatinine on a timed urine collection may be used to estimate 24-hour excretion [1]. A dipstick protein measurement of 2+ or greater also may suggest proteinuria in excess of 300 mg over 24 hours, but this measurement varies with urine concentration and may be unreliable [3]. A definitive diagnosis of gestational hypertension is impossible until the pregnancy is completed because women with apparent isolated increases in blood pressure initially may develop systemic disease later. In contrast to the substantial risks (reviewed subsequently) associated with preeclampsia, women who have only hypertension, without systemic manifestations, throughout their course tend to do well in pregnancy.

Hypertensive disorders of pregnancy also include hypertension antedating the pregnancy. Chronic hypertension is defined as a blood pressure

---

* Corresponding author. Endocrinology, Diabetes, and Hypertension Division, Harvard Medical School, Brigham and Women's Hospital, 221 Longwood Avenue, Boston, MA 02115.

E-mail address: eseely@partners.org (E.W. Seely).

0889-8529/06/$ - see front matter © 2005 Elsevier Inc. All rights reserved.
doi:10.1016/j.ecl.2005.09.003
endo.theclinics.com

Box 1. Classification of hypertension in pregnancy

Preeclampsia
- Systolic blood pressure ≥ 140 mm Hg or diastolic blood pressure ≥ 90 mm Hg occurring ≥ 20 weeks' gestation in a previously normotensive woman
  Proteinuria ≥ 300 mg in a 24-hour urine collection

Gestational hypertension
- Systolic blood pressure ≥ 140 mm Hg or diastolic blood pressure ≥ 90 mm Hg ≥ 20 weeks' gestation in a previously normotensive woman, but without proteinuria

Chronic hypertension
- Systolic blood pressure ≥ 140 mmHg or diastolic blood pressure ≥ 90 mm Hg that is documented < 20th week of gestation

Preeclampsia superimposed on chronic hypertension
- New-onset or greatly increased proteinuria
- Sudden exacerbation of hypertension or other signs of multisystem involvement such as thrombocytopenia or transaminitis in a woman with prior hypertension

---

Data from Gifford RW, August PA, Cunningham G. Report of the National High Blood Pressure Education Program Working group on high blood pressure in pregnancy. Am J Obstet Gynecol 2000;183:S1–22.

---

greater than 140/90 mm Hg before pregnancy or before the 20th week of gestation. Most women with chronic hypertension do well in pregnancy except when proteinuria or superimposed preeclampsia occurs [4]. It may be difficult in some cases to distinguish new-onset hypertension from chronic hypertension; blood pressure typically decreases in the late first and early second trimesters, then increases to prepregnancy levels in the third trimester [5]. In women for whom prepregnancy blood pressures are not available, this return to baseline blood pressure may be misdiagnosed as new-onset hypertension. The possibility of secondary hypertension also should be considered in women with hypertension in pregnancy, particularly when severe. A history of symptoms or signs suggesting secondary causes (eg, hypokalemia suggesting hyperaldosteronism or episodic hypertension and symptoms suggesting pheochromocytoma) should prompt further evaluation.

Two severe complications of preeclampsia are (1) the HELLP syndrome, characterized by the constellation of hemolysis, elevated liver enzymes, and low platelets, and (2) eclampsia, characterized by the development of seizures. Both conditions are rare, but associated with a particularly poor prognosis.

Clinical manifestations of preeclampsia

Maternal

In addition to the elevated blood pressure and proteinuria required for the diagnosis of preeclampsia, women with this condition often have signs or symptoms indicating dysfunction of any of several organ systems, including the renal, gastrointestinal, coagulation, and central nervous systems. Cardiac complications are rare in preeclampsia, but heart failure may occur, generally in women with preexisting heart disease.

Renal

Involvement of the renal system is characteristic of preeclampsia, and the presence of proteinuria is part of the definition of the disorder. Histologically, the kidneys show glomerular endotheliosis [6] (ie, swelling of the glomerular endothelium resulting primarily from hypertrophy of endothelial and mesangial cells). With increasing severity of disease, creatinine clearance declines; acute tubular necrosis and frank renal failure may occur. Because in normal pregnancy, creatinine clearance increases, serum creatinine levels in the "normal "range for nonpregnant women (eg, creatinine > 0.8 mg/dL) may suggest clinically significant renal dysfunction in pregnancy.

Other manifestations of renal involvement in preeclampsia include reduced urinary excretion of uric acid [7] and calcium [8]. The hypouricosuria results in serum uric acid levels that, as with creatinine, are often still within the normal nonpregnant range but are elevated for pregnancy. Hypocalciuria seems to result from insufficient circulating levels of 1,25-dihydroxyvitamin D_3, likely owing to insufficient placental 1-hydroxylation of 25-hydroxyvitamin D_3 and relative secondary hyperparathyroidism [9].

Hepatic

Pathologic changes in the liver in women with preeclampsia reflect ischemic damage. Transaminase elevations are well described and indicate hepatocellular necrosis. Severe liver involvement occurs as part of the HELLP syndrome.

Hematologic

Low platelet counts may complicate preeclampsia, along with or as part of the HELLP syndrome. Microangiopathic hemolytic anemia may be present and is believed to be secondary to endothelial damage. In severe disease, disseminated intravascular coagulopathy may occur.

Neurologic

The most severe complication of preeclampsia is eclampsia. Headache, blurred vision, photophobia, or mental status changes may be early signs of impending eclampsia, but eclampsia also may occur in the absence of these manifestations. There are no reliable predictors for development of eclampsia in women with preeclampsia. Only about 50% of women who have a seizure have severe hypertension (defined as $\geq$ 160/110 mm Hg) [10], and the absence of severe hypertension does not exclude the possibility of seizure.

Fetal/neonatal

Preeclampsia is associated with decreased fetoplacental perfusion, which frequently results in intrauterine growth restriction and small-for-gestational-age infants. Preeclampsia is one of the leading causes of prematurity because of the frequent need for early delivery in affected women.

Risk factors for preeclampsia

Several risk factors are recognized for the development of preeclampsia (Box 2) [11,12]. Primiparity is considered one of the most powerful predictors of increased risk, increasing the likelihood of preeclampsia by 5- to 10-fold [13]; a proposed explanation for this observation is that it may represent a maternal immunologic reaction to paternal antigens. Although extremes of age have been suggested to be risk factors for preeclampsia, the relationship between young age and increased risk for preeclampsia seems to be explained by the association between younger age and first pregnancy. The higher risk that has been observed in older women may be explained at least in part by other age-related risk factors for preeclampsia, including obesity and chronic hypertension.

Box 2. Established risk factors for preeclampasia

- Primiparity
- Prior personal or family history of preeclampsia
- Obesity
- Hypertension
- Diabetes mellitus
- Renal disease
- Collagen vascular disease
- Thrombophilia
- Multiple gestation

Data from Roberts JN, Pearson GD, Cutler JA, Lindheimer MD. Summary of the NHLBI Working Group on Research on Hypertension in Pregnancy. Hypertension Preg 2003;22:109–27; and Duckitt K, Harrington D. Risk factors for preeclampsia at antenatal booking: systematic review of controlled studies. BMJ 2005;330:565.

Even in the absence of frank obesity, increasing body mass index (BMI) is associated with increased risk for preeclampsia [13]; similarly, increased blood pressure even within the normal range is a recognized risk factor [14]. Black race also may predispose, although the association between black race and preeclampsia may be explained by the high prevalence of obesity and chronic hypertension in this population.

Other recognized risk factors for preeclampsia include a prior personal or family history of preeclampsia [12]. A maternal history of preeclampsia increases the risk of preeclampsia in a woman's daughter and her son's female partner [15]. There may be several susceptibility genes for preeclampsia. Associations have been described between risk for preeclampsia and polymorphisms the genes for factor V Leiden, angiotensinogen, and endothelial nitric oxide synthase, although these have not been confirmed consistently in other populations [16]. Conditions linked to preeclampsia, in addition to preexisting hypertension, include diabetes mellitus, renal disease, collagen vascular disease [1], and possibly polycystic ovary syndrome [17].

An increased risk of preeclampsia also has been reported in multiparous women when there is a change in paternity [18], with shorter length of sexual relationship, and with prior use of barrier contraceptives; these observations have been suggested to support a possible immunologic cause of the disorder. More recent data have suggested, however, that relationships between these factors and preeclampsia may be explained by other confounding factors [19]. The risk associated with a change in paternity may be explained by the length of the interval between pregnancies; longer intervals seem to predispose to preeclampsia regardless of paternity [20].

Women who are current cigarette smokers during pregnancy seem to have a decreased risk of developing preeclampsia, even after adjustment for BMI [21]; in contrast, women who stop smoking before pregnancy do not have decreased risk. Possible mediators of the risk reduction associated with cigarette smoking include increase in nitric oxide production, decrease in thromboxane production, or alteration in cell immunity; better understanding of these factors might lead to preventive strategies without the hazards of smoking.

Decreased placental perfusion is considered a central feature of preeclampsia (see section on pathophysiology later). Conditions associated with increased placental size, such as multiple gestation [22], increase the risk for preeclampsia. The risk for severe preeclampsia was reported to be significantly greater with triplet pregnancy compared with twin pregnancy [23].

Assessment of risk factors for preeclampsia should be a part of routine prenatal care. Women who have identified risk factors may benefit from closer surveillance during pregnancy [24].

Pathophysiology of preeclampsia

Despite decades of research, the cause of preeclampsia remains uncertain. Many theories have been proposed.

Maternal factors

Endothelial dysfunction is a hallmark of preeclampsia and involves the placental and systemic circulations [25]. It is unclear whether endothelial dysfunction is primary (causal) or a secondary manifestation of disease. Signs of endothelial dysfunction include hypertension, proteinuria, microangiopathic hemolytic anemia, and organ hypoperfusion. Several laboratory abnormalities consistent with abnormal endothelial function have been observed in women with preeclampsia, including decreased levels of prostacyclin (with an increased ratio of thromboxane to prostacyclin) [26] and increased levels of endothelin-1 [27] (a growth factor derived from endothelial cells that causes vasoconstriction). Increased pressor responsiveness to angiotensin II (in contrast to the refractoriness to this substance observed in normal pregnancy) also is characteristic of preeclampsia.

Insulin resistance is a well-recognized correlate of endothelial dysfunction and may play a role in the pathogenesis of preeclampsia [28]. In normal pregnancy, insulin resistance increases with gestation, and insulin resistance is greater in women with preeclampsia. Studies of women with established preeclampsia revealed higher levels of insulin and glucose, increased levels of triglycerides and free fatty acids [29], and elevated levels of cytokines (eg, tumor necrosis factor-α [30]) associated with the insulin-resistant state.

Although abnormalities observed in cross-sectional studies of preeclampsia could be a result rather than a cause of disease, several of these abnormalities have been shown to precede the development of preeclampsia. Prospective studies of pregnant women who subsequently developed preeclampsia have shown higher levels of glucose [31], insulin [32], triglycerides, free fatty acids [33], and tumor necrosis factor-α [34] and lower levels of high-density lipoprotein [35] and sex hormone–binding globulin [36] than in women who remain normotensive through pregnancy [28]. More recently, elevated levels of the cytokine soluble fms-like tyrosine kinase-1(sflt-1) and lower levels of placental growth factor (PlGF) were reported to antedate the development of preeclampsia [37]; high levels of sflt-1 are proposed to antagonize vasodilatory effects of PlGF-1 and vascular endothelium-derived growth factor, resulting in placental vascular insufficiency and other systemic effects.

Follow-up studies of women with a history of preeclampsia have revealed several metabolic abnormalities, including increased insulin resistance [38] and abnormal endothelial relaxation [39]. These observations, coupled with the abnormalities observed in women before the development of preeclampsia, have suggested the importance of underlying maternal factors and factors specific to the pregnancy in the pathogenesis of disease.

Fetoplacental factors

During normal pregnancy, fetal trophoblasts transform maternal spiral arteries from resistance muscular vessels to low-resistance vessels by replacing endothelial cells and smooth muscle cells of the media [40]. Several factors (eg, nitric oxide and vascular adhesion molecules) seem to play a role in successful trophoblastic transformation. In preeclampsia, the trophoblastic invasion is incomplete such that spiral arteries maintain increased vascular tone, leading to decreased placental perfusion. It is currently uncertain which mediators of trophoblastic invasion are defective in preeclampsia.

Predictors of preeclampsia

Given the increased maternal and fetal morbidity and mortality associated with preeclampsia, attempts have been made to identify markers predictive of the development of preeclampsia. Several purported markers (eg, hyperinsulinemia and hypocalciuria) have been associated with a higher risk of preeclampsia, but the overlap in levels between women who have and have not developed the disease is too great for them to serve as useful discriminators in practice. Assessments of vascular function also have been proposed as discriminatory markers; however, assessment of angiotensin II pressor response [41] is too invasive and impractical and Doppler assessment of uterine artery blood flow is too nonspecific [42] for clinical use. It is currently uncertain whether serum levels of sflt-1 or serum or urinary levels of PlGF [43] will prove to be useful in distinguishing between pregnant women who will and will not develop preeclampsia.

Prevention of preeclampsia

The lack of predictive markers for the development of preeclampsia has complicated efforts to prevent the disease. Nonetheless, several interventions have been studied in populations considered to be at increased risk based on historical factors, such as primiparity.

Aspirin

Based on the observation of relative increases in thromboxane relative to prostacylin levels in women with preeclampsia, aspirin or other antiplatelet agents have been proposed as preventive agents. Although several small trials suggested a benefit to aspirin, a large multicenter, placebo-controlled, randomized trial [44] including 6927 women at increased risk for preeclampsia found no significant reduction overall in the risk of preeclampsia with aspirin therapy (60 mg/d). Subgroup analyses indicated a possible benefit in reducing risk in women who delivered before 32 weeks' gestation, but such women could not be reliably identified prospectively. Another large randomized trial of low-dose aspirin (60 mg/d) in high-risk women also showed no significant benefit [45].

Calcium

Similar to aspirin, calcium supplementation seemed to be a promising preventive strategy in small studies. In a multicenter, placebo-controlled, randomized trial of 4589 healthy nulliparous women [46], supplementation with 2 g of elemental calcium daily did not reduce significantly the risks of preeclampsia or pregnancy-associated hypertension among the group overall or among women with low calcium intake or low urinary calcium levels at baseline.

Antioxidants

Because preeclampsia has been considered to reflect a state of increased oxidant stress, it has been hypothesized that supplementation with antioxidants might reduce risk for this disorder. A randomized trial of supplementation with vitamins E and C was terminated early, however, after the rates of preeclampsia did not differ materially between women receiving and not receiving supplementation [47]. Low levels of ω-3 fatty acids have been associated with increased rates of preeclampsia [48], but it is not known whether supplementation reduces this risk.

Lifestyle modifications

Women who are lean before pregnancy have a lower risk of preeclampsia than women with higher pregravid BMI [12]. It is not known, however, if weight loss before pregnancy in obese women reduces risk. Some retrospective data have indicated that higher levels of leisure-time physical activity in the first 20 weeks of pregnancy are associated with a significantly reduced risk for preeclampsia [49]. However, another retrospective report found no significant reduction in the risk for preeclampsia with greater leisure-time or non–leisure-time physical activity [50].

Management of preeclampsia

Women with established or suspected preeclampsia require close clinical surveillance. The goal is to avoid the development of eclampsia or other complications in the mother, but prolong the pregnancy as long as possible, as long as the mother and fetus are stable. Indications for immediate delivery have been outlined by the Working Group on High Blood Pressure in Pregnancy and include maternal and fetal factors [1]. Maternal indications include gestational age 38 weeks or greater; platelet count less than 100,000 cells/mm^3; progressive decline in either liver or renal function; signs of placental abruption; or symptoms of persistent severe headaches, visual changes, severe epigastric pain, nausea, or vomiting. Fetal indications for delivery include abnormal nonstress testing or ultrasound scans indicating severe growth restriction, unfavorable biophysical profile, or oligohydramnios.

Maternal and fetal monitoring

Clinical monitoring of the mother includes frequent blood pressure determinations, questioning for symptoms (eg, abdominal pain, headache, visual changes, or photophobia), and laboratory testing (urine protein measurement, preferably on a 24-hour urine sample, platelet count, creatinine, and transaminases). Laboratory testing is recommended on at least a weekly basis in patients considered to have mild stable disease. Monitoring of the fetus includes fetal ultrasound (to assess fetal size and amniotic fluid volume) and nonstress testing (to assess fetal heart rate reactivity) or determination of biophysical profile (to assess fetal well-being). Intervals for maternal and fetal testing are not well defined, but more frequent testing is recommended when disease is more severe.

In women who develop preeclampsia at less than 34 weeks' gestation, an approach of expectant management has been advocated [51]. Women are admitted to the hospital for close maternal and fetal monitoring, and antihypertensive therapy is initiated when indicated (see later). In a randomized trial comparing this approach with immediate delivery, expectant management prolonged pregnancy 2 weeks and resulted in fewer days in the neonatal intensive care unit and higher birth weight, although there was an increased rate of infants small for gestational age [51]. Other trials have suggested similar benefits to expectant management involving close monitoring of the mother and the fetus under supervision of physicians experienced in managing such pregnancies [52,53].

Antihypertensive therapy

Antihypertensive medications are used in women with severe chronic hypertension or severe preeclampsia to decrease the maternal risk of stroke and intracerebral hemorrhage. A possible risk of lowering the mother's blood pressure is hypoperfusion of the fetoplacental unit, which already is compromised in severely hypertensive pregnancy. Studies of women with mild preeclampsia [54,55] have shown no benefit to pharmacologic therapy (either labetalol or calcium channel blockers) and suggested that antihypertensive therapy may increase the risk of intrauterine growth restriction. Recommended thresholds for starting pharmacologic therapy for elevated blood pressure levels are higher than the thresholds outside of pregnancy. The Working Group Report on High Blood Pressure in Pregnancy recommends initiation of antihypertensive therapy for a diastolic blood pressure 105 mm Hg or greater [1].

No antihypertensive medication is specifically approved by the US Food and Drug Administration (FDA) for use in pregnant women, although the FDA classifies medications based on available data regarding safety in pregnancy. Medications commonly used in pregnancy and their FDA classifications are reviewed in Table 1.

Table 1
Pharmacologic therapy for hypertensive pregnancy

Agent	Route of administration	Contraindications	FDA classification[a]
Chronic treatment of hypertension[b]			
Methyldopa	By mouth	—	B
Beta-blockers	By mouth	May exacerbate asthma and heart failure	C
Labetalol	By mouth	May exacerbate asthma and heart failure	C
Calcium channel blockers	By mouth	Caution when used with magnesium sulfate	C
Acute management of severe hypertension[c]			
Hydralazine	IV	—	C
Labetolol	IV	May exacerbate asthma and heart failure	C
Nitroprusside	IV	Risk of cyanide toxicity to mother and fetus	C

[a] *Categories:* **A** (not listed), adequate and well-controlled studies have failed to show a risk to the fetus in the first trimester of pregnancy (and there is no evidence of risk in later trimesters); **B**, animal reproduction studies have failed to show a risk to the fetus and there are no adequate and well-controlled studies in pregnant women; **C**, animal reproduction studies have shown an adverse effect on the fetus and there are no adequate and well-controlled studies in humans, but potential benefits may warrant use of the drug in pregnant women despite potential risks; **D** (not listed), positive evidence of human fetal risk based on adverse reaction data from investigational or marketing experience or studies in humans, but potential benefits may warrant use of the drug in pregnant women despite potential risks; and **X** (not listed), studies in animals or humans have showed fetal abnormalities and/or there is positive evidence of human fetal risk based on adverse reaction data from investigational or marketing experience, and the risks involved in use of the drug in pregnant women clearly outweigh potential benefits.

[b] ACEIs and ARBs are contraindicated in the second and third trimesters of pregnancy because of the risk of fetal or neonatal renal failure and other complications (category D).

[c] Short-acting calcium channel blockers have been used in this setting, but are not approved for treating hypertensive crisis even in nonpregnant patients, and may increase risk for cardiovascular events.

There is no evidence that antihypertensive therapy in women with mild-to-moderate chronic hypertension reduces the risk for developing preeclampsia. A meta-analysis of randomized trials of the treatment of mild-to-moderate hypertension in pregnancy (including 17 that compared different pharmacologic therapies with one another and 24 that compared pharmacologic therapy with placebo) showed no reduction in the rate of preeclampsia with antihypertensive therapy overall or with any specific agent [56].

For women who require antihypertensive medication in pregnancy, methyldopa has the longest record of use of pregnancy and often is considered a first-line choice for management. Follow-up of children born to mothers who took methyldopa during pregnancy revealed no negative effects on development at 7.5 years of age [57]. β-Blockers and labetalol also are used, but may increase risk of intrauterine growth restriction [54,58]. Calcium channel blockers are considered an alternative, although data also are limited for this class.

Angiotensin-converting enzyme inhibitors are considered contraindicated in the management of hypertension in pregnancy as a result of the observation of cases of fetal and neonatal renal failure in infants of mothers treated with these agents [59]. Based on their similar mechanisms of action and case reports describing adverse outcomes (including oligohydramnios, fetal growth restriction, stillbirth or neonatal death, and neonatal renal failure) in offspring of exposed women, angiotensin receptor blockers likewise are contraindicated in the management of hypertension in pregnancy [60].

Emergency treatment of hypertension in pregnancy

For severe hypertension (defined as sustained systolic blood pressure $\geq$ 160 mm Hg or diastolic blood pressure $\geq$ 105 mm Hg [1]) unresponsive to oral medications, intravenous therapy is warranted. Medications recommended in this setting include hydralazine and labetalol [61,62]. Nitroprusside has been used, specifically in cases unresponsive to these medications, but its use may be complicated by cyanide toxicity in the fetus or mother. Short-acting oral nifedipine has been suggested as an alternative to intravenous medication, however, reports of cardiovascular events after its administration [63] argue against its use. An additional concern with use of calcium channel blockers is the increased risk for neuromuscular depression when used in combination with magnesium sulfate, which may result in paralysis or cardiac failure (see Table 1) [64].

Seizure prophylaxis

Magnesium sulfate is the agent of choice for the prevention of seizures in women with preeclampsia [65]. In a randomized, placebo-controlled trial including more than 10,000 women with preeclampsia, the group assigned to magnesium sulfate had a 58% reduction in the risk for eclampsia (0.8% versus 1.9%). Randomized trials also have confirmed the superiority of magnesium sulfate to phenytoin [66] and nimodipine [67] in seizure prevention.

Implications of preeclampsia for later life risks

Although the clinical manifestations of preeclampsia resolve after delivery, women who have had this disorder may be at increased cardiovascular risk later in life [68]. A study of 406 women with severe preeclampsia or eclampsia in their first pregnancy showed a 2.6-fold increased risk for hypertension over 2 to 24 years of follow-up compared with 409 women with a history of normotensive pregnancy [69]. In a population-based cohort study, women with preeclampsia and preterm delivery (which is considered to indicate more severe disease) had an 8-fold increased risk of cardiovascular mortality compared with women who were normotensive and gave birth at term [70]. Studies of long-term risks may be biased, however, by possible misdiagnosis of chronic hypertension as preeclampsia, and further research is needed to better understand the long-term risks associated with a history of preeclampsia and to identify effective interventions. Currently, lifestyle interventions to control BMI and reduce insulin resistance—including dietary changes and increased physical activity—are reasonable and should be encouraged.

Summary

New-onset hypertension complicates 5% to 10% of pregnancies. Preeclampsia is associated with substantial risk to the mother and the fetus. Recognized risk factors include primiparity and preexisting chronic hypertension. Many biochemical abnormalities (eg, hyperinsulinemia, hyperlipidemia, elevated levels of tumor necrosis factor-α, and, more recently, elevated levels of sflt-1 and reduced levels of PlGF) also have been recognized to predispose to disease. Currently, there is no marker for disease that has proved sufficiently discriminatory to be used in practice, and no interventions are known to be effective in preventing the disease. The "cure" for preeclampsia is delivery of the fetus, but delivery earlier than necessary poses major risks to the fetus; management involves close follow-up of the mother and the fetus to prolong the pregnancy as long as is safely possible. Although no antihypertensive medications are approved for use in pregnancy, clinical experience has supported certain choices (including methyldopa, β-blockers, and calcium channel blockers for long-term management and hydralazine, labetalol, and nitroprusside for acute management). Angiotensin-converting enzyme inhibitors and angiotensin receptor blockers are contraindicated in the second and third trimesters of pregnancy. Women with a history of preeclampsia are at increased risk of preeclampsia in subsequent pregnancies and may be at increased risk for subsequent hypertension and cardiovascular disease. Further research is needed to understand causes of preeclampsia better and to identify interventions that can prevent its occurrence and reduce subsequent risks in women who have had preeclampsia.

References

[1] Gifford RW, August PA, Cunningham G. Report of the National High Blood Pressure Education Program Working Group on High Blood Pressure in Pregnancy. Am J Obstet Gynecol 2000;183:S1–22.

[2] Sibai B, Kupferminc M. Pre-eclampsia. Lancet 2005;365:785–99.

[3] Waugh JJ, Clark TJ, Divakaran TG, et al. Accuracy of urinalysis dipstick technique in predicting significant proteinuria in pregnancy. Obstet Gynecol 2004;103:769–77.

[4] Sibai BM, Lindheimer M, Hauth J, et al. Risk factors for preeclampsia, abruptio placentae, and adverse neonatal outcomes among women with chronic hypertension. National Institute

of Child Health and Human Development Network of Maternal-Fetal Medicine Units. N Engl J Med 1998;339:667–71.

[5] Wilson M, Morganti AA, Zervoulakis D, et al. Blood pressure, the renin-angiotensin system and sex steroids throughout normal pregnancy. Am J Med 1980;68:97–104.

[6] Spargo BH, McCartney C, Winemiller R. Glomerular capillary endotheliosis in toxemia of pregnancy. Arch Pathol 1959;13:593–9.

[7] Fadel HE, Northrup G, Misenhimer HR. Hyperuricemia in pre-eclampsia: a reappraisal. Am J Obstet Gynecol 1976;125:640–7.

[8] Taufield PA, Ales KL, Resnick LM, et al. Hypocalciuria in preeclampsia. N Engl J Med 1987;316:715–8.

[9] Seely EW, Wood RJ, Brown EM, et al. Lower serum ionized calcium and abnormal calciotropic homrone levels in preeclampsia. J Clin Endocrinol Metab 1992;74: 1436–40.

[10] Sibai BM. Diagnosis, prevention, and management of eclampsia. Obstet Gynecol 2005;105: 402–10.

[11] Roberts JN, Pearson GD, Cutler JA, et al. Summary of the NHLBI Working Group on Research on Hypertension in Pregnancy. Hypertension Preg 2003;22:109–27.

[12] Duckitt K, Harrington D. Risk factors for preeclampsia at antenatal booking: systematic review of controlled studies. BMJ 2005;330:565.

[13] Eskenazi B, Fenster L, Sidney S. A multivariate analysis of risk factors for preeclampsia. JAMA 1991;266:237–41.

[14] Solomon CG, Graves SW, Greene MF, et al. Glucose intolerance as a predictor of hypertension in pregnancy. Hypertension 1994;23:717–21.

[15] Esplin MS, Fausett MB, Fraser A. Paternal and maternal components of the predisposition to preeclampsia. N Engl J Med 2001;344:867–72.

[16] Consortium GOPEC. Disentangling fetal and maternal susceptibility for pre-eclampsia: a British multicenter candidate-gene study. Am J Hum Genet 2005;77(1):127–31.

[17] DeVries MJ, Dekker GA, Shoemaker J. Higher risk of preeclampsia in the polycystic ovary syndrome: a case control study. Eur J Obstet Gynaecol Reprod Biol 1998;76:91–5.

[18] Trupin LS, Simon LP, Eskenazi B. Change in paternity: a risk factor for preeclampsia in multiparas. Epidemiology 1996;7:240–4.

[19] Ness RB, Markovic N, Harger G, et al. Barrier methods, length of preconception intercourse, and preeclampsia. Hypertens Pregnancy 2004;23:227–35.

[20] Skjaerven R, Wilcox AJ, Lie RT. The interval between pregnancies and the risk of preeclampsia. N Engl J Med 2002;346:33–8.

[21] Conde-Aqudelo A, Althabe F, Balizan JM, et al. Cigarette smoking during pregnancy and risk of preeclampsia: a systematic review. Am J Obstet Gynecol 1999;181:1026–35.

[22] Sibai BM, Hauth J, Caritis S, et al. Hypertensive disorders in twin versus singleton gestations. National Institute of Child Health and Human Development Network of Maternal-Fetal Medicine Units. Am J Obstet Gynecol 2000;182:938–42.

[23] Mastrobattista JM, Skupski DW, Monga M, et al. The rate of severe preeclampsia is increased in triplet as compared to twin gestations. Am J Perinatol 1997;14:263–5.

[24] Milne F, Redman C, Walker J, et al. The pre-eclampsia community guideline (PRECOG): how to screen for and detect onset of preeclampsia in the community. BMJ 2005; 330(7491):576–80.

[25] Roberts JM, Taylor RN, Musci TJ, et al. Preeclampsia: an endothelial cell disorder. Am J Obstet Gynecol 1989;161:1200–4.

[26] Friedman SA. Preeclampsia: a review of the role of prostaglandins. Obstet Gynecol 1988;71: 122–37.

[27] Fiore G, Florio P, Micheli L, et al. Endothelin 1 triggers placental oxidative stress pathways: putative role in pre-eclampsia. J Clin Endocrinol Metab 2005;90(7):4205–10.

[28] Seely EW, Solomon CG. Insulin resistance and its potential role in pregnancy-induced hypertension. J Clin Endocrinol Metab 2003;88:2393–8.

[29] Lorentzen B, Birkeland KI, Endresen MJ, et al. Glucose intolerance in women with pre-eclampsia. Acta Obstet Gynecol Scand 1998;77:22–7.

[30] Vince GC, Startkey PM, Austgulen R, et al. Interkleukin-6, tumor necrosis factor and soluble tumor factor receptors in women with pre-eclampsia. Br J Obstet Gynaecol 1995;102:20.

[31] Solomon CG, Graves SW, Greene MF, et al. Glucose intolerance as a predictor of hypertension in pregnancy. Hypertension 1994;23:717–21.

[32] Solomon CG, Carroll JS, Okumura K, et al. Higher cholesterol and insulin levels are associated with increased risk for pregnancy-induced hypertension. Am J Hypertens 1999;12:276–82.

[33] Lorentzen B, Endresen MJ, Clausen T, et al. Fasting serum free fatty acids and triglycerides are increased before 20 weeks of gestation in women who later develop preeclampsia. Hypertens Pregnancy 1994;13:103–9.

[34] Serin YS, Ozcelik B, Bapbou M, et al. Predictive value of tumor necrosis factor-[alpha] (TNF-[alpha]) in preeclampsia. Eur J Obstet Gynecol Reprod Biol 2002;100:143–5.

[35] Kaaje R, Laivuori H, Laasko M, et al. Evidence of a state of increased insulin resistance in preeclampsia. Metabolism 1999;48:892–6.

[36] Wolf M, Sandler L, Muniz K, et al. First trimester insulin resistance and subsequent preeclampsia: prospective study. J Clin Endocrinol Metab 2002;87:1563–8.

[37] Levine RJ, Maynard SE, Qian C, et al. Circulating angiogenic factors and risk of preeclampsia. N Engl J Med 2004;350:672–83.

[38] Fuh MMT, Yin C-S, Pei D, et al. Resistance to insulin-mediated glucose uptake and hyperinsulinemia in women who had preeclampsia during pregnancy. Am J Hypertens 1995;8:768–71.

[39] Chambers JC, Fusi L, Malik I, et al. Association of maternal endothelial dysfunction with preeclampsia. JAMA 2001;285:1607–12.

[40] Kaufmann P, Black S, Huppertz B. Endovascular trophoblast invasion: implications for the pathogenesis of intrauterine growth retardation and preeclampsia. Biol Reprod 2003;69:1–7.

[41] Gant NF, Daley GL, Chand S, et al. A study of angiotensin II pressor response throughout primigravid pregnancy. J Clin Invest 1973;52:2682–9.

[42] Irion O, Masse J, Forest J-C, et al. Prediction of pre-eclampsia, low birthweight for gestation, and prematurity by uterine blood flow velocuite waveform analysis in low risk nulliparous women. Br J Obstet Gynaecol 1998;105:422–9.

[43] Levine RJ, Thadani R, Qian C, et al. Urinary placental growth factor and risk of preeclampsia. JAMA 2005;293:77–85.

[44] CLASP (Collaborative Low-dose Aspirin Study in Pregnancy) Collaborative group. CLASP: a randomized trial of low-dose aspirin for the prevention and treatment of preeclampsia among 9364 pregnant women. Lancet 1994;343:619–29.

[45] Caritis S, Sibai B, Hauth J, et al. Low dose aspirin to prevent preeclampsia in women at high risk. N Engl J Med 1998;338:701–5.

[46] Levine RJ, Hauth JC, Curet LB, et al. Trial of calcium to prevent preeclampsia. N Engl J Med 1997;337:69–76.

[47] Beazley D, Ahokas R, Livingston J, et al. Vitamin C and E supplementation in women at high risk for preeclampsia: a double-blind, placebo-controlled trial. Am J Obstet Gynecol 2005;192:520–1.

[48] Williams MA, Zigheim RW, King IB, et al. Omega three fatty acids in maternal erythrocytes and risk of preeclampsia. Epidemiology 1995;6:232–7.

[49] Marcoux S, Brisson J, Fabia J. Effect of leisure time physical activity on the risk of preeclampsia and gestational hypertension. J Epidemiol Community Health 1989;43:147–52.

[50] Saftlas AF, Logsden-Sackett N, Wang W, et al. Work, leisure-time physical activity, and risk of preeclampsia and gestational hypertension. Am J Epidemiol 2004;160:758–65.

[51] Sibai BM, Mercer BM, Schiff E, et al. Aggressive versus expectant management of severe preeclampsia at 28 to 32 weeks' gestation: a randomized controlled trial. Am J Obstet Gynecol 1994;171:818–22.

[52] Visser W, Wallenburg HC. Maternal and perinatal outcome of temporizing management in 254 consecutive patients with severe pre-eclampsia remote from term. Eur J Obstet Gynaecol Reprod Biol 1995;63:147–54.

[53] Oettle C, Hall D, Roux A, et al. Early onset severe pre-eclampsia: expectant management at a secondary hospital in close association with a tertiary institution. Br J Obstet Gynaecol 2005;112:84–8.

[54] Sibai BM, Gonzalez AR, Mabie WC, et al. A comparison of labetalol plus hospitalization versus hospitalization alone in the management of preeclampsia remote from term. Obstet Gynecol 1987;70.323 7.

[55] Sibai BM, Barton JR, Akl S, et al. A randomized prospective comparison of nifedipine and bed rest versus bed rest alone in the management of preeclampsia remote from term. Am J Obstet Gynecol 1992;167:879–84.

[56] Ablalos E, Duley L, Steyn W. Antihypertensive drug therapy for mild to moderate hypertension in pregnancy. Cochrane Database System Review 2001:CD002252.

[57] Ounsted M, Cockburn J. Maternal hypertension with superimposed preeclampsia: effect in child development at 7.5 years. Br J Obstet Gynaecol 1983;90:644–9.

[58] Butters L, Kennedy S, Rubin PC. Atenolol in essential hypertension during pregnancy. BMJ 1990;301:587–9.

[59] Hanssens M, Keirse MJ, Vankelecom F, et al. Fetal and neonatal effects of treatment with angiotensin-converting enzyme inhibitors in pregnancy. Obstet Gynecol 1991;78:128–35.

[60] Alwan S, Polifka JE, Friedman JM. Angiotensin II receptor antagonist treatment during pregnancy. Birth Defects Res A Clin Mol Teratol 2005;73(2):123–30.

[61] Mabie WC, Gonzalez AR, Sibai BM, et al. A comparative trial of labetalol and hydralazine in the acute management of severe hypertension complicating pregnancy. Obstet Gynaecol 1987,70:328 33.

[62] Paterson-Brown S, Robson SC, Redfern N, et al. Hydralazine boluses for the treatment of severe hypertension in pre-eclampsia. Br J Obstet Gynaecol 1994;101:409–13.

[63] Grossman E, Messerli FH, Grodzicki T, et al. Should a moratorium be placed on sublingual nifedipine capsules given for hypertensive emergencies and pseudoemergencies? JAMA 1996;276:1328–31.

[64] Davis WB, Wells SR, Kuller JA, et al. Analysis of the risks associated with calcium channel blockade: implications for the obstetrician-gynecologist. Obstet Gynecol Surv 1999; 54(Suppl):179–82.

[65] Do women with pre-eclampsia and their babies benefit from magnesium sulfate? The Magpie Trial: a randomised placebo-controlled trial. Lancet 2002;359:1877–90.

[66] Lucas MJ, Leveno KJ, Cunningham FG. A comparison of magnesium sulfate with phenytoin for the prevention of eclampsia. N Engl J Med 1995;333:201–5.

[67] Belford MA, Anthony J, Saade GR, et al. A comparison of magnesium sulfate and nimodipine for the prevention of eclampsia. N Engl J Med 2003;348:304–11.

[68] Seely EW. Hypertension in pregnancy: a potential window into long-term cardiovascular risk in women. J Clin Endocrinol Metab 1999;84:1858–61.

[69] Sibai BM, el-Nazer A, Gonzalez-Ruiz A. Severe preeclampsia-eclampsia in young primigravid women: subsequent pregnancy outcome and remote prognosis. Am J Obstet Gynecol 1986;155:1011–6.

[70] Irgens HU, Reisaeter L, Irgens LM, et al. Long term mortality of mothers and fathers after pre-eclampsia: population based cohort study. BMJ 2001;323:1213–7.

ELSEVIER
SAUNDERS

Endocrinol Metab Clin N Am
35 (2006) 173–191

ENDOCRINOLOGY
AND METABOLISM
CLINICS
OF NORTH AMERICA

Endocrinology of Parturition

Victoria Snegovskikh, MD[a],[*],
Joong Shin Park, MD, PhD[b],
Errol R. Norwitz, MD, PhD[a]

[a]*Department of Obstetrics, Gynecology, and Reproductive Sciences,
Yale University School of Medicine, New Haven, CT, USA*
[b]*Department of Obstetrics and Gynecology, Seoul National University
College of Medicine, Seoul, Korea*

Reproductive success is critical for survival of the species. The timely on-set of labor and delivery is an important determinant of perinatal outcome. Preterm birth (defined as delivery before 37 weeks' gestation) and post-term pregnancy (defined as pregnancy continuing beyond 42 weeks) are both as-sociated with a significant increase in perinatal morbidity and mortality. The factors responsible for the timing of labor in the human are complex and, as yet, are not completely understood. This article reviews the current under-standing of the parturition cascade responsible for the spontaneous onset of labor at term and discusses preterm labor and post-term pregnancy.

Historical context

Considerable evidence suggests that the fetus is in control of the timing of labor. Horse–donkey crossbreeding experiments in the 1950s resulted in a gestational length intermediate between that of horses (340 days) and that of donkeys (365 days) [1–3], suggesting a role for the fetal genotype in the initiation of labor. The mechanism by which the fetus triggers labor at term has been demonstrated elegantly in domestic ruminants such as sheep and cows and involves the activation at term of the fetal hypothalamic-pituitary-adrenal (HPA) axis, leading to a surge in adrenal cortisol produc-tion. Fetal cortisol then acts to up-regulate directly the activity of placental 17α-hydroxylase/17,20-lyase (CYP17) enzyme, which catalyzes the conver-sion of pregnenolone to 17β-estradiol. The switch in progesterone:estrogen

---

* Corresponding author.
E-mail address: vica@inbox.ru (V. Snegovskikh).

0889-8529/06/$ - see front matter © 2005 Elsevier Inc. All rights reserved.
doi:10.1016/j.ecl.2005.09.012
endo.theclinics.com

ratio at term provides the impetus for uterine prostaglandin production and labor [4–9]. However, human placentae lack the CYP17 enzyme, which is critical to this pathway [2], and, as such, this mechanism does not apply in humans. During the Hippocratic period, it was believed that the fetus presented head down so that it could kick its legs up against the fundus of the uterus and propel itself through the birth canal. Although we have moved away from this simple and mechanical view of labor, the factors responsible for the initiation and maintenance of labor at term are not well defined. The slow progress in our understanding of labor in humans is the result, in large part, of the absence of an adequate animal model. Parturition in most animals results from changes in circulating hormone levels in the maternal and fetal circulations at the end of pregnancy (endocrine events), whereas labor in humans results from a complex dynamic biochemical dialog that exists between the fetoplacental unit and the mother (paracrine and autocrine events).

Diagnosis of labor

Labor is the physiologic process by which a fetus is expelled from the uterus and is common to all viviparous species. Labor remains a clinical diagnosis. It requires the presence of regular painful uterine contractions, which increase in frequency and intensity, leading to progressive cervical effacement and dilatation. In normal labor, there appears to be a time-dependent relationship between these elements: the biochemical connective tissue changes in the cervix usually precede uterine contractions that, in turn, precede cervical dilatation. All of these events occur usually before spontaneous rupture of the fetal membranes [10]. The mean duration of human singleton pregnancy is 280 days (40 weeks) from the first day of the last normal menstrual period. "Term" is defined as the period from 37.0 to 42.0 weeks of gestation.

Parturition cascade at term

It is likely that a parturition cascade exists at term that removes the mechanisms maintaining uterine quiescence and recruits factors promoting uterine activity (Fig. 1) [8,9]. Given its teleologic importance, such a cascade would likely have multiple redundant loops to ensure a fail-safe system of securing pregnancy success and ultimately the preservation of the species. In such a model, each element is connected to the next in a sequential fashion, and many of the elements demonstrate positive feed-forward characteristics typical of a cascade mechanism. The sequential recruitment of signals that serve to augment the labor process suggests that it may not be possible to single out any one signaling mechanism as being responsible for the initiation of labor. It may therefore be prudent to describe such mechanisms as being responsible for promoting, rather than initiating, the process of labor [11].

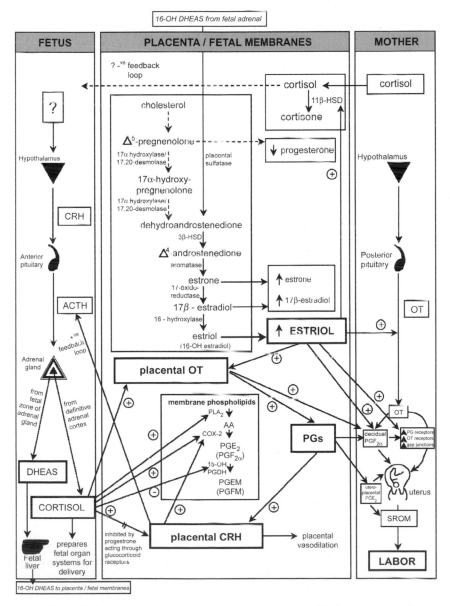

Fig. 1. Proposed parturition cascade for labor induction at term. The spontaneous induction of labor at term in the human is regulated by a series of paracrine-autocrine hormones acting in an integrated parturition cascade responsible for promoting uterine contractions. COX-2, cyclooxygenase 2; OT, oxytocin; PGDH, prostaglandin dehydrogenase; PGEM, 13,14-dihydro-15-keto-PGE$_2$, PGFM, 13,14-dihydro-15-keto-PGF$_{2\alpha}$; PLA$_2$, phospholipase A; SROM, spontaneous rupture of the fetal membranes; 11β-HSD, 11β-hydroxysteroid dehydrogenase; 16-OH DHEAS, 16-OH-dehydroepiandrostendione sulfate.

Regardless of whether the trigger for labor begins within or outside the fetus, the final common pathway for labor ends in the maternal tissues of the uterus and is characterized by the development of regular phasic uterine contractions. As in other smooth muscles, myometrial contractions are mediated through the ATP-dependent binding of myosin to actin. In contrast to vascular smooth muscle, however, myometrial cells have a sparse innervation, which is further reduced during pregnancy [12]. The regulation of the contractile mechanism of the uterus is therefore largely humoral or dependent on intrinsic factors within the myometrial cells.

Autocrine and paracrine mediators of parturition

Labor at term may be regarded best physiologically as a release from the inhibitory effects of pregnancy on the myometrium rather than as an active process mediated by uterine stimulants [13]. For example, strips of quiescent term myometrial tissue placed in an isotonic water bath will contract vigorously and spontaneously without added stimuli [13,14]. In vivo, however, it is likely that both mechanisms are important. A comprehensive analysis of each of the individual paracrine-autocrine pathways implicated in the process of labor has been reviewed in detailed elsewhere [8,9,11,15,16]. Briefly, human labor at term is a multifactorial physiologic event involving an integrated set of changes within the maternal tissues of the uterus (myometrium, decidua, and uterine cervix), which occur gradually over a period of days to weeks. Such changes include but are not limited to an increase in prostaglandin synthesis and release within the uterus, an increase in the myometrial gap junction formation, and up-regulation of myometrial oxytocin receptors. Once the myometrium and cervix are prepared, endocrine or paracrine-autocrine factors from the fetoplacental unit bring about a switch in the pattern of myometrial activity from irregular to regular contractions. The fetus may coordinate this switch in myometrial activity through its influence on placental steroid hormone production, through the mechanical distention of the uterus and through the secretion of neurohypophyseal hormones and other stimulators of prostaglandin synthesis. The final common pathway toward labor appears to be the activation of the fetal HPA axis and is probably common to all viviparous species.

Role of the fetal hypothalamic-pituitary-adrenal axis in the onset of labor

Activation of the fetal HPA axis results in enhanced fetal pituitary adrenocorticotropin hormone (ACTH) secretion that leads, in turn, to the release of abundant C19 estrogen precursor dehydroepiandrosterenedione sulfate (DHEAS) from the intermediate (fetal) zone of the fetal adrenal. This is because the human placenta is an incomplete steroidogenic organ, and estrogen synthesis by the human placenta has an obligate need for C19 steroid precursor (see Fig. 1) [16]. DHEAS is converted in the fetal liver to 16-hydroxy DHEAS and then travels to the placenta where it is metabolized into estradiol (E_2), estrone (E_1), and estriol (E_3). In the rhesus monkey, an infusion of C19 precursor (androstenedione) leads to preterm delivery [17]. This effect is blocked by the concurrent infusion of an aromatase inhibitor [18], demonstrating that conversion to estrogen is important. However, a systemic infusion of estrogen failed to induce delivery, suggesting that the action of estrogen is likely paracrine-autocrine [17,19,20]. In addition to DHEAS, the fetal adrenal glands also produce copious amounts of cortisol. Cortisol acts to prepares fetal organ systems for extrauterine life and to promote expression of a number of placental genes, including corticotropin releasing hormone (CRH), oxytocin, and prostaglandins (especially prostaglandin E_2 [PGE_2]).

CRH is a peptide hormone released by the hypothalamus but is also expressed by placental and chorionic trophoblasts and amnionic and decidual cells [21–23]. CRH stimulates pituitary ACTH secretion and adrenal cortisol production. In the mother, cortisol inhibits hypothalamic CRH and pituitary ACTH release, creating a negative feedback loop. In contrast, cortisol stimulates CRH release by the decidual, trophoblastic, and fetal membranes [23–26]. CRH, in turn, further drives maternal and fetal HPA activation, thereby establishing a potent positive feed-forward loop. In normal pregnancy, the increased production of CRH from decidual, trophoblastic, and fetal membranes leads to an increase in circulating cortisol beginning in midgestation [27]. The effects of CRH are enhanced by a fall in maternal plasma CRH-binding protein near term [28]. CRH also enhances prostaglandin production by amnionic, chorionic, and decidual cells [23]. Prostaglandins, in turn, stimulate CRH release from the decidual and fetal membranes [24]. The rise in prostaglandins ultimately results in parturition [29]. CRH also can directly affect myometrial contractility [30]. Taken together, these factors suggest that placental CRH serves as a placental clock that controls the timing of labor [31,32]. A longitudinal measurement of CRH throughout pregnancy suggests that the placental clock may be set to run fast or slow as early as the first or second trimester of pregnancy [31,33–35]. Once the speed of the placental clock is set, the timing of delivery may be predetermined.

Role of estrogens in the onset of labor

Human pregnancy is characterized by a hyperestrogenic state of unparallel magnitude in the entire mammalian kingdom. The placenta is the primary source of estrogens, and concentrations of estrogens increase in the maternal circulation with increasing gestational age. Placental estrone and 17β-estradiol are derived primarily from maternal C19 androgens (testosterone and androstenedione), whereas estriol is derived almost exclusively from the fetal C19 estrogen precursor (DHEAS). Estrogens do not themselves cause uterine contractions but do promote a series of myometrial changes, including increasing the number of prostaglandin receptors, oxytocin receptors, and gap junctions, and up-regulating the enzymes responsible for muscle contractions (myosin light chain kinase, calmodulin) [36–39] that enhance the capacity of the myometrium to generate contractions.

Role of progesterone in the onset of labor

The administration of a progesterone receptor antagonist such as RU-486 readily induces abortion if given before 7 weeks (49 days) of gestation [40]. Similarly, the surgical removal of the corpus luteum, the source of progesterone, before 7 weeks results in pregnancy loss [41]. Taken together, these data suggest that adequate production of progesterone by the corpus luteum is critical to the maintenance of early pregnancy until the placenta takes over this function at approximately 7 to 9 weeks of gestation (hence, its name: *pro-gest*ational st*e*roid horm*one*). The role of progesterone in later pregnancy, however, is less clear.

In contrast to most animal species, the circulating levels of progesterone during human labor are similar to levels measured 1 week prior [2,42], suggesting that the systemic withdrawal of progesterone is not a prerequisite for labor in humans. This is in contrast to most laboratory animals (with the noted exceptions of the guinea pig and armadillo) in which progesterone withdrawal is an essential component of parturition. However, circulating hormone levels do not necessarily reflect tissue levels, and there is increasing evidence from both in vitro [43–45] and in vivo studies [46–48] that the spontaneous onset of labor at term may be preceded by a physiologic (functional) withdrawal of progesterone activity at the level of the uterus. In one clinical trial, Meis and colleagues [47] randomly assigned 459 patients at high risk for preterm delivery by virtue of a previous preterm birth to receive a weekly intramuscular injection of 17α-hydroxyprogesterone caproate (250 mg) or a matching placebo, beginning at 16 to 20 weeks of gestation and continuing until 36 weeks. Prophylaxis with 17α-hydroxyprogesterone significantly reduced the risk of delivery at less than 37 weeks (36% versus 55% in the placebo group [relative risk [RR], 0.66; 95% CI, 0.54%–0.81%]), less than 35 weeks (21% versus 31% [RR, 0.67; 95% CI, 0.48%–0.93%]), and less than 32 weeks (11% versus 20% [RR, 0.58; 95% CI, 0.37%–0.91%]). Progesterone likely maintains uterine quiescence during the latter half of pregnancy by limiting the production of stimulatory prostaglandins and inhibiting the expression of contraction-associated protein genes (ion channels, oxytocin and prostaglandin receptors, and gap junctions) within the myometrium [9,49]. The molecular mechanisms by which progesterone maintains uterine quiescence are not known, but the progesterone receptor is likely critical to its action. In support of this hypothesis, the administration of the progesterone receptor antagonist RU-486 at term leads to increased uterine activity and the induction of labor [50].

Cortisol and progesterone appear to have antagonistic actions within the fetoplacental unit. For example, cortisol increases prostaglandin production by the placental and fetal membranes by up-regulating cyclooxygenase-2 (amnion and chorion) and down-regulating 15-hydroxyprostaglandin dehydrogenase (15-OH-PGDH) (chorionic trophoblast), thereby promoting cervical ripening and uterine contractions. Progesterone has the opposite effect [51]. In addition, cortisol has been shown to compete with the inhibitory action of progesterone in the regulation of placental CRH gene expression in primary cultures of human placenta [52]. It is likely, therefore, that the cortisol-dominant environment of the fetoplacental unit just before the onset of labor may act through a series of autocrine-paracrine pathways to overcome the efforts of progesterone to maintain uterine quiescence and prevent myometrial contractions.

Role of other autocrine-paracrine hormones in the onset of labor

Placental oxytocin acts directly on the myometrium to cause contractions and indirectly by up-regulating prostaglandin production, especially prostaglandin $F_{2\alpha}$ ($PGF_{2\alpha}$) by the decidua [53]. $PGF_{2\alpha}$, in turn, is produced primarily by the maternal decidua and acts on the myometrium to up-regulate oxytocin receptors and gap junctions, thereby promoting uterine contractions. PGE_2 is primarily of fetoplacental origin and is likely more important in promoting cervical ripening (maturation) and spontaneous rupture of the fetal membranes.

Preterm labor and birth

Preterm (premature) birth, defined as delivery between 20 and 37 weeks, complicates 7% to 10% of all deliveries [54,55]. Despite intense efforts, the ability of obstetric care providers to prevent preterm labor and birth is limited. Instead of decreasing, the incidence of preterm birth in the United States has continued to rise over the past 2 decades, reaching a peak of 12.1% in 2002 (Fig. 2) [56]. Based on these data, there are approximately 460,000 preterm births in the United States each year. Prematurity is the leading cause of perinatal death in nonanomalous newborns in the United States. Even at gestational ages in which survival is relatively assured, significant morbidity is still common. For example, Robertson and colleagues [57] reported that, at 30 weeks' gestation, the risk of respiratory distress syndrome in surviving infants is 50%, and necrotizing enterocolitis will develop in 11% and intraventricular hemorrhage in 5%.

Causes of preterm birth

Preterm labor likely represents a syndrome rather than a single diagnosis because the causes are varied. Approximately 20% of all preterm deliveries are iatrogenic and are performed for maternal or fetal indications, including intrauterine growth restriction, preeclampsia, placenta previa, and nonreassuring fetal testing [8]. Of the remaining cases of preterm birth,

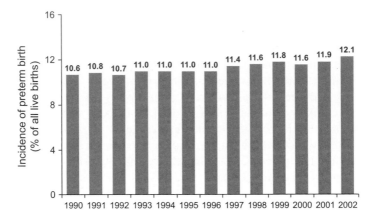

Fig. 2. Preterm births in the United States, 1990–2002. (*Data from* the National Center for Health Statistics, final natality data, and the March of Dimes Perinatal Data Center, 2003. Available at http://marchofdimes.com/peristats.)

approximately 30% occur in the setting of preterm premature rupture of the membranes (pPROM), 20% to 25% result from intra-amniotic infection, and the remaining 25% to 30% are caused by spontaneous (unexplained) preterm labor (Fig. 3) [8,58].

Preterm labor may reflect a breakdown of the normal mechanisms responsible for maintaining uterine quiescence throughout gestation. For example, the choriodecidua is enriched selectively with 15-OH-PGDH, the enzyme responsible for degrading the primary (biologically active) prostaglandins. A deficiency in choriodecidual 15-OH-PGDH activity may impair the ability of the fetal membranes to metabolize the primary prostaglandins, thereby allowing PGE_2 to reach the myometrium and initiate contractions. Such a deficiency has been described and may account for up to 15% of idiopathic preterm labor [59]. Alternatively, premature labor may represent a

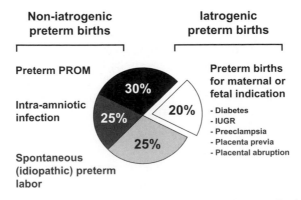

Fig. 3. Causes of preterm births. (*Data from* Tucker JM, Goldenberg RL, Davis RO, et al. Etiologies of preterm birth in an indigent population: is prevention a logical expectation? Obstet Gynecol 1991;77:343–7.)

short-circuiting or overwhelming of the normal parturition cascade. Indeed, a feature of the proposed parturition cascade would be the ability of the fetoplacental unit to trigger labor prematurely if the intrauterine environment became hostile and threatened the well being of the fetus. For example, up to 30% of preterm labors are believed to result from intra-amniotic infection [58]. In many patients with infection, elevated levels of lipoxygenase and cyclooxygenase pathway products can be demonstrated [58,60]. There are also increased concentrations of cytokines (including interleukin [IL]-1β, IL-6, and tumor necrosis factor [TNF]-α) in the amniotic fluid of such women [61]. Cytokines and eicosanoids appear to accelerate each other's production in a cascade-like fashion, which may act to overwhelm the normal parturition cascade, resulting in preterm labor. Recently, thrombin has been shown to be a powerful uterotonic agent [62,63], providing a physiologic mechanism for preterm labor secondary to placental abruption.

Molecular mechanisms of preterm labor

Clinical and experimental evidence links most preterm births to four distinct pathogenic processes. Although these four pathogenic processes can and often do occur simultaneously, each has a unique biochemical and biophysical signature with variable temporal manifestations and distinct epidemiologic profiles. Regardless of the initiating event, these processes converge on a final common biologic pathway characterized by cervical and fetal membrane extracellular matrix degradation and myometrial activation, leading to uterine contractions that increase in frequency and intensity cervical change (preterm labor) with or without pPROM.

Premature activation of the maternal or fetal
hypothalamic-pituitary-adrenal axis

Premature activation of the fetal or maternal HPA axes is evident in up to 33% of preterm births [64]. Maternal physical and psychologic stress leads to the premature activation of the maternal HPA axis and has been linked consistently to preterm birth [65–67]. The activation of the fetal HPA axis has been associated with preterm delivery, and uteroplacental insufficiency is a source of fetal stress [64,68,69]. Indeed, chronic hypertension and severe pregnancy-induced hypertension are associated with an increase of 36% and 300%, respectively, in spontaneous preterm birth [70]. Both maternal and fetal stress likely cause preterm labor by increasing the release of placental CRH, which, in turn, programs the placental clock (Fig. 4) [71,72]. Recent studies have noted elevated second trimester maternal serum CRH concentrations among patients who deliver preterm [33,73,74].

Decidual and amniochorionic inflammation

Laboratory and clinical data show a consistent association between spontaneous preterm labor and genital tract infections [75,76]. The final common

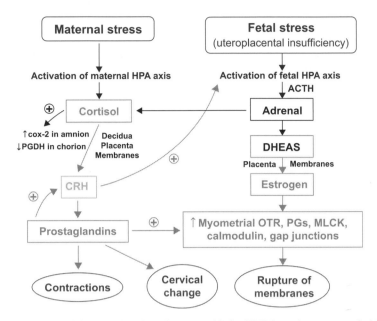

Fig. 4. Maternal and fetal HPA axis and preterm birth. COX-2, cyclooxygenase 2; MLCK, myosin light chain kinase; OTR, oxytocin receptors; PGDH, prostaglandin dehydrogenase.

pathway is a maternal or fetal inflammatory response that is likely triggered by infection in the decidua or amniochorion, with release of inflammatory mediators (cytokines, matrix metalloproteinases [MMPs]) by activated macrophages and granulocytes. In one histopathologic study [77], for example, evidence of chorioamnionitis was observed in 70% of patients with preterm birth associated with pPROM. IL-1, IL-6, and TNF-α directly stimulate PGE_2 and $PGF_{2\alpha}$ production and inhibit their metabolism in the chorion [78,79]. Cytokines also induce MMPs (collagenase, gelatinase, and stromelysins) that weaken the fetal membranes and ripen the cervix by disrupting the normally rigid collagen extracellular matrix (Fig. 5). TNF-α may play an additional role because it can induce apoptosis. Elevated circulating levels of TNF-α have been associated with pPROM [80].

Midtrimester cervicovaginal IL-6 [81] and plasma granulocyte colony-stimulating factor levels [82] also are elevated in asymptomatic women who subsequently deliver preterm, but the sensitivity and positive predictive values of these tests are only approximately 50%. The fetus can also initiate a systemic inflammatory cytokine response leading to labor. One study of 41 women who had pPROM showed that microbial invasion of the uterine cavity elicited an increase in fetal IL-6 levels that was associated with impending preterm labor and birth [83]. Taken together, these data support the hypothesis that many instances of spontaneous preterm labor results from an inflammatory process associated with the activation of the genital tract

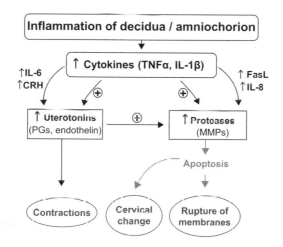

Fig. 5. Inflammation of decidua-amniochorion and preterm labor. FasL, fas ligand.

cytokine network and the presence of cytokines in the maternal or fetal compartment several weeks before delivery.

Decidual hemorrhage

Decidual hemorrhage (abruption) presenting as vaginal bleeding in more than one trimester of pregnancy is associated with a three- and sevenfold increased risk, respectively, of preterm birth [84] and pPROM [85]. The risk of preterm birth is even higher (100-fold) in such women if they also had a previous pregnancy complicated by pPROM [86]. The causes of decidual hemorrhage-associated preterm birth include older, parous, married, and college-educated women [87], a profile quite distinct from that of both infection- and stress-mediated preterm labor.

Thrombin, a plasma protease that converts fibrinogen into fibrin, is formed from prothrombin by the action of prothrombinase (factor Xa). Recent studies have shown that thrombin stimulates myometrial contractions by activating phosphatidylinositol-signaling pathways in a dose-dependent fashion [88]. Thrombin also increases expression of plasminogen activators and MMPs (Fig. 6) [89,90]. The release of thrombin associated with placental abruption may therefore directly initiate the final common pathway leading to preterm labor.

Pathologic uterine distention

Excessive uterine stretching caused by multiple-birth pregnancy or polyhydramnios is associated with preterm labor. Preterm birth rates exceed 50% for twin pregnancies, 80% for triplet pregnancies, and 90% for quadruplet pregnancies. The mechanism is not clear but appears to involve a signal initiated by the mechanical stretching of uterine myometrial, cervical, and fetal membrane cells that is transmitted through the cellular

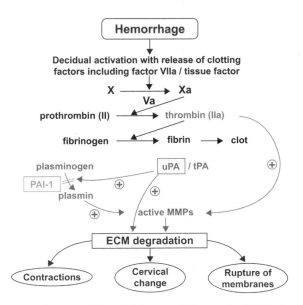

Fig. 6. Hemorrhage and preterm labor. ECM, extracellular matrix; PAI-1, plasminogen activator inhibitor 1; tPA, tissue-type plasminogen activator; uPA, urokinase plasminogen activator.

cytoskeleton and leads to the activation of cellular protein kinases (Fig. 7) [91]. Three genes have recently been identified whose expression in the membranes is up-regulated by acute distention in vitro and in association with labor: an interferon-stimulated gene encoding a 54-kD protein, the gene for Huntington-interacting protein 2 (an ubiquitin-conjugating enzyme), and a novel as yet unidentified transcript [92]. The precise role of these factors in parturition is not known.

Post-term pregnancy

Post-term (prolonged) pregnancy is defined as a pregnancy that has extended to or beyond 42 weeks (294 days) from the first day of the last normal menstrual period or 14 days beyond the best obstetric estimate of the date of delivery [93]. Because of the heterogeneity of populations, definitions, the use of ultrasonography, and local practice patterns (such as the routine induction of labor at term and the management of parturients who previously have undergone cesarean delivery), the reported incidence of pregnancies continuing beyond the estimated date of delivery varies widely. In the United States, approximately 18% of all births occur after 41 weeks, 3% to 14% (mean 10%) occur after 42 weeks and are therefore post-term, and 4% of pregnancies will continue to or beyond 43 weeks in the absence of obstetric intervention [94,95]. The routine early use of ultrasonography to accurately date pregnancies can reduce the rate of false-positive diagnoses and thereby

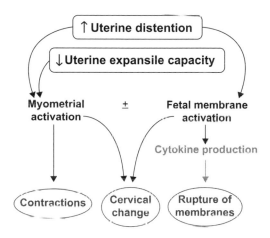

Fig. 7. Uterine distension and preterm labor.

the overall rate of post-term pregnancy from 10% to approximately 1% to 3% [96–99].

Causes of post-term pregnancy

As discussed previously, the most common cause of prolonged pregnancy is an error in gestational age dating. In most cases, the cause of true post-term pregnancy is not known. Risk factors include nulliparity and a previous post-term pregnancy [100,101]. Recent data have also shown an association with male fetuses [102]. Rarer causes include placental sulfatase deficiency, fetal adrenal insufficiency, or fetal anencephaly (in the absence of polyhydramnios). The increased risk of post-term pregnancy in women who have had previous post-term pregnancy suggests an underlying biologic or genetic cause, which has yet to be defined adequately [101,103].

Complications of post-term pregnancy

Recent studies have shown that the risks to the fetus [104–108] and mother [107,109,110] of continuing the pregnancy beyond the estimated date of delivery is greater than appreciated originally. Antepartum stillbirths account for more perinatal deaths than either complications of prematurity or sudden infant death syndrome [106]. Once a fetus is delivered, it is no longer at risk of intrauterine fetal demise (stillbirth). When pregnancies exceed 42 weeks, perinatal mortality (stillbirths plus early neonatal deaths) increases to 4 to 7 per 1000 deliveries compared with 2 to 3 per 1000 deliveries at 40 weeks [111,112]. Perinatal mortality at 43 weeks' gestation is fourfold higher than that at 40 weeks and is five- to sevenfold higher at 44 weeks [112]. Post-term pregnancy is also an independent risk factor for neonatal encephalopathy [113] and for death in the first year of life [105–107]. Since the risks of the routine induction of labor (primarily failed induction leading to cesarean delivery) are lower than reported previously [114,115], recent consensus opinions recommend the routine induction of labor at an earlier gestation age, specifically 41 weeks' gestation [93,107].

Summary

Labor is a complex physiologic process involving fetal, placental, and maternal signals. The timely onset of labor and birth is an important determinant of perinatal outcome. Both preterm labor and delivery and post-term pregnancy are associated with increased perinatal morbidity and mortality. Considerable evidence suggests that the fetus is in control of the timing of labor and, thus, its birth, but exactly how this is achieved in the human is still unknown. A better understanding of the mechanisms responsible for the process of labor will further our knowledge about disorders of parturition, such as preterm labor, and improve the ability of obstetric care providers to secure a successful pregnancy outcome.

References

[1] Liggins GC. The onset of labour: an overview. In: McNellis D, Challis JRG, MacDonald PC, et al, editors. The onset of labor: cellular and integrative mechanisms: a National Institute of Child Health and Human Development research planning workshop (November 29–December 1, 1987). Ithaca (NY): Perinatology Press; 1988. p. 1–3.

[2] Liggins GC. Initiation of labor. Biol Neonate 1989;55:366–94.

[3] Turnbull AC, Anderson AB. Evidence of a foetal role in determining the length of gestation. Postgrad Med J 1969;45:65–7.

[4] Liggins BJ, Fairclough RJ, Grieves SA, et al. The mechanism of initiation of parturition in the ewe. Recent Prog Horm Res 1973;29:111–59.

[5] Flint APF, Anderson ABM, Steele PA, et al. The mechanism by which fetal cortisol controls the onset of parturition in the sheep. Biochem Soc Trans 1975;3:1189–94.

[6] Thorburn GD, Hollingworth SA, Hooper SB. The trigger for parturition in sheep: fetal hypothalamus or placenta? J Dev Physiol 1991;15:71–9.

[7] Matthews SG, Challis JRG. Regulation of the hypothalamo-pituitary-adreno-cortical axis in fetal sheep. Trends Endocrinol Metab 1996;4:239–46.

[8] Norwitz ER, Robinson JN, Challis JR. The control of labor. N Engl J Med 1999;341:660–6.

[9] Challis JRG, Matthews SG, Gibb W, et al. Endocrine and paracrine regulation of birth at term and preterm. Endocr Rev 2000;21:514–50.

[10] Duff P, Huff RW, Gibbs RS. Management of premature rupture of membranes and unfavorable cervix in term pregnancy. Obstet Gynecol 1984;63:697–702.

[11] Myers DA, Nathanielsz PW. Biologic basis of term and preterm labor. Clin Perinatol 1993; 20:9–28.

[12] Pauerstein CJ, Zauder HL. Autonomic innervation, sex steroids and uterine contractility. Obstet Gynecol Surv 1970;25:617–30.

[13] López Bernal A, Rivera J, Europe-Finner GN, et al. Parturition: activation of stimulatory pathways or loss of uterine quiescence? Adv Exp Med Biol 1995;395:435–51.

[14] Garrioch DB. The effect of indomethacin on spontaneous activity in the isolated human myometrium and on the response to oxytocin and prostaglandin. Br J Obstet Gynaecol 1978;85:47–52.

[15] Honnebier MB, Nathanielsz PW. Primate parturition and the role of the maternal circadian system. Eur J Obstet Gynecol Reprod Biol 1994;55:193–203.

[16] Nathanielsz PW. Comparative studies on the initiation of labor. Eur J Obstet Gynecol Reprod Biol 1998;78:127–32.

[17] Mecenas CA, Giussani DA, Owiny JR, et al. Production of premature delivery in pregnant rhesus monkeys by androstenedione infusion. Nat Med 1996;2:442–8.

[18] Giussani DA, Jenkins SL, Mecenas CA, et al. Daily and hourly temporal association between delta4-androstenedione-induced preterm myometrial contractions and maternal plasma estradiol and oxytocin concentrations in the 0.8 gestation rhesus monkey. Am J Obstet Gynecol 1996;174:1050–5.

[19] Figueroa JP, Honnebier MBOM, Binienda Z, et al. Effect of 48 hour intravenous Δ^4-androstenedione infusion on pregnant rhesus monkeys in the last third of gestation: Changes in maternal plasma estradiol concentrations and myometrial contractility. Am J Obstet Gynecol 1989;161:481–6.

[20] Nathanielsz PW, Jenkins SL, Tame JD, et al. Local paracrine effects of estradiol are central to parturition in the rhesus monkey. Nat Med 1998;4:456–9.

[21] Zoumakis E, Makrigiannakis A, Margioris AN, et al. Endometrial corticotropin-releasing hormone: its potential autocrine and paracrine actions. Ann N Y Acad Sci 1997;828:84–94.

[22] Petraglia F, Potter E, Cameron VA, et al. Corticotropin-releasing factor-binding protein is produced by human placenta and intrauterine tissues. J Clin Endocrinol Metab 1993;77:919–24.

[23] Jones SA, Brooks AN, Challis JR. Steroids modulate corticotropin-releasing hormone production in human fetal membranes and placenta. J Clin Endocrinol Metab 1989;68:825–30.

[24] Petraglai F, Coukos G, Volpe A, et al. Involvement of placental neurohormones in human parturition. Ann N Y Acad Sci 1991;622:331–40.

[25] Smith R, Mesiano S, Chan EC, Brown S, et al. Corticotropin-releasing hormone directly and preferentially stimulates dehydroepiandrosterone sulfate secretion by human fetal adrenal cortical cells. J Clin Endocrinol Metab 1998;83:2916–20.

[26] Chakravorty A, Mesiano S, Jaffe RB. Corticotropin-releasing hormone stimulates P450 17alpha- hydroxylase/17,20-lyase in human fetal adrenal cells via protein kinase C. J Clin Endocrinol Metab 1999;84:3732–8.

[27] Lockwood CJ, Radunovic N, Nastic D, et al. Corticotropin-releasing hormone and related pituitary-adrenal axis hormones in fetal and maternal blood during the second half of pregnancy. J Perinat Med 1996;24:243–51.

[28] Perkins AV, Eben F, Wolfe CD, et al. Plasma measurements of corticotrophin-releasing hormone-binding protein in normal and abnormal human pregnancy. J Endocrinol 1993; 138:149–57.

[29] Gibb W. The role of prostaglandins in human parturition. Ann Med 1998;30:235–41.

[30] Grammatopoulos DK, Hillhouse EW. Role of corticotropin-releasing hormone in onset of labor. Lancet 1999;354:1546–9.

[31] McLean M, Bisits A, Davies J, et al. A placental clock controlling the length of human pregnancy. Nat Med 1995;1:460–3.

[32] Korebrits C, Ramirez MM, Watson L, et al. Maternal corticotropin-releasing hormone is increased with impending preterm birth. J Clin Endocrinol Metab 1998;83:1585–91.

[33] Hobel CJ, Dunkel-Schetter C, Roesch SC, et al. Maternal plasma corticotropin-releasing hormone associated with stress at 20 weeks' gestation in pregnancies ending in preterm delivery. Am J Obstet Gynecol 1999;180(1 Pt 3):S257–63.

[34] Wadhwa PD, Porto M, Garite TJ, et al. Maternal corticotropin-releasing hormone levels in the early third trimester predicts length of gestation in human pregnancy. Am J Obstet Gynecol 1998;179:1079–85.

[35] Leung TN, Chung TK, Madsen G, et al. Elevated mid-trimester maternal corticotrophin-releasing hormone levels in pregnancies that delivered before 34 weeks. Br J Obstet Gynaecol 1999;106:1041–6.

[36] Lye SJ, Nicholson BJ, Mascarenhas M, et al. Increased expression of connexin-43 in the rat myometrium during labor is associated with an increase in the plasma estrogen:progesterone ratio. Endocrinology 1993;132:2380–6.

[37] Bale TL, Dorsa DM. Cloning, novel promoter sequence, and estrogen regulation of a rat oxytocin receptor gene. Endocrinology 1997;138:1151–8.

[38] Windmoller R, Lye SJ, Challis JR. Estradiol modulation of ovine uterine activity. Can J Physiol Pharmacol 1983;61:722–8.

[39] Matsui K, Higashi K, Fukunaga K, et al. Hormone treatments and pregnancy alter myosin light chain kinase and calmodulin levels in rabbit myometrium. J Endocrinol 1983;97:11–9.

[40] Peyron R, Aubeny E, Targosz V, et al. Early termination of pregnancy with mifepristone (RU 486) and the orally active prostaglandin misoprostol. N Engl J Med 1993;328:1509–13.

[41] Csapo AI, Pulkkinen M. Indispensability of the human corpus luteum in the maintenance of early pregnancy: luteectomy evidence. Obstet Gynecol Surv 1978;33:69–81.

[42] Hanssens MC, Selby C, Symonds EM. Sex steroid hormone concentrations in preterm labour and the outcome of treatment with ritodrine. Br J Obstet Gynaecol 1985;92:698–702.

[43] Madsen G, Zakar T, Ku CY, et al. Prostaglandins differentially modulate progesterone receptor-A and -B expression in human myometrial cells: evidence for prostaglandin-induced functional progesterone withdrawal. J Clin Endocrinol Metab 2004;89:1010–3.

[44] Grazzini E, Guillon G, Mouillac B, et al. Inhibition of oxytocin receptor function by direct binding of progesterone. Nature 1998;392:509–12.

[45] Condon JC, Jeyasuria P, Faust JM, et al. A decline in the levels of progesterone receptor coactivators in the pregnant uterus at term may antagonize progesterone receptor function and contribute to the initiation of parturition. Proc Natl Acad Sci U S A 2003;100:9518–23.

[46] Keirse MJNC. Progestogen administration in pregnancy may prevent preterm delivery. Br J Obstet Gynaecol 1990;97:149–54.

[47] Meis PJ, Klebanoff M, Thom E, et al. National Institute of Child Health and Human Development Maternal-Fetal Medicine Units Network. Prevention of recurrent preterm delivery by 17 alpha-hydroxyprogesterone caproate. N Engl J Med 2003;348:2379–85.

[48] Da Fonseca EB, Bittar RE, Carvalho MH, et al. Prophylactic administration of progesterone by vaginal suppository to reduce the incidence of spontaneous preterm birth in women at increased risk: a randomized placebo-controlled double-blind study. Am J Obstet Gynecol 2003;188:419–24.

[49] Norwitz ER, Schust DJ, Fisher SJ. Implantation and the survival of early pregnancy. N Engl J Med 2001;345:1400–8.

[50] Neilson JP. Mifepristone for induction of labour. Cochrane Database Syst Rev 2000:(4); CD002865.

[51] Challis JR, Sloboda DM, Alfaidy N, et al. Prostaglandins and mechanisms of preterm birth. Reproduction 2002;124:1–17.

[52] Karalis K, Goodwin G, Majzoub JA. Cortisol blockade of progesterone: a possible molecular mechanism involved in the initiation of human labor. Nat Med 1996;2:556–60.

[53] Wilson T, Liggins GC, Whittaker DJ. Oxytocin stimulates the release of arachidonic acid and prostaglandin F2 alpha from human decidual cells. Prostaglandins 1988;35:771–80.

[54] Rush RW, Keirse MJNC, Howat P, et al. Contribution of preterm delivery to perinatal mortality. BMJ 1976;2:965–8.

[55] Villar J, Ezcurra EJ, de la Fuente VG, et al. Preterm delivery syndrome: the unmet need. Res Clin Forums 1994;16:9–33.

[56] Martin JA, Hamilton BE, Sutton PD, et al. Births: final data for 2002. Natl Vital Stat Rep 2003;52:1.

[57] Robertson PA, Sniderman SH, Laros RK Jr, et al. Neonatal morbidity according to gestational age and birth weight from five tertiary care centers in the United States, 1983 through 1986. Am J Obstet Gynecol 1992;166:1629–41.

[58] Romero R, Avila C, Brekus CA, et al. The role of systemic and intrauterine infection in preterm parturition. Ann N Y Acad Sci 1991;662:355–75.

[59] Matthews SG, Challis JRG. Regulation of the hypothalamo-pituitary-adreno-cortical axis in fetal sheep. Trends Endocrinol Metab 1996;4:239.

[60] Dudley DJ. Preterm labor: an intra-uterine inflammatory response syndrome? J Reprod Immunol 1997;36:93–109.

[61] Romero R, Emamian M, Wan M, et al. Prostaglandin concentrations in amniotic fluid of women with intra-amniotic infection and preterm labor. Am J Obstet Gynecol 1987;157: 1461–7.

[62] Elovitz MA, Saunders T, Ascher-Landsberg J, et al. Effects of thrombin on myometrial contractions in vitro and in vivo. Am J Obstet Gynecol 2000;183:799–804.

[63] Elovitz M, Baron J, Phillippe M. The role of thrombin in preterm parturition. Am J Obstet Gynecol 2001;185:1059–63.

[64] Arias F, Rodriquez L, Rayne SC, et al. Maternal placental vasculopathy and infection: two distinct subgroups among patients with preterm labor and preterm ruptured membranes. Am J Obstet Gynecol 1993;168:585–91.

[65] Berkowitz GS, Kasl SV. The role of psychosocial factors in spontaneous preterm delivery. J Psychosom Res 1983;27:283–90.

[66] Lobel M, Dunkel-Schetter C, Scrimshaw SC. Prenatal maternal stress and prematurity: a prospective study of socioeconomically disadvantaged women. Health Psychol 1992;11: 32–40.

[67] Copper RL, Goldenberg RL, Das A, et al, for the National Institute of Child Health and Human Development Maternal-Fetal Medicine Units Network. The preterm prediction study: maternal stress is associated with spontaneous preterm birth at less than thirty-five weeks' gestation. Am J Obstet Gynecol 1996;175:1286–92.

[68] Ott WJ. Intrauterine growth retardation and preterm delivery. Am J Obstet Gynecol 1993; 168:1710–5

[69] Salafia CM, Ghidini A, Lopez-Zeno JA, et al. Uteroplacental pathology and maternal arterial mean blood pressure in spontaneous prematurity. J Soc Gynecol Investig 1998,5: 68–71.

[70] Kramer MS, McLean FH, Eason EL, et al. Maternal nutrition and spontaneous preterm birth. Am J Epidemiol 1992;136:574–83.

[71] McLean M, Bisits A, Davies J, et al. A placental clock controlling the length of human pregnancy. Nat Med 1995;1:460–3.

[72] Korebrits C, Ramirez MM, Watson L, et al. Maternal corticotropin-releasing hormone is increased with impending preterm birth. J Clin Endocrinol Metab 1998;83:1585–91.

[73] Wadhwa PD, Porto M, Garite TJ, et al. Maternal corticotropin-releasing hormone levels in the early third trimester predict length of gestation in human pregnancy. Am J Obstet Gynecol 1998;179:1079–85.

[74] Leung TN, Chung TK, Madsen G, et al. Elevated mid-trimester maternal corticotrophin-releasing hormone levels in pregnancies that delivered before 34 weeks. Br J Obstet Gynaecol 1999;106:1041–6.

[75] Lockwood CJ, Kuczynski E. Markers of risk for preterm delivery. J Perinat Med 1999;27: 5–20.

[76] Goldenberg RL, Hauth JC, Andrews WW. Intrauterine infection and preterm delivery. N Engl J Med 2000;342:1500–7.

[77] Moretti M, Sibai BM. Maternal and perinatal outcome of expectant management of premature rupture of membranes in the midtrimester. Am J Obstet Gynecol 1988;159:390–6.

[78] Romero R, Durum S, Dinarello CA, et al. Interleukin-1 stimulates prostaglandin biosynthesis by human amnion. Prostaglandins 1989;37:13–22.

[79] Van Mier CA, Sangha RK, Walton JC, et al. Immunoreactive 15-hydroxyprostaglandin dehydrogenase (PGDH) is reduced in fetal membranes from patients at preterm delivery in the presence of infection. Placenta 1996;17:291–7.

[80] Lei H, Furth EE, Kalluri R, et al. A program of cell death and extracellular matrix degradation is activated in the amnion before the onset of labor. J Clin Invest 1996;98:1971–8.

[81] Lockwood CJ, Ghidini A, Wein R, et al. Increased interleukin-6 concentrations in cervical secretions are associated with preterm delivery. Am J Obstet Gynecol 1994;171:1097–102.

[82] Goldenberg RL, Andrews WW, Mercer BM, et al, for the National Institute of Child Health and Human Development Maternal-Fetal Medicine Units Network. The preterm prediction study: granulocyte colony-stimulating factor and spontaneous preterm birth. Am J Obstet Gynecol 2000;182:625–30.

[83] Yoon BH, Romero R, Jun JK, et al. Amniotic fluid cytokines (interleukin-6, tumor necrosis factor-alpha, interleukin-1 beta, and interleukin-8) and the risk for the development of bronchopulmonary dysplasia. Am J Obstet Gynecol 1997;177:825–30.

[84] Williams MA, Mittendorf R, Lieberman E, et al. Adverse infant outcomes associated with first-trimester vaginal bleeding. Obstet Gynecol 1991;78:14–8.

[85] Harger JH, Hsing AW, Tuomala RE, et al. Risk factors for preterm premature rupture of fetal membranes: a multicenter case-control study. Am J Obstet Gynecol 1990;163: 130–7.

[86] Ekwo EE, Gosselink CA, Moawad A. Unfavorable outcome in penultimate pregnancy and premature rupture of membranes in successive pregnancy. Obstet Gynecol 1992;80:166–72.

[87] Strobino B, Pantel-Silverman J. Gestational vaginal bleeding and pregnancy outcome. Am J Epidemiol 1989;129:806–15.

[88] Elovitz MA, Ascher-Landsberg J, Saunders T, et al. The mechanisms underlying the stimulatory effects of thrombin on myometrial smooth muscle. Am J Obstet Gynecol 2000;183: 674–81.

[89] Rosen T, Schatz F, Kuczynshi E, et al. Thrombin-enhanced matrix metalloproteinase-1 expression: a mechanism linking placental abruption with premature rupture of the membranes. J Matern Fetal Neonatal Med 2002;11:11–7.

[90] Lockwood CJ, Krikun G, Aigner S, et al. Effects of thrombin on steroid-modulated cultured endometrial stromal cell fibrinolytic potential. J Clin Endocrinol Metab 1996;81: 107–12.

[91] Ou CW, Orsino A, Lye SJ. Expression of connexin-43 and connexin-26 in the rat myometrium during pregnancy and labor is differentially regulated by mechanical and hormonal signals. Endocrinology 1997;138:5398–407.

[92] Nemeth E, Millar LK, Bryant-Greenwood G. Fetal membrane distention: II. differentially expressed genes regulated by acute distention in vitro. Am J Obstet Gynecol 2000;182:60–7.

[93] American College of Obstetricians and Gynecologists. Management of postterm pregnancy. ACOG Practice Bulletin No. 55. 2004.

[94] Ventura SJ, Martin JA, Curtin SC, et al. Births: final data for 1998. Natl Vital Stat Rep 2000;48:1–100.

[95] Bakketeig LS, Bergsjo P. Post-term pregnancy: magnitude of the problem. In: Chalmers I, Enkin M, Keirse M, editors. Effective care in pregnancy and childbirth. Oxford: Oxford University Press; 1991.

[96] Boyd ME, Usher RH, McLean FH, et al. Obstetric consequences of postmaturity. Am J Obstet Gynecol 1988;158:334–8.

[97] Gardosi J, Vanner T, Francis A. Gestational age and induction of labor for prolonged pregnancy. Br J Obstet Gynaecol 1997;104:792–7.

[98] Taipale P, Hiilermaa V. Predicting delivery date by ultrasound and last menstrual period on early gestation. Obstet Gynecol 2001;97:189–94.

[99] Neilson JP. Ultrasound for fetal assessment in early pregnancy. Cochrane Database Syst Rev 2000; CD000182.

[100] Alfirevic Z, Walkinshaw SA. Management of post-term pregnancy: to induce or not? Br J Hosp Med 1994;52:218–21.

[101] Mogren I, Stenlund H, Hogberg U. Recurrence of prolonged pregnancy. Int J Epidemiol 1999;28:253–7.

[102] Divon MY, Ferber A, Nisell H, et al. Male gender predisposes to prolongation of pregnancy. Am J Obstet Gynecol 2002;187:1081–3.

[103] Olesen AW, Basso O, Olsen J. Risk of recurrence of prolonged pregnancy. BMJ 2003;326: 476.

[104] Herabutya Y, Prasertsawat PO, Tongyai T, et al. Prolonged pregnancy: the management dilemma. Int J Gynecol Obstet 1992;37:253–8.

[105] Hilder L, Costeloe K, Thilaganathan B. Prolonged pregnancy: evaluating gestation-specific risks of fetal and infant mortality. Br J Obstet Gynaecol 1998;105:169–73.

[106] Cotzias CS, Paterson-Brown S, Fisk NM. Prospective risk of unexplained stillbirth in singleton pregnancies at term: population based analysis. BMJ 1999;319:287–8.

[107] Rand L, Robinson JN, Economy KE, et al. Post-term induction of labor revisited. Obstet Gynecol 2000;96:779–83.

[108] Smith GC. Life-table analysis of the risk of perinatal death at term and post term in singleton pregnancies. Am J Obstet Gynecol 2001;184:489–96.

[109] Alexander JM, McIntire DD, Leveno KJ. Forty weeks and beyond: pregnancy outcomes by week of gestation. Obstet Gynecol 2000;96:291–4.

[110] Treger M, Hallak M, Silberstein T, et al. Post-term pregnancy: should induction of labor be considered before 42 weeks? J Matern Fetal Neonatal Med 2002;11:50–3.

[111] Bakketeig LS, Bergsjo P. Post-term pregnancy: magnitude of the problem. In: Enkin M, Keirse MJ, Chalmers I, editors. Effective care in pregnancy and childbirth. Oxford: Oxford University Press; 1989.

[112] Feldman GB. Prospective risk of stillbirth. Obstet Gynecol 1992;79:547–53.

[113] Badawi N, Kurinczuk JJ, Keogh JM, et al. Antepartum risk factors for newborn encephalopathy: the Western Australian case-control study. BMJ 1998;317:1549–53.

[114] Hannah ME, Hannah WJ, Hellmann J, et al for the Canadian Multicenter Post-Term Pregnancy Trial Group. Induction of labor as compared with serial antenatal monitoring in post term pregnancy: a randomized controlled trial. N Engl J Med 1992;326:1587–92.

[115] Hannah ME, Hannah WJ, Willan A. Comment on the effectiveness of induction of labor for postterm pregnancy. Am J Obstet Gynecol 1994;170:716–23.

ELSEVIER
SAUNDERS

Endocrinol Metab Clin N Am
35 (2006) 193–204

ENDOCRINOLOGY
AND METABOLISM
CLINICS
OF NORTH AMERICA

Developmental Origins of Adult Metabolic Disease

Rebecca Simmons, MD[a,b,*]

[a]*Department of Pediatrics, Children's Hospital of Philadelphia, Philadelphia, PA, USA*
[b]*University of Pennsylvania, Philadelphia, PA, USA*

The combined epidemiologic, clinical, and animal studies clearly demonstrate that the intrauterine environment influences growth and development of the fetus and the subsequent development of adult diseases. There are critical specific windows during development, often coincident with periods of rapid cell division, during which a stimulus or insult may have long-lasting consequences on tissue or organ function after birth. Birth weight is only one marker of an adverse fetal environment, and confining studies to this population only may lead to erroneous conclusions regarding etiology. Studies using animal models of uteroplacental insufficiency suggest that mitochondrial dysfunction and oxidative stress play an important role in the pathogenesis of the fetal origins of adult disease.

Low birth weight

It is becoming increasingly apparent that the in utero environment in which a fetus grows and develops may have long-term effects on subsequent health and survival [1,2]. The landmark cohort study of 300,000 men by Ravelli and colleagues [3] showed that exposure to the Dutch famine of 1944 through 1945 during the first half of pregnancy resulted in significantly higher obesity rates at the age of 19 years. Subsequent studies demonstrated a relation between low birth weight and the later development of cardiovascular disease [4] and impaired glucose tolerance [5–8] in men in England. Other studies of populations in the United States [9–11], Sweden [12], France [13,14], Norway [15], and Finland [16] have all demonstrated

* University of Pennsylvania, 421 Curie Boulevard, BRB II/III, Room 1308, Philadelphia, PA 19104.
  E-mail address: rsimmons@mail.med.upenn.edu

0889-8529/06/$ - see front matter © 2005 Elsevier Inc. All rights reserved.
doi:10.1016/j.ecl.2005.09.006   *endo.theclinics.com*

a significant correlation between low birth weight and the later development of adult diseases. The associations with low birth weight and increased risk of coronary heart disease, stroke, and type 2 diabetes remain strong even after adjusting for lifestyle factors, such as smoking, physical activity, occupation, income, dietary habits, and childhood socioeconomic status, and occur independent of the current level of obesity or exercise [17].

High birth weight

Higher birth weight is associated with higher body mass index (BMI) and increased prevalence of obesity in adult life, although the effect size is relatively small [18]. The impact of intrauterine life in relation to later obesity may be in determining the vulnerability of individuals to increased body mass in childhood or adult life. Those who become obese as adults tend to have been heavier at birth and to have had an accelerated gain in body mass through childhood and adolescence. Factors in early childhood may lead to obesity through metabolic programming (discussed elsewhere in this article) or establishment of lifestyle behaviors. During infancy, breastfeeding may protect against the development of excess weight during childhood. Most but not all epidemiologic studies demonstrate this protective effect, which could be mediated by behavioral or physiologic mechanisms. Confounding cultural factors associated with the decision to breastfeed and later obesity are possible, however. Recent data also suggest that rapid weight gain during infancy is associated with obesity later in childhood, perhaps reflecting a combination of genetically determined catch-up growth and postnatal environmental factors [18].

Role of catch-up growth

The highest risk for the development of type 2 diabetes is among adults who were born small and became overweight during childhood [19–21]. Insulin resistance is most prominent in Indian children and in Indian men and women who were born small for gestational age (SGA) but had a high fat mass between the ages of 2 and 12 years [20,21]. Similar findings were reported in 10-year-old children in the United Kingdom [22]. In contrast, in two recent preliminary studies from the United Kingdom, catch-up growth in the first 6 months of life was not clearly related to blood pressure as a young adult, although birth weight was [23,24]. Interpretation of these studies is complicated by the vague definitions of catch-up growth. Catch-up growth can refer to the first 6 to 12 months of life to as late as 2 years after birth and usually refers to realignment of one's genetic growth potential after intrauterine growth retardation (IUGR). This definition allows for fetal growth retardation at any birth weight—even large fetuses can be growth retarded relative to their genetic potential. Although it is likely that accelerated growth confers an additional risk to the growth-retarded fetus, these conflicting results demonstrate the need for additional carefully designed studies to determine just how childhood growth rates influence the later development of cardiovascular disease and type 2 diabetes.

Size at birth and insulin secretion and insulin action

The mechanisms underlying the association between size at birth and impaired glucose tolerance or type 2 diabetes are unclear. A number of studies in children and adults have shown that non- or prediabetic subjects with low birth weight are insulin resistant and thus predisposed to the development of type 2 diabetes [9,12–14,19–27]. IUGR is known to alter the fetal development of adipose tissue, which is closely linked to the development of insulin resistance [28,29]. In a well-designed case-control study of 25-year-old adults, individuals born SGA at 37 weeks or later had a significantly higher percentage of body fat [14]. Insulin sensitivity, even after adjusting for BMI or total fat mass, was markedly impaired in these SGA subjects. There were no significant differences between the SGA and control groups with respect to parental history of type 2 diabetes, cardiovascular disease, hypertension, or dyslipidemia. Of importance to generalizing the findings to other populations, the causes of IUGR were gestational hypertension (50%), smoking (30%), maternal short stature (7%), congenital anomalies (7%), and unknown (6%).

It was originally thought that the adverse effect of IUGR on glucose homeostasis was mediated through programming of the fetal endocrine pancreas [1]. Growth-retarded fetuses and newborns have been shown to have a reduced population of pancreatic β-cells [30]. Low birth weight has been associated with a reduced insulin response after glucose ingestion in young nondiabetic men; however, a number of other studies have found no impact of low birth weight on insulin secretion in human beings [12,26,27]. None of these earlier studies adjusted for the corresponding insulin sensitivity, however, which has a profound impact on insulin secretion. Therefore, Jensen and colleagues [31] measured insulin secretion and insulin sensitivity in a well-matched white population of 19-year-old glucose-tolerant men with birth weights below the 10th percentile (SGA) or between the 50th and 75th percentiles (controls). To eliminate the major confounders, such as "diabetes genes," none of the participants had a family history of diabetes, hypertension, or ischemic heart disease. There was no difference between the groups with regard to current weight, BMI, body composition, or lipid profile. When controlled for insulin sensitivity, insulin secretion was reduced by 30%. Insulin sensitivity was normal in the SGA subjects, however. The investigators hypothesized that defects in insulin secretion may precede defects in insulin action and that once SGA individuals accumulate body fat, they develop insulin resistance [31].

Epidemiologic challenges

These data suggest that low birth weight is associated with glucose intolerance, type 2 diabetes, and cardiovascular disease. The question remains as to whether these associations reflect fetal nutrition or other factors that contribute to birth weight and the observed glucose intolerance. Because of the retrospective nature of the cohort identification, many confounding variables were not always recorded, such as lifestyle, socioeconomic status, education, maternal age, parental build, birth order, obstetric complications, smoking, and maternal health. Maternal nutritional status, directly in the form of diet history or indirectly in the form of BMI, height, and pregnancy weight gain, were usually not recorded. Instead, birth anthropometric measures were used as proxies for presumed undernutrition in pregnancy.

Genetics versus environment

Several epidemiologic and metabolic studies of twins and first-degree relatives of patients with type 2 diabetes have demonstrated an important genetic component of diabetes [32–35]. The association between low birth weight and risk of type 2 diabetes in some studies could theoretically be explained by a genetically determined reduced fetal growth rate. In other words, the genotype responsible for type 2 diabetes may itself cause retarded fetal growth in utero. This forms the basis for the fetal insulin hypothesis, which suggests that genetically determined insulin resistance could result in low insulin-mediated fetal growth in utero as well as insulin resistance in childhood and adulthood [36]. Insulin is one of the major growth factors in fetal life, and monogenic disorders that affect fetal insulin secretion or fetal insulin resistance also affect fetal growth. Mutations in the gene encoding glucokinase that result in low birth weight and maturity onset diabetes of the young have been identified [37,38]. Such mutations are rare, however, and no analogous common allelic variation has yet been discovered.

Recent genetic studies suggest that the increased susceptibility to type 2 diabetes of subjects who are born SGA results from the combination of genetic factors and an unfavorable fetal environment. Polymorphisms of PPARγ2, a gene involved in the development and metabolic function of adipose tissue, have been shown to modulate the susceptibility of subjects who are born SGA to develop insulin resistance later in life [39,40]. The polymorphism is only associated with a higher risk of type 2 diabetes if birth weight is reduced [39,40].

There is obviously a close relation between genes and the environment. Not only can maternal gene expression alter the fetal environment; the maternal intrauterine environment also affects fetal gene expression.

What animal models can tell us

Animal models have a normal genetic background on which environmental effects during gestation or early postnatal life can be tested for their role in inducing diabetes. The most commonly used animal models are caloric or protein restriction, glucocorticoid administration, or induction of uteroplacental insufficiency in the pregnant rodent. In the rat, maternal dietary protein restriction (approximately 40%–50% of normal intake) throughout gestation and lactation has been reported to alter glucose homeostasis and hypertension in the adult offspring [41–46]. Offspring are significantly growth retarded, remain growth retarded throughout life, and develop mild β-cell secretory abnormalities in some cases [41–45] and insulin resistance in others [43,46–50]. Aged rats develop hyperglycemia, which is characterized by defects in insulin signaling in muscle, adipocytes, and liver [47–50].

Fetal overexposure to glucocorticoids via maternal administration or by inhibition of placental 11β–hydroxysteroid dehydrogenase–1 in the rat induces hypertension, glucose intolerance, and abnormalities in hypothalamo-pituitary-adrenocortical (HPA) function after birth [51–54].

To extend these experimental studies of growth retardation, we developed a model of uteroplacental insufficiency (IUGR) in the rat that restricts fetal growth [55,56]. Growth-retarded fetal rats have critical features of a metabolic profile characteristic of growth-retarded human fetuses: decreased levels of glucose, insulin, insulin-like growth factor-I (IGF-I), amino acids, and oxygen [57–59]. By 6 months of age, IUGR rats develop diabetes with a phenotype remarkably similar to that observed in the human being with type 2 diabetes: progressive dysfunction in insulin secretion and insulin action. Thus, the studies in various animal models support the hypothesis that an abnormal intrauterine milieu can induce permanent changes in glucose homeostasis after birth and lead to type 2 diabetes in adulthood.

Cellular mechanisms: mitochondrial dysfunction and oxidative stress

The intrauterine environment influences development of the fetus by modifying gene expression in pluripotential cells or terminally differentiated and poorly replicating cells. The long-range effects on the offspring (into adulthood) depend on the cells undergoing differentiation, proliferation, or functional maturation at the time of the disturbance in maternal fuel economy. The fetus also adapts to an inadequate supply of substrates (eg, glucose, amino acids, fatty acids, oxygen) by metabolic changes, redistribution of blood flow, and changes in the production of the fetal and placental hormones that control growth.

The fetus' immediate metabolic response to placental insufficiency is catabolism—it consumes its own substrates to provide energy. A more prolonged reduction in availability of substrates leads to a slowing in growth. This enhances the fetus' ability to survive by reducing the use of substrates and lowering the metabolic rate. Slowing of growth in late gestation leads to disproportion in organ size, because organs and tissues that are growing rapidly at the time are affected the most.

Uteroplacental insufficiency caused by such disorders as preeclampsia, maternal smoking, and abnormalities of uteroplacental development is one of the most common causes of fetal growth retardation. The resultant abnormal intrauterine milieu restricts the supply of crucial nutrients to the fetus, thereby limiting fetal growth. Multiple studies have now shown that IUGR is associated with increased oxidative stress in the human fetus [60–66]. A major consequence of limited nutrient availability is an alteration in the redox state in susceptible fetal tissues, leading to oxidative stress. In particular, low levels of oxygen, evident in growth-retarded fetuses, decrease the activity of complexes of the electron transport chain, which generates increased levels of reactive oxygen species (ROS). Overproduction of ROS initiates many oxidative reactions that lead to oxidative damage not only in the mitochondria but in cellular proteins, lipids, and nucleic acids. Increased ROS levels inactivate the iron-sulfur centers of the electron transport chain complexes and tricarboxylic acid cycle aconitase, resulting in shutdown of mitochondrial energy production.

A key adaptation enabling the fetus to survive in a limited energy environment may be the reprogramming of mitochondrial function [67,68]. These alterations in mitochondrial function can have deleterious effects, however, especially in cells that have a high-energy requirement, such as the β-cell. The β-cell depends on the normal production of ATP for nutrient-induced insulin secretion [69–76] and proliferation [77]. Thus, an interruption of mitochondrial function can have profound consequences for the β-cell.

Mitochondrial dysfunction can also lead to increased production of ROS, which leads to oxidative stress if the defense mechanisms of the cell are overwhelmed. β-Cells are especially vulnerable to attack by ROS, because the expression of antioxidant enzymes in pancreatic islets is low [78,79] and β-cells have a high oxidative energy requirement. Increased ROS impair glucose-stimulated insulin secretion [80,81], decrease gene expression of key β-cell genes [82–86], and induce cell death [87–91].

We have found that uteroplacental insufficiency induces mitochondrial dysfunction in the fetal β-cell, leading to increased production of ROS, which, in turn, damage mitochondrial DNA (mtDNA). A self-reinforcing cycle of progressive deterioration in mitochondrial function leads to a corresponding decline in β-cell function. Finally, a threshold in mitochondrial dysfunction and ROS production is reached, and diabetes ensues [92].

Mitochondrial dysfunction is not limited to the β-cell in the IUGR animal. IUGR animals exhibit marked insulin resistance early in life (before the onset of hyperglycemia), which is characterized by blunted whole-body glucose disposal in response to insulin and impaired insulin suppression of hepatic glucose output [93]. Basal hepatic glucose production is also increased [93]. Oxidation rates of pyruvate, glutamate, succinate, and α-ketoglutarate are significantly blunted in isolated hepatic mitochondria from IUGR pups (before the onset of diabetes) [94]. This derangement in oxidative phosphorylation predisposes the IUGR rat to increased hepatic glucose production by suppressing pyruvate oxidation and increasing gluconeogenesis [94].

Mitochondria in muscle of IUGR young adult rats, before the onset of hyperglycemia, exhibit significantly decreased rates of state-3 oxygen consumption with pyruvate, glutamate, α-ketoglutarate, and succinate [95]. Decreased pyruvate oxidation in IUGR mitochondria is associated with decreased ATP production, decreased pyruvate dehydrogenase activity, and increased expression of pyruvate dehydrogenase kinase 4 (PDK4). Such a defect in IUGR mitochondria leads to a chronic reduction in the supply of ATP available from oxidative phosphorylation. Impaired ATP synthesis in muscle compromises energy-dependent GLUT4 recruitment to the cell surface, glucose transport, and glycogen synthesis, which contributes to insulin resistance and hyperglycemia of type 2 diabetes [95].

Our studies are likely to have important clinical applicability as well. A recent study in young adult offspring of patients with type 2 diabetes demonstrated that those subjects with insulin resistance had a 30% reduction in mitochondrial phosphorylation compared with age-matched controls [96]. The investigators speculated that insulin resistance in the skeletal muscle of insulin-resistant offspring of patients with type 2 diabetes was attributable to an inherited defect in mitochondrial oxidative phosphorylation [96]. Thus, our studies elucidate the molecular mechanisms underlying the link between mitochondrial dysfunction, whether hereditary or secondary to an environmental insult, and the later development of type 2 diabetes.

Summary

The combined epidemiologic, clinical, and animal studies clearly demonstrate that the intrauterine environment influences growth and development of the fetus and the subsequent development of adult diseases. There are critical specific windows during development, often coincident with periods of rapid cell division, during which a stimulus or insult may have long-lasting consequences on tissue or organ function after birth. Birth weight is only one marker of an adverse fetal environment, and confining studies to this population only may lead to erroneous conclusions regarding etiology. Studies using animal models of uteroplacental insufficiency suggest that mitochondrial dysfunction and oxidative stress play an important role in the pathogenesis of the fetal origins of adult disease.

References

[1] Hales CN, Barker DJP. Type 2 diabetes mellitus: the thrifty phenotype hypothesis. Diabetologia 1992;35:595–601.

[2] Kermack WO. Death rates in Great Britain and Sweden. Lancet 1934;1:698–703.

[3] Ravelli GP, Stein ZA, Susser MW. Obesity in young men after famine exposure in utero and early infancy. N Engl J Med 1976;295:349–53.

[4] Barker DJP, Winter PD, Osmond C, et al. Weight in infancy and death from ischaemic heart disease. Lancet 1989;ii:577–80.

[5] Hales CN, Barker DJP, Clark PMS, et al. Fetal and infant growth and impaired glucose tolerance at age 64. BMJ 1991;303:1019–22.

[6] Phipps K, Barker DJ, Hales CN, et al. Fetal growth and impaired glucose tolerance in men and women. Diabetologia 1993;36:225–8.

[7] Fall CHD, Osmond C, Barker DJP, et al. Fetal and infant growth and cardiovascular risk factors in women. BMJ 1995;310:428–32.

[8] Barker DJP, Hales CN, Fall CHD, et al. Type 2 diabetes mellitus, hypertension, and hyperlipidemia (syndrome X): relation to reduced fetal growth. Diabetologia 1993;36:62–7.

[9] Hales CN, Barker DJ. The thrifty phenotype hypothesis. Br Med Bull 2001;60:5–20.

[10] Valdez R, Athens MA, Thompson GH, et al. Birthweight and adult health outcomes in a biethnic population in the USA. Diabetologia 1994;37:624–31.

[11] Curhan GC, Willett WC, Rimm EB, et al. Birthweight and adult hypertension, diabetes mellitus and obesity in US men. Circulation 1996;94:3246–50.

[12] Lithell HO, McKeigue PM, Berglund L, et al. Relation of size at birth to non-insulin dependent diabetes and insulin concentrations in men aged 50–60 years. BMJ 1996;312:406–10.

[13] Leger J, Levy-Marchal C, Bloch J, et al. Reduced final height and indications for insulin resistance in 20 year olds born small for gestational age: regional cohort study. BMJ 1997;315:341–7.

[14] Jaquet D, Gaboriau A, Czernichow P, et al. Insulin resistance early in adulthood in subjects born with intrauterine growth retardation. J Clin Endocrinol Metab 2000;85:1401–6.

[15] Egeland GM, Skjaerven R, Irgrens LM. Birth characteristics of women who develop gestational diabetes: population based study. BMJ 2000;321:546–7.

[16] Forsen T, Eriksson J, Tuomilehto J, et al. The fetal and childhood growth of persons who develop type 2 diabetes. Ann Intern Med 2000;133:176–82.

[17] Rich-Edwards JW, Colditz GA, Stampfer MJ, et al. Birthweight and the risk for type 2 diabetes mellitus in adult women. Ann Intern Med 1999;130:278–84.

[18] St. Jeor ST, Hayman LL, Daniels SR, et al. American Heart Association. Prevention Conference VII: obesity, a worldwide epidemic related to heart disease and stroke: group II: age-dependent risk factors for obesity and comorbidities. Circulation 2004;110:471–5.

[19] Eriksson J, Forsen T, Tuomilehto J, et al. Fetal and childhood growth and hypertension in adult life. Hypertension 2000;36:790–4.

[20] Bavdekar A, Sachdev HS, Fall CHD, et al. Relation of serial changes in childhood body-mass index to impaired glucose tolerance in young adulthood. N Engl J Med 2004;350:865–75.

[21] Bavdekar A, Yajnik CS, Fall CH, et al. Insulin resistance syndrome in 8-year-old Indian children: small at birth, big at 8 years, or both? Diabetes 1999;48:2422–9.

[22] Hoffman PL, Cutfield WS, Robinson EM, et al. Insulin resistance in short children with intrauterine growth retardation. J Clin Endocrinol Metab 1997;82:402–6.

[23] Li C, Johnson MS, Goran MI. Effects of low birth weight on insulin resistance syndrome in Caucasian and African-American children. Diabetes Care 2001;24:2035–42.

[24] Yajnik CS, Fall CH, Vaidya U, et al. Fetal growth and glucose and insulin metabolism in four-year-old Indian children. Diabet Med 1995;12:330–6.

[25] Clausen JO, Borch-Johnsen K, Pedersen O. Relation between birth weight and the insulin sensitivity index in a population sample of 331 young, healthy Caucasians. Am J Epidemiol 1997;146:23–31.

[26] Flanagan DE, Moore VM, Godsland IF, et al. Fetal growth and the physiological control of glucose tolerance in adults: a minimal model analysis. Am J Physiol Endocrinol Metab 2000;278:E700–6.

[27] Phillips DI, Barker DJ, Hales CN, et al. Thinness at birth and insulin resistance in adult life. Diabetologia 1994;37:150–4.

[28] Widdowson EM, Southgate DAT, Hey EN. Nutrition and metabolism of the fetus and infant. In: Visser HKA, editor. Body composition of the fetus and infant in nutrition and metabolism of the fetus and infant. The Hague: Martinus Nijhoff; 1979. p. 169–77.

[29] Lapillonne A, Braillon P, Chatelain PG, et al. Body composition in appropriate and small for gestational age infants. Acta Paediatr 1997;86:196–200.

[30] Van Assche FA, De Prins F, Aerts L, et al. The endocrine pancreas in small for dates infants. Br J Obstet Gynaecol 1977;84:751–3.

[31] Jensen CB, Storgaard H, Dela F, et al. Early differential defects of insulin secretion and action in 19-year-old Caucasian men who had low birth weight. Diabetes 2002;51.1271–80.

[32] Barnett AH, Eff C, Leslie RDG, et al. Diabetes in identical twins. Diabetologia 1981;20: 87–93.

[33] Newman B, Selby JV, King MC, et al. Concordance for type 2 diabetes mellitus in male twins. Diabetologia 1987,30:763 8.

[34] Warram JH, Martin BC, Krolewski AS, et al. Slow glucose removal rate and hyperinsulinemia precede the development of type II diabetes in the offspring of diabetic parents. Ann Intern Med 1990;113:909–15.

[35] Vaag A, Henricksen JE, Madsbad S, et al. Insulin secretion, insulin action, and hepatic glucose production in identical twins discordant for NIDDM. J Clin Invest 1995;95:690–8.

[36] Hattersley AT, Tooke JE. The fetal insulin hypothesis: an alternative explanation of the association of low birthweight with diabetes and vascular disease. Lancet 1999;353: 1789–92.

[37] Froguel P, Zouali H, Vionnet N. Familial hyperglycemia due to mutations in glucokinase: definition of a subtype of diabetes mellitus. N Engl J Med 1993;328:697–702.

[38] Hattersley AT, Beards F, Ballantyne E, et al. Mutations in the glucokinase gene of the fetus result in reduced birth weight. Nat Genet 1998;19:268–70.

[39] Kubaszek A, Markkanen A, Eriksson JG, et al. The association of the K121Q polymorphism of the plasma cell glycoprotein-1 gene with type 2 diabetes and hypertension depends on size at birth. J Clin Endocrinol Metab 2004;89:2044–7.

[40] Eriksson JG, Lindi V, Uusitupa M, et al. The effects of the Pro12Ala polymorphism of the peroxisome proliferator-activated receptor-gamma2 gene on insulin sensitivity and insulin metabolism interact with size at birth. Diabetes 2002;517:2321–4.

[41] Dahri S, Snoeck A, Reusens-Billen B, et al. Islet function in off-spring of mothers on low-protein diet during gestation. Diabetes 1991;40:115–20.

[42] Snoeck A, Remacle C, Reusens B, et al. Effect of a low protein diet during pregnancy on the fetal rat endocrine pancreas. Biol Neonate 1990;57:107–18.

[43] Ozanne SE, Wang CL, Coleman N, et al. Altered muscle insulin sensitivity in the male offspring of protein-malnourished rats. Am J Physiol 1996;271:E1128–34.

[44] Berney DM, Desai M, Palmer DJ, et al. The effects of maternal protein deprivation on the fetal rat pancreas: major structural changes and their recuperation. J Pathol 1997;183: 109–15.

[45] Wilson MR, Hughes SJ. The effect of maternal protein deficiency during pregnancy and lactation on glucose tolerance and pancreatic islet function in adult rat offspring. J Endocrinol 1997;154:177–85.

[46] Burns SP, Desai M, Cohen RD, et al. Gluconeogenesis, glucose handling, and structural changes in livers of the adult offspring of rats partially deprived of protein during pregnancy and lactation. J Clin Invest 1997;100:1768–74.

[47] Ozanne SE, Jensen CB, Tingey KJ, et al. Low birthweight is associated with specific changes in muscle insulin-signaling protein expression. Diabetologia 2005;48:547–52.

[48] Ozanne SE, Olsen GS, Hansen LL, et al. Early growth restriction leads to down regulation of protein kinase C zeta and insulin resistance in skeletal muscle. J Endocrinol 2003;177: 235–41.

[49] Petry CJ, Dorling MW, Pawlak DB, et al. Diabetes in old male offspring of rat dams fed a reduced protein diet. Int J Exp Diabetes Res 2001;2:139–43.

[50] Fernandez-Twinn DS, Wayman A, Ekizoglou S, et al. Maternal protein restriction leads to hyperinsulinemia and reduced insulin-signaling protein expression in 21-mo-old female rat offspring. Am J Physiol Regul Integr Comp Physiol 2005;288:R368–73.

[51] Benediktsson R, Lindsay R, Noble J, et al. Glucocorticoid exposure *in utero*; a new model for adult hypertension. Lancet 1993;341:339–41.

[52] Lindsay RS, Lindsay RM, Edwards CRW, et al. Inhibition of 11β-hydroxysteroid dehydrogenase in pregnant rats and the programming of blood pressure in the offspring. Hypertension 1996;27:1200–4.

[53] Lindsay RS, Lindsay RM, Waddell B, et al. Programming of glucose tolerance in the rat: role of placental 11β-hydroxysteroid dehydrogenase. Diabetologia 1996;39:1299–305.

[54] Niyirenda MJ, Seckl JR. Intrauterine events and the programming of adulthood disease: the role of fetal glucocorticoid exposure. Int J Mol Med 1998;2:607–14.

[55] Simmons RA, Templeton L, Gertz S, et al. Intrauterine growth retardation leads to type II diabetes in adulthood in the rat. Diabetes 2001;50:2279–86.

[56] Boloker J, Gertz S, Simmons RA. Offspring of diabetic rats develop obesity and type II diabetes in adulthood. Diabetes 2002;51:1499–506.

[57] Ogata ES, Bussey M, Finley S. Altered gas exchange, limited glucose, branched chain amino acids, and hypoinsulinism retard fetal growth in the rat. Metabolism 1986;35:950–77.

[58] Simmons RA, Gounis AS, Bangalore SA, et al. Intrauterine growth retardation: fetal glucose transport is diminished in lung but spared in brain. Pediatr Res 1991;31:59–63.

[59] Unterman T, Lascon R, Gotway M, et al. Circulating levels of insulin-like growth factor binding protein-1 (IGFBP-1) and hepatic mRNA are increased in the small for gestational age fetal rat. Endocrinology 1990;127:2035–7.

[60] Myatt L, Eis ALW, Brockman DE, et al. Differential localization of superoxide dismutase isoforms in placental villous tissue of normotensive, pre-eclamptic, and intrauterine growth-restricted pregnancies. J Histochem Cytochem 1997;45:1433–8.

[61] Karowicz-Billinska A, Suzin J, Sieroszewski P. Evaluation of oxidative stress indices during treatment in pregnant women with intrauterine growth retardation. Med Sci Monit 2002; 8(3): CR211–CR6.

[62] Ejima K, Nanri H, Toki N, et al. Localization of thioredoxin reductase and thioredoxin in normal human placenta and their protective effect against oxidative stress. Placenta 1999;20: 95–101.

[63] Kato H, Yoneyama Y, Araki T. Fetal plasma lipid peroxide levels in pregnancies complicated by preeclampsia. Gynecol Obstet Invest 1997;43:158–61.

[64] Bowen RS, Moodley J, Dutton MF, et al. Oxidative stress in pre-eclampsia. Acta Obstet Gynecol Scand 2001;80:719–25.

[65] Wang Y, Walsh SW. Increased superoxide generation is associated with decreased superoxide dismutase activity and mRNA expression in placental trophoblast cells in pre-eclampsia. Placenta 2001;22:206–12.

[66] Wang Y, Walsh SW. Placental mitochondria as a source of oxidative stress in pre-eclampsia. Placenta 1998;19:581–6.

[67] Peterside IE, Selak MA, Simmons RA. Impaired oxidative phosphorylation in hepatic mitochondria of growth retarded rats alters glucose metabolism. Am J Physiol 2003;285: E1258–64.

[68] Selak MA, Storey BT, Peterside IE, et al. Impaired oxidative phosphorylation in skeletal muscle contributes to insulin resistance and hyperglycemia. Am J Physiol 2003;285: E130–7.

[69] Panten U, Zielman S, Langer J, et al. Regulation of insulin secretion by energy metabolism in pancreatic β-cell mitochondria. Biochem J 1984;219:189–96.

[70] Newgard CB, McGarry JD. Metabolic coupling factors in pancreatic β-cell signal transduction. Annu Rev Biochem 1995;64:689–719.

[71] Schuit F. Metabolic fate of glucose in purified islet cells. Glucose regulated anaplerosis in β-cells. J Biol Chem 1997;272:18572–9.

[72] Mertz RJ, Worley JF, Spencer B, et al. Activation of stimulus-secretion coupling in pancreatic β-cells by specific products of glucose metabolism. J Biol Chem 1996;271(9):4838–45.

[73] Ortsater H, Liss P, Akerman KEO. Contribution of glycolytic and mitochondrial pathways in glucose-induced changes in islet respiration and insulin secretion. Pflugers Arch Eur J Physiol 2002;444:506–12.

[74] Antinozzi PA, Ishihara H, Newgard CB, et al. Mitochondrial metabolism sets the maximal limit of fuel-stimulated insulin secretion in a model pancreatic beta cell. A survey of four fuel secretagogues. J Biol Chem 2002;277:11746–55.

[75] Malaisse WJ, Hutton JC, Carpinelli AR, et al. The stimulus-secretion coupling of amino acid-induced insulin release. Metabolism and cationic effects of leucine. Diabetes 1980;29:431–7.

[76] Lenzen S, Schmidt W, Rustenbeck I, et al. 2-Ketoglutarate generation in pancreatic β-cell mitochondria regulates insulin secretory action of amino acids and 2-keto acids. Biosci Rep 1986;6:163–9.

[77] Noda M, Yamashita S, Takahashi N, et al. Switch to anaerobic glucose metabolism with NADH accumulation in the beta-cell model of mitochondrial diabetes. Characteristics of beta HC9 cells deficient in mitochondrial DNA transcription. J Biol Chem 2002;277:41817–26.

[78] Lenzen S, Drinkgern J, Tiedge M. Low antioxidant enzyme gene expression in pancreatic islets compared with various other mouse tissues. Free Radic Biol Med 1996;20:463–6.

[79] Tiedge M, Lortz S, Drinkgern J, et al. Relationship between antioxidant enzyme gene expression and antioxidant defense status of insulin-producing cells. Diabetes 1997;46:1733–42.

[80] Maechler P, Jornot L, Wollheim CB. Hydrogen peroxide alters mitochondrial activation and insulin secretion in pancreatic beta cells. J Biol Chem 1999;274:27905–13.

[81] Sakai K, Matsumoto K, Nishikawa T, et al. Mitochondrial reactive oxygen species reduce insulin secretion by pancreatic β-cells. Biochem Biophys Res Commun 2003;300:216–22.

[82] Kaneto H, Xu G, Fujii N, et al. Involvement of c-Jun N-terminal kinase in oxidative stress-mediated suppression of insulin gene expression. J Biol Chem 2002;277:30010–8.

[83] Kaneto HH, Xu G, Fujii N, et al. Involvement of protein kinase C beta 2 in c-myc induction by high glucose in pancreatic beta-cells. J Biol Chem 2002;277:3680–5.

[84] Kaneto H, Xu G, Song KH, et al. Activation of the hexosamine pathway leads to deterioration of pancreatic beta-cell function through the induction of oxidative stress. J Biol Chem 2001;276:31099–104.

[85] Kaneto H, Kajimoto Y, Fujitani Y, et al. Oxidative stress induces p21 expression in pancreatic islet cells: possible implication in beta-cell dysfunction. Diabetologia 1999;42:1093–7.

[86] Jonas JC, Laybutt DR, Steil GM, et al. High glucose stimulates early response gene c-Myc expression in rat pancreatic beta cells. J Biol Chem 2001;276:35375–81.

[87] Jonas JC, Sharma A, Hasenkamp W, et al. Chronic hyperglycemia triggers loss of pancreatic beta cell differentiation in an animal model of diabetes. J Biol Chem 1999;274:14112–21.

[88] Efanova IB, Zaitsev SV, Zhivotovsky B, et al. Glucose and tolbutamide induce apoptosis in pancreatic β-cells. J Biol Chem 1998;273:22501–7.

[89] Moran A, Zhang HJ, Olson LK, et al. Differentiation of glucose toxicity from β-cell exhaustion during the evolution of defective insulin gene expression in the pancreatic islet cell line, HIT-T15. J Clin Invest 2000;99(3):534–9

[90] Donath MY, Gross DJ, Cerasi E, et al. Hyperglycemia-induced β-cell apoptosis in pancreatic islets of Psammomas obesus during development of diabetes. Diabetes 1999;48:738–44.

[91] Silva JP, Kohler M, Graff C, et al. Impaired insulin secretion and β-cell loss in tissue specific knockout mice with mitochondrial diabetes. Nat Genet 2000;26:336–40.

[92] Park J, Suponitsky-Kroyer I, Simmons RA. Epigenetic silencing of Pdx-1 in growth retarded [IUGR] rats. Endocrinology, in press.

[93] Vuguin P, Raab E, Liu B, et al. Hepatic insulin resistance precedes the development of diabetes in a model of intrauterine growth retardation. Diabetes 2004;53:2617–22.

[94] Peterside IE, Selak MA, Simmons RA. Impaired oxidative phosphorylation in hepatic mitochondria of growth retarded rats alters glucose metabolism. Am J Physiol 2003;285(6): E1258–64.
[95] Selak MA, Storey BT, Peterside IE, et al. Impaired oxidative phosphorylation in skeletal muscle contributes to insulin resistance and hyperglycemia. Am J Physiol 2003;285:E130–7.
[96] Petersen KF, Dufour S, Befroy D, et al. Impaired mitochondrial activity in the insulin-resistant offspring of patients with type 2 diabetes. N Engl J Med 2004;350:664–71.

ELSEVIER
SAUNDERS

Endocrinol Metab Clin N Am
35 (2006) 205–218

ENDOCRINOLOGY
AND METABOLISM
CLINICS
OF NORTH AMERICA

Index

Note: Page numbers of article titles are in **boldface** type.

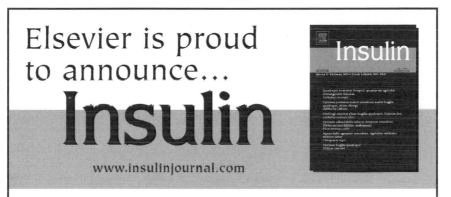

Changing Your Address?

Make sure your subscription changes too! When you notify us of your new address, you can help make our job easier by including an exact copy of your Clinics label number with your old address (see illustration below.) This number identifies you to our computer system and will speed the processing of your address change. Please be sure this label number accompanies your old address and your corrected address—you can send an old Clinics label with your number on it or just copy it exactly and send it to the address listed below.

We appreciate your help in our attempt to give you continuous coverage. Thank you.

W. B. Saunders Company

SHIPPING AND RECEIVING DEPTS.
151 BENIGNO BLVD.
BELLMAWR, N.J. 08031

SECOND CLASS POSTAGE
PAID AT BELLMAWR, N.J.

This is your copy of the
_____ **CLINICS OF NORTH AMERICA**

00503570 DOE—J32400   101   NH   8102

JOHN C DOE MD
324 SAMSON ST
BERLIN   NH   03570

XP-D11494

JAN ISSUE

Your Clinics Label Number
Copy it exactly or send your label along with your address to:
W.B. Saunders Company, Customer Service
Orlando, FL 32887-4800
Call Toll Free 1-800-654-2452

Please allow four to six weeks for delivery of new subscriptions and for processing address changes.